Basic Aspects of Blood Trauma

# Basic Aspects of Blood Trauma

A Workshop Symposium on Basic Aspects of Blood Trauma in
Extracorporeal Oxygenation held at Stolberg near Aachen,
Federal Republic of Germany, November 21-23, 1978

Sponsored by the Commission of the European Communities,
as advised by the Committee on Medical and Public Health Research

*edited by*

## H. Schmid-Schönbein

*Department of Physiology,
Rhenish-Westphalian Technical University,
Aachen, Federal Republic of Germany*

## P. Teitel

*Department of Physiology,
Rhenish-Westphalian Technical University,
Aachen, Federal Republic of Germany*

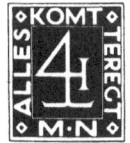

Martinus Nijhoff Publishers
The Hague/Boston/London 1979

for

The Commission of the European Communities

The distribution of this book is handled by the following team of publishers:

*for the United States and Canada*

Kluwer Boston, Inc.
160 Old Derby Street
Hingham, MA 02043
USA

*for all other countries*

Kluwer Academic Publishers Group
Distribution Center
P.O. Box 322
3300 AH  Dordrecht
The Netherlands

*For further information:*

Martinus Nijhoff Publishers B.V.,
P.O.B. 566
2501 CN  The Hague
The Netherlands

---

**Library of Congress Cataloging in Publication Data**                    CIP

Workshop Symposium on Basic Aspects of Blood Trauma in Extracorporeal Oxygenation, Stolberg, Ger., 1978.

Basic aspects of blood trauma.

1.   Blood – Circulation, Artificial – Complications and sequelae – Congresses.
2.   Oxygenators – Congresses.   3.   Blood – Coagulation, Disorders of – Congresses.
4.   Hemolysis and hemolysins – Congresses.   I.   Schmid-Schönbein, H.   II.   Teitel, P.
III.   Commission of the European Communities.

QP110.A7W67            1978            617'.412            79-26407

ISBN-13: 978-90-247-2279-2            e-ISBN: 978-94-009-9337-2
DOI: 10.1007/978-94-009-9337-2

---

Cover photograph: courtesy of Mr. H. K. Koerten, Laboratory for Electron Microscopy, Leiden University, The Netherlands


Publication arranged by:
Commission of the European Communities, Directorate-General Scientific
and Technical Information and Information Management, Luxembourg


EUR 6467EN

© ECSC, EEC, EAEC, Brussels-Luxembourg, 1979

Softcover reprint of the hardcover 1st edition 1999

TABLE OF CONTENTS

# F O R E W O R D

It may strike someone why forewords ever are written when so few people bother to read them. Naturally the reader is more interested in the contents of the book than in its wrapping and circumstances. Nevertheless, a note is necessary for the record on how this book has come to be.

In 1977 the Council of the European Communities signed a document on the first European Concerted Action under the auspices of CREST (Commitee on Scientific and Technical Research) and CRM (Commitee on Medical Research), originally proposed by SWG/BME (Specialized Working Group on Biomedical Engineering). The Concerted Action should concern itself with problems in extracorporal oxygenation for the duration of 4 years.

A Concerted Action Committee (COMAC) was formed and consisted of nationally appointed delegates. A project leader was elected the following year.

The aim of a Concerted Action is to promote dissemination of knowledge and new techniques thereby gradually bringing about a cordination of the national scientific programmes in the member countries. The financial support from the Council enables COMAC and the project leader, inter alia, to support meetings, study groups and sojourns for scientists in the member countries. It is hoped that efforts in the European Community will lead to a closer contact and corporation between European scientific groups.

The present book is the result of the dynamic and diligent work of Professor, dr.med H.Schmid-Schönbein (German member of the COMAC) and is based on a small meeting held 21-23 November 1978 in Stolberg near Aachen. The experience of the participants reached from the clinical despair when diffuse bleeding endangers the patient, to rheological aspects and advanced methods of molecular analysis of coagulation factors. This book indicates the realization that advanced technology cannot improve long term survival of patients with failing lung function, and that extracorporal oxygenation appears to induce severe alterations in the patient's "safety" mechanism. The devoted therapist (or better a group of therapists) must have a broad knowledge, ranging from technical aspects over haemodynamics, pathophysiology to the coagulation aspects covered in this book to improve the therapy.

It is a pleasant opportunity on behalf of COMAC to express admiration and gratitude to Professor Schmid-Schönbein on his efforts which resulted in this book.

Steen Gamwell Dawids
project leader

# ACKNOWLEDGEMENTS

This book contains the proceedings of the workshop on "Blood Trauma in Extracorporeal Oxygenation" sponsered by the European Commission through the "Concerted Action" on Extracorporeal Oxygenation in Stolberg/Aachen, November 21-23, 1978, organized by members of the Sonderforschungsbereich 109 of the Deutsche Forschungsgemeinschaft at the RWTH Aachen.

The papers presented were accepted as submitted by the authors, the discussion was transcribed and edited by the participants. Later, the remarks were slightly modified and condensed by the editors, who, however, made a special effort to preserve the spirit of the actual meeting. The introductory chapter on "unspecific defense system activation" was condensed from various discussion remarks during the meeting. It was presented in full to the general assembly of the Concerted Action at its meeting in Milan, March 6-8, 1979. The closing session of the workshop was devoted to a general discussion aiming at a reappraisal of the concepts presented and at formulating "practical consequences". The contents of this session were condensed from the record. Very soon, general agreement evolved that it is presently premature to formulate detailed guidelines for the prophylaxis, diagnosis, prevention or cure of blood trauma in extracorporeal oxygenators available to date. This topic was deferred to future meetings of the "Concerted Action" focussing on such topics as the rationale, the practice and the supervision of anticoagulation with heparin, but also on platelet inhibition, hemodilution and defibrinogenation during extracorporeal circulation.

This book became possible through the untiring and devoted efforts of Ms. Maria Brendt, Ms. Magda Munstra-Zuidema and Ms. Christine Weiland.

Ms. Weiland later single-handedly collected the missing discussion remarks, collected the figures in the discussion and layed out and typed the entire discussion. The technical help of our colleagues Mr. Blasberg, Dr. Fischer, Dr. Mottaghy and Dr. Wurzinger who served as technical moderators during the actual session and of Mr. Franz Keutgen is gratefully acknowledged. The photographes were kindly prepared by Mr. Franz-Joseph Kaiser.

Basic Aspects of Blood Trauma

# 1. BIOLOGICAL ANALYSIS OF BLOOD TRAUMA: THE RESPONSE OF THE UNSPECIFIC DEFENSE SYSTEM TO FOREIGN TECHNICAL APPARATUS[1]

H. Schmid-Schönbein[2], Department of Physiology, Medical Faculty, RWTH Aachen, Melatener Str. 211, D-5100 Aachen, West Germany

ABSTRACT

In the past, the "trauma" inflicted to blood by artificial organs has been mechanistically explained by passive mechanical damage and by passive deposition of thrombotic material to "artificial" surfaces. However, from a biological standpoint, the haematological complications or artificial organs have to be considered as the consequence of an activation of the unspecific defense system (U.D.S.) of the blood, i.e. an *active* response of *living cells* and activated *enzymes*.

The U.D.S. system is phylogenetically old and responds *indiscriminately* but *actively* to unspecific stimuli. Therefore, changes in the physical and chemical environment of its constituents, i.e. changes in the mechanical, thermal, osmotic conditions and chemical composition must act as *adequate stimulus* to the U.D.S. In defense to microbial stimulation, it *always* cooperates with the phylogentically new *specific* defense system (the immune system in the strict sense). Thence, in most clinical cases requiring extracorporeal oxygenation, the U.D.S. is either activated beforehand or by the oxygenator itself.

---

1   Presented as a lecture to the plenary assembly of the "Concerted Action on Extracorporeal Oxygenation", Milan, March 6, 1979

2   Supported by Deutsche Forschungsgemeinschaft, Sonderforschungsbereich 109, (*Künstliche Organe*) RWTH Aachen, Projekt $C_2$ and $C_5$.

# 1. INTRODUCTION

The contact between the human blood and foreign technical apparatus (circulatory) and respiratory assist devices, artificial kidneys) leads to changes in the plasmatic and cellular components of the blood, which have often only been taken as signs of gross but passive blood destruction. There is much evidence to support this notion in parts (mechanical cellolysis of erythrocytes and thrombocytes), however, these changes have to be seen in a broader biological context as an organ-specific *reaction* of the blood.

It is an unjustified oversimplification to simply treat the blood as transport organ for respiratory gases ($O_2$ and $CO_2$) and metabolites. The blood is rather also an organ system for specific and unspecific defense mechanisms, directed against the hazards of mechanical, microbiological and toxicological risks posed to multicellular macro-organisms in an environment in which trauma and other disturbances of the physical integrity are common. The two defense systems of the blood are based on humural and cellular constituents; the latter have to be considered as "excitable cells", capable of responding in a predictable and automatic fashion to adequate stimuli. The response of the cellular constituents in controlled and coordinated by chemical mediators. The immunological research of the last century has distinguished two separate defense systems of the blood:

I. The highly *specific defense system* (immune system sensustrictori) which is *phylogenetically new* and is *ontogenetically learned*. It is reacting to molecular stimuli ("immunogen") on the surface of the viruses, fungi and bacteria but also to molecules secreted by other cells. The response with the selective recruitment of a limited number of "committed cells" (immunocytes = lymphocytes and plasma cells). The immune system recognizes "non-self-properties" also in transplanted organs and therefore reacts with a typical defense resulting in transplant "rejection".

The *constituents* of the U.D.S. include *cells* (thrombocytes, granulocytes and erythrocytes), *plasmatic proenzymes*
(e.g. prothrombin, plasminogen, complement, the HAGEMAN-
factor and prekallikrein) as well as plasmatic *substrates*
(e.g. fibrinogen, kininogens). The *efferent limb* of the
U.D.S. consists of a cellular and enzymatic activation by
adequate stimuli (abnormal pH or temperature, abnormal surfaces or flow conditions). The *afferent limb* includes
cellular responses such as activation of contractile proteins, leading to *shape changes* and *secretion* of biological mediators (e.g. serotonin, histamin, heparin). In
addition, a cascade activation of various cross reacting
enzymes such as activated HAGEMAN-factor, thrombin, plasmin, kallikrein and properdin activated complement.

As the biological mediators and activated proenzymes not
only act on the substrates (leading to fibrin and bradykinin) but also act back on the enzymes and cells, the
U.D.S. shows pronounced "*interactive amplification*". When
activated fully and for prolonged periods, the unspecific
defense system may even be autocatalytically directed
against the patient's organism.

The control and suppression of the specific defense system
was a prerequisite for successful *organ transplantation*.
It may be predicted, that the success of artificial organs
will stand and fall with the removal of stimuli and the
depression of the response and most of all of the interactive amplification of the U.D.S.

II. The *unspecific defense system* is phylogenetically old
    and represents an inborn reaction of blood cells and
    plasma constituents (various pro-enzymes) which react
    indiscriminately to many physical and chemical stimuli,
    involving many cells (in number and type) and mole-
    cules of the plasma. The blood trauma occurring in the
    application of artificial organs is the consequence of
    its activation - since adequate stimuli to many of its
    constituents occur.

Today, it is generally accepted that the success of *organ
transplantation* is often limited due to the fact that
transplanted organs act as adequate and specific stimuli
to the immune system (T-lymphocytes or "Killer-cells") and
are therefore attacked by lymphocate clones which execute
a typical "delayed type" immune reaction (see Textbooks of
Immunology). The effect of their multiple defense actions
against this iatrogenically inflicted challenge to the
immune system is called "organ rejection". This is a ste-
reotyped acquired reaction of certain lymphocytes and
limits or aestroys the function of a surgically competent
graft.

It is helpful to face the fact that the contact between
blood and foreign *artificial organs* inflicts a similar
challenge to the other, the unspecific defense system of
the blood. Whether or not the prolonged contact and thus
the prolonged challenge of the unspecific defense system
by various adequate stimuli can be tolerated not only
depends on nature and magnitude of the stimuli as such,
but also on the active response of living cells and on the
equilibrium between activation and inhibition of biologically active plasmatic mediators.

In the past, blood trauma has not received the necessary
biological analysis. Since obviously the understanding of
the reaction between artificial organ and unspecific defense system (U.D.S.) is of equal importance for the future of prolonged application of artificial internal organs, research into the biology of this system is highly

desirable. The following communication attempts to familiarize the reader with the present knowledge about the constituents, the individual physiological properties and the coordinated reaction of the unspecific defense system.

## 2. CONSTITUENTS OF THE U.D.S.: *"Inflammatory"* cells and molecules

The constituents of the U.D.S. are listed in table I, they are cellular and plasmatic ("humoral") reaction partners in physiological functions of the blood that were historically considered separate but are now recognized as partners cooperating in defense against injury.

### 2.1. CELLS

The granulocytes (polymorpho-nucleated neutrophiles (P.M.N.'s) and basophiles) and monocytes in the circulating blood, but also the macrophages and the mast-cells of the interstitial tissue are the typical mono-nuclear, mono-cellular constituents of the unspecific defense system since they share archaic properties of animal cells: excitability, motility, ability for phagocytosis and secretion of stored material. These fundamental cellular functions are not only found in protozoa but also in the cells constituting the phylogenetically oldest metazoa (pluri-cellular) organisms; for this reason it is justified to call the U.D.S. "old"(or even archaic)(see Textbooks of Biology). All these cellular responses are the result of a typical excitation process: The cell membrane interacts with external stimuli, permits the passage of ions ($Na^+$, $Ca^{++}$), which activate the various metabolic pathways within the cytoplasma, resulting in the activation of contractile proteins, the secretory apparatus and/or phagocytosis.

In addition, thrombocytes as cell fragments of the blood share most of these typical cellular functions with the true cells, i.e. they can show motility ("shape-change"), phagocytosis (see COPLEY and WITTE) and secretion in response to external stimuli. The red cells, the other important but least viable cell fragment found in the circulating blood, is possibly participating passively in the U.D.S. To understand the full dynamics of the U.D.S.

6

it is necessary to include not only the blood cells but
also the endothelial cells, (with the likewise typical
biological variability and function) but also all cells
of the interstitial tissue (mast-cells, macrophages, fibro-
blastes etc.) in the U.D.S.

| Cells | Mediators (tissue hormones) | Enzymes and Proenzymes |
|---|---|---|
| Blood cells | | Cellular enzymes |
| neutrophilic and eosi- nophilic granulocytes | | |
| basophilic granulo- cytes and mast-cells | Histamin, Heparin | Lysosomal enzymes |
| Monocytes and Macro- phages | | |
| Thrombocytes | Serotonin, Histamin | |
| Erythrocytes (passive) | Adenosin-Diphosphate | |
| Blood vessel cells | | Plasmatic enzymes |
| vascular smooth muscle | | Coagulation proenzymes (e.g. Hageman Faktor, Prothrombin, Faktor V, VII, IX, X, XIII) |
| endothelial cells | | |
| Interstitial cells | | Fibrinolytic proenzymes |
| Macrophages | | (e.g. Plasminogen) |
| Mast cells | Histamin, Heparin | |
| Histiocytes | Bradykinin | Kininogens Complement |

Table I: Components of the U.D.S.

## 2.2. PLASMA PROTEINS

There are several classes of plasma proteins involved in
the U.D.S.; most of them are produced by the hepatocytes
and circulate not only in the plasma but also in the
lymph  and interstitial fluid spaces. According to their
function we have to differentiate three different protein
classes:

a) *Pro-enzymes*

There is a vast multitute of pro-enzymes, i.e. protein
molecules which acquire enzymatic properties following
physical or chemical change of their configuration.
Among these are noteworthy the so-called HAGEMAN-factor
and other pro-enzymes of the coagulation cascade, pre-
kallikreins, the various components of the complement
system including properdin and proteins such as kinino-
gen and plasminogen.

b) *Acute-Phase-Proteins*

The so-called acute-phase-proteins (unified into one
group due to their fairly rapid appearance following
mechanical, thermal, toxic or bacteriological challenge)
include various different proteins such as fibrinogen
(as a substrate for coagulation enzymes), $\alpha$-II-macro-
globuline (as a specific inhibitor of various enzymes),
transport globulines such as haptoglobine and acid
oromucoid, but also plasma lysosomal enzymes.

c) *Inhibitory Proteins*

Inhibitory proteins such as antithrombin III, antiplasmin, antitrypsin and complement inactivators have to
be mentioned because they are probably pivotal for the
actual control of the plasmatic events of the U.D.S.

## 2.3. MEDIATORS

In addition to these cellular and macromolecular consti-
tuents-in-waiting, there are other chemical agents which
participate in the U.D.S. when it is active. Most of
these act on many constituents of the U.D.S. and can thus
be taken as transmitters or mediators.

a) *Secretory Mediators*

When activated cells secrete material previously syn-
thetized and/or stored into their environment. Many of
these secreted agents such as serotonin (secreted by
platelets), histamin (secreted by basophiles, mast-cells

8

and platelets), heparin (secreted by mast-cells), cate-
cholamines (secreted by platelets) have extremely
potent effects on other cells and act as mediators that
transmit information from one cell to the other. Lysosomal-enzymes (secreted by macrophages and granulocytes)
also act on cells and molecules (proenzymes and substrates) and can help in spreading the activation.

b) *Cytoplasmatic Mediators*

The U.D.S. also depends on mediators liberated by cellolysis, which include lysosomal-enzymes (from macrophages and granulocytes) phospholipids (from destroyed
platelets and other cellular elements), adenosindi-
phosphate (liberated from destroyed red cells) and
most importantly arachidonic acid derivatives, liberated from the  membranal compartments (plasma membrane
and/or organelle membrane) following challenge or
destruction of cells and the activation of phospho-
lipases.

c) *Activated Plasma Enzymes as Mediators*

Activated pro-enzymes, i.e. enzymes capable of binding
to their substrates following partial cleavage act as
mediators of activation spreaders, these include
thrombin, plasmin, activated complement and kallikrein.
Also fibrinopeptides, fibrin degradation products,
prostaglandines and a multitude of other molecules
which appear during the course of an U.D.S. response
are capable of effecting the function of other cellular
and/or enzymatic component of the U.D.S.


2.4. INHIBITORS

The inhibitors of the U.D.S. include these specific pro-
tease inhibitors such as $\alpha_1$-antithrombin, $\alpha_1$-antitrypsin,
$\alpha_2$-antichymotrypsin and $\alpha_2$-macroglobulin, a pluripotent
enzymatic inhibitor exhibiting for example antiplasmin
activity. There also numerous inactivators of comple-

ment, notably $C_3$-inactivator. Heparin, the secretion product of mast-cells, acts as an inhibitor of thrombin in cooperation with antithrombin III. Inhibitory mechanisms can also be triggered into action by certain stimuli, the precise interaction between activated constituents of the U.D.S. and their specific or general inhibitors is not yet clearly understood in a quantitative manner.

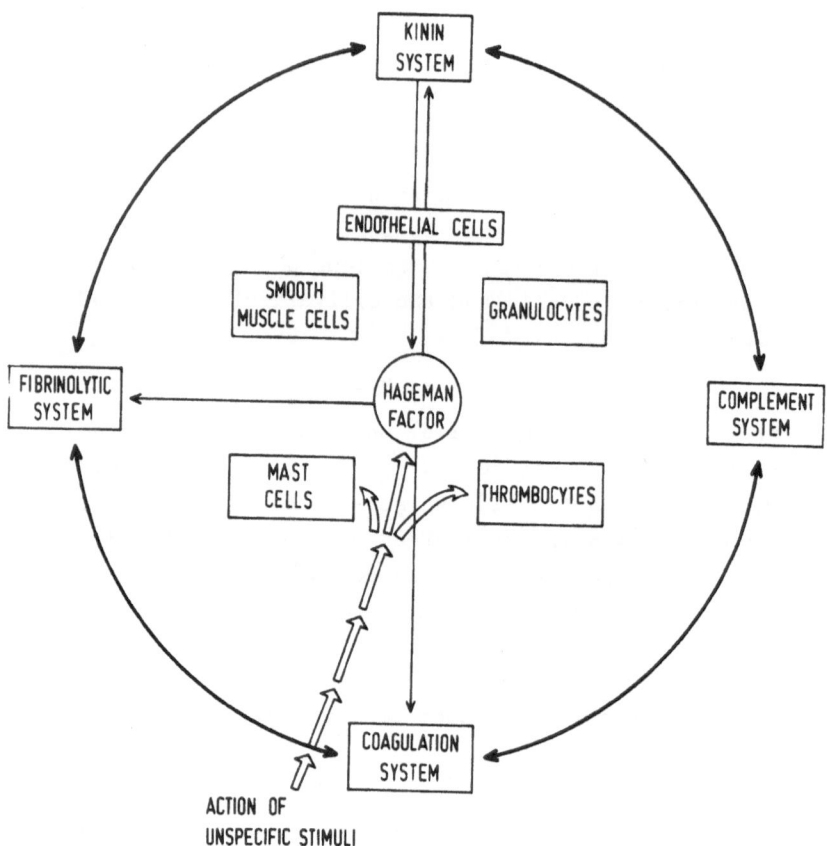

Fig. 1: Schematic representation of the encymatic and cellular systems comprising the unspecific defense system. Unspecific stimuli act on the Hageman factor, on mast-cells or thrombocytes and trigger responses by activated encymes and cells.

10

# 3. PHYSIOLOGY OF THE U.D.S.

The U.D.S. is a biological system capable of greatly variable response to wide selection of stimuli. The response is governed:

I.   by the strength and duration of stimuli.

II.  by the general and/or local concentration of reactive constituents of the U.D.S., a factor not only governed by the production and break-down by the constituents but also by local accumulation and/or dilution. The latter factors depend on the presence or absence of blood and transmural exchange of the constituents of the U.D.S. The *intravascular* local concentration of U.D.S.-constituents depends on the intervascular flow, or flow retardation or even flow-stop. The extravascular concentration of cells, macromolecules and micromolecules also depends on the "permeability of the vessel-wall", parameters primarily governed by the physiological state of endothelial cells.

III. by the time of exposure, namely the duration of the stimulus, the fate of the stimulated constituents and the turnover (synthesis and breakdown) of the U.D.S.-constituents.

IV.  by inhibitory reactions.

The paramount role of the time of exposure becomes evident if one realizes that the U.D.S., like any excitable system of many cells in the body, and especially the specific defense system, comprises

a) an afferent limb
b) an efferent limb and most significantly
c) interactive amplification (and/or inhibition).


## 3.1. AFFERENT LIMB

The afferent limb of the U.D.S. consists of the "excitation" of the cellular and an "activation" of the molecular constituents of the U.D.S. here, we have to differentiate between

1. the stimulus as such, defined as any change in the
   environmental conditions sufficient to elicit a
   response and
2. the interaction between stimulus and the receptor in
   cells or the reactive site in enzymes.

Environmental changes assume the nature of a "stimulus"
and thence of an "information" to biological systems
that have an apparatus for the perception of changes in
the physical characteristics (temperature, pressure and
flow) of the blood, als well as of the changes of the surface characteristics of the blood conduits. Chemical
stimuli can be unspecific (pH and osmolarity) or specific
changes in the "milieu intérieur" of the blood such as
the appearance of stimulating enzymes or mediators which
interact with molecular "receptors" on the surface of
cells or with the "active site" of an enzyme.

Many details about the physiology of "receptors" (simply
defined as any apparatus capable of receiving any kind of
information from the environment) in the cells of the
U.D.S. are not yet clear. It can be assumed, however, that
proteins in the membrane of the cells of the U.D.S. experience conformational changes. These may for example
change the gate characteristics of cation transporting
protein systems or a change in the activity of membrane
adenylate cyclase activity. As a consequence, ional or
hormonal "second messengers" penetrate or appear in the
intercellular cytoplasma and trigger metabolic activities
within the cells. In this respect, the rôles of $Ca^{++}$ and
cyclic adenosine-monophosphate (cAMP) are especially con-
spicuous. The rôle of these two mediators in platelet
physiology is especially well documented, but basically
similar events must be assumed to take place in any other
living cell. The efferent limb of the cellular U.D.S.-
reactions therefore depends on three distinct but coopera-
tive cell organelle-systems:

12

1. on the appropriate information receiving system,
   capable of sensing environmental changes in extracellular space,
2. on an information exchange system from the extracellular to the intracellular system and
3. an apparatus for triggering metabolic changes within
   the intracellular space.

It is important to keep in mind that the driving forces
for transmembranal ion transport are supplied by the
resting metabolism (ionic pumps etc.), which by their
very action supply steep electrochemical gradients for
such ion species as $Ca^{++}$ and $Na^+$. The stimulus thus only
acts on the *gating* mechanism which allows a passive
potential driven action to take place.

## 3.2. EFFERENT LIMB

The efferent limb consists of the typical response
effector of the excitable cells to these stimuli. The
response of the cellular U.D.S. constituents consists
in an overall change in the shape function or integrity
of the membrane of cells, subsequent passive transmembranal transport of ions ($Na^+$ and $Ca^{++}$ moving into the cell,
potassium moving out of the cell) along preexisting concentration gradients but also in the enzymatic production
of so-called "second messengers", e.g. (cAMP). These in
turn, lead to changes in the cell metabolism such as an
activation of the contractile proteins leading to a cell
mobility, phagocytosis and secretion.

The activation of pro-enzymes in the plasma, e.g. a
change in their configuration as in Hageman-factor or by
cleavage of molecular fragment allows their genetically
programmed action to be triggered following which subsequent enzymatic cleavages of other enzymes and substrates
as well as of the enzymes themselves (and thus autocata-
lytic enhancement of enzyme cascades) takes place.

In the case of exposure to the set of stimuli presented

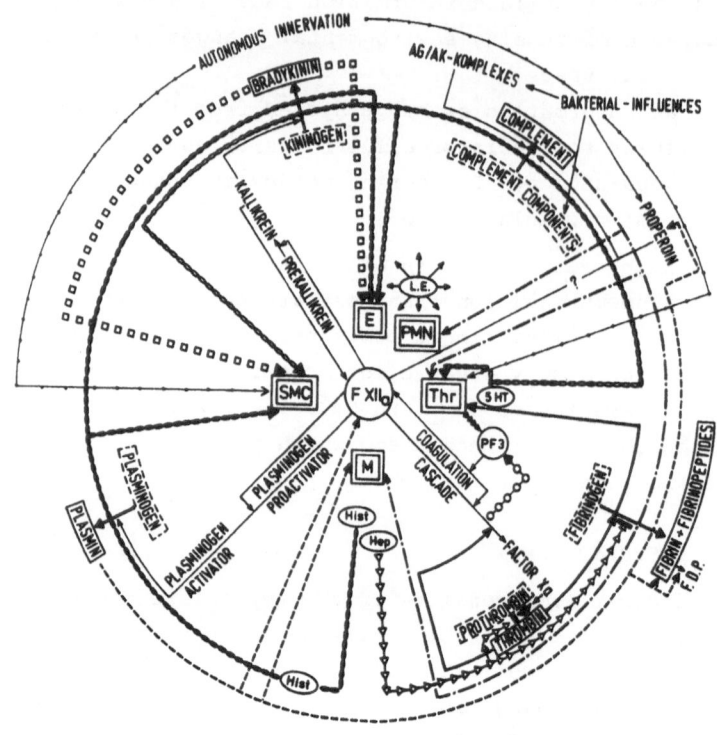

Thr = THROMBOCYTES
M   = MASTCELLS
SMC = SMOOTH MUSCLE CELLS
E   = ENDOTHELIUM
PMN = GRANULOCYTES
PF3 = PLATELET FACTOR 3 ∘∘∘∘
L.E. = LYSOSOMAL ENZYMES
Hist = HISTAMIN ━━━━
Hep = HEPARIN ➤➤➤➤
5HT = SEROTONIN ━━━━
BRADYKININ □ □ □ □
F XII₍ₐ₎ = ACTIVATED HAGEMAN-FACTOR

Fig. 2: Schematic representation of some interactions between
different cellular and encymatic components of the U.D.S.
Unspecific stimuli act on factor XII, which triggers the
activation of the coagulation cascade, the fibrinolytic
system, the kinin-system and the properdin-system. Cellular
components are activated directly or via activated encymes.
Amplification occurs through the release of cellular mediators
(histamin, 5HT, platelet-factor 3 or lysosomal encymes.
Besides unspecific stimuli, the system can be activated
(or coactivated) by various bacterial influences or auto-
nomous innervation.

14

to the blood during the perfusion of an extracorporeal circulatory device, the *cellular* efferent limbs of the U.D.S. therefore is triggered by mechanical and chemical stimuli leading to the activation of the contractile and the secretory apparatus in thrombocytes and granulocytes. But, in addition and beyond this, activation, a passive straining of all types of blood cells, occurs, eventually leading to total rupture of the cell (cellolysis) with all its consequences. Extracorporeal perfusion also activates plasmatic pro-enzymes, the *enzymatic* efferent limb consisting in the activity of coagulatory, fibrinolytic kinin-forming and complement enzymes. Once activated, a co-activation of subsequent pro-enzymes of the coagulatory and fibrinolytic system is achieved and also a cross-reaction between coagulatory, fibrinolytic kinin-forming and complement enzymes. The haemodynamic effects of the U.D.S. largely depends on its products, and thus on the kinetics of its action upon the substrates. Efferent limb substrates such as fibrinogen, kininogens as well as lipids from activated cells (arachidonic acids) are acted upon by the efferent limb enzymes, resulting in the formation of such products as fibrin, but also fibrin degradation products (F.D.P.'s), bradykinine as well as prostaglandines. In addition, the activated complement enzymes act on cellular proteins located in the membranes, thereby changing the configuration of these important biological structures. As a consequence, cells not only change their biochemical structure but also their biological function. Anything from a moderate change in cell activity to total cell lysis can occur.

## 3.3. INTERACTIVE AMPLIFICATION

The action of activated complement upon granulocytes is a good example of the interactive amplification of the U.D.S.; due to changes in the cellular activity, the cells undergo a change which transforms them from their resting to their activated state during which they not only become

more susceptable to any other stimuli but produce products
(e.g. lysosomes, histamin) which themselves act upon other
cells. In addition, an interaction between the many lysosomal enzymes and the activated pro-enzymes of the plasma
can occur. As a consequence, proteases in high concentration become available and act on the coagulatory, fibrinolytic, complement and bradykinin system, the efferent limb
becoming overactive by a cascade type amplification. The
coagulatory enzymes have especially many positive feedback loops. The overall activity is, however, also enhanced by liberation by thromboplastic phospholipids from
cells which are activated and/or destroyed. The progressive
release of mediators by active secretion as well as by
passive cellolysis results in an recruitment of more and
more cells, pro-enzymes and substrates in the overall
U.D.S. response.

There are, in addition, many cross-reactions: among these,
the action of thrombine on platelets, the action of complement on PMN's, mast-cells and platelets are most noteworthy. Another type of act again involves platelets, which
may become exposed to ADP released by mechanically strained
red cells.

A most important aspect of interactive amplification is
related to *flow-depended local accumulation* of activated
cells (thrombocytes), enzymes (HAGEMAN-factor, thrombin)
or the product of the enzymatic action (fibrin, plasmin,
bradykinin and prostaglandines). If, due to a change in
the vascular or extravascular flow conditions these constituents are of the U.D.S., are localized either in an
artificial organ or in an important natural organ (e.g.
the lung), where localized interactive amplification becomes drastically more effective, leading to a gross in-
terferance with the function of the tissue (e.g. the
lungs) or the artificial organs (e.g. an oxygenator).

# 4. INTERFERENCE WITH THE ACTIVATION OF THE UNSPECIFIC DEFENSE SYSTEM

The theoretical scheme outlined above can also be extended
to identify mechanisms of interference. The research stra-
tegies in the development of artificial organs should be
directed towards the afferent limb, the efferent limb and
the interactive amplification. Today, the use of heparin
as an antithrombin is the primary mode of interference,
sufficient to keep alive the physiological entity consisting of a human organism and extracorporeal oxygenation
systems for limited time periods.

## 4.1. INTERFERENCE WITH AFFERENT LIMB

The most significant mode of interference with the U.D.S.
activation must direct itself towards the removal of the
stimulus. By careful maintenance of temperature, pH, osmolarity and ionic concentration of the blood, all *unspecific stimuli* can be reduced substantially. Improving the
surface characteristics and the flow conditions in all
parts of the artificial organs is certainly the most important means of interference or avoidance of afferent
limb activation.

The afferent limb of the U.D.S. system can also be atte-
nuated by drugs: Acetyl-Salicylic Acid (ASA), Persantin,
Prostacyclin and other platelet inhibitory drugs might
interfere successfully with the efferent limb stimulation
and most of all with the interactive amplification. Red
cell membrane stabilisation (by Chlorpromazin), suggested
to reduce the mechanical lysis of erythrocytes, might act
in the same manner.

## 4.2. EFFERENT LIMB INTERFERENCE

The administration of a powerful antithrombin (heparin)
is presently the most popular measure to interfere with
efferent limb activation. However, while there is an efferent limb interference with the enzymes (primarily factor
IIa and Xa) there might be simultaneous activation of

platelets. At least in some species, a heparin has an activation rather than an inhibiting effect upon the platelets. A very successful interference with the efferent limb of the U.D.S. micht be seen in the dilution and/or removal of the substrates for cells and enzymes. Here, the liberal infusion of protein-free electrolyte solutions (haemodilution) or the defibrinogenation (e.g. by ANCROD) has been shown to improve the overall performance of the artificial organs and the physiology of experimental animals connected to them.

## 4.3. DEPRESSION OF INTERACTIVE AMPLIFICATION

Not only the afferent limb but also the efferent limb antagonists discussed above, might be seen capable of interfering with the interactive amplification. In this respect, the most important physical factor is the maintenance of adequate flow and therefore the avoidance of localized thrombi or coagulae. If the localized interactive amplification can be avoided or depressed the reticulo-endothelial system of the experimental animal or the patient should have a better chance to cope with the products of the U.D.S. system by phagocytosis or inactivation. Since, the phagocytotic capacity of the RES is limited, reduced activation of the afferent and efferent limb might remove the load on the RES, therfore giving it a better chance to counteract interactive amplification.

## 5. CONSEQUENCES FOR THE CLINICAL APPLICATION OF OXYGENATORS

It is well known, that the mere contact of a healthy human
body with the presently available extracorporeal oxygenators, expecially when extended over periods of more
than 4 hours, leads to a severe blood trauma and therefore such severe activation of the U.D.S. This fact alone
can lead to respiratory failure, producing an "iatrogenic"
indication for the very use of membrane oxygenators (which
are used in treatment with the so-called "pump-lung-syn-
drome"). This important established fact should be kept in
mind when a prolonged extracorporeal oxygenation is
planned for treatment of any other disease state. The basic underlying diseases, such as viral and bacterial pneu-
monia, burn, toxic lung failure and the so-called "shock-
lung syndrome" are a priori characterized by activation
of the U.D.S. It must be kept in mind that the very syn-
dromes which provide the indication for extracorporeal
oxygenation are in themselves most adequate, potent and
"natural" pre-stimulators of the U.D.S. Consequently, all
patient-candidates for extracorporeal oxygenation start
with a maximally activated U.D.S. system at the time of
their connection to the extracorporeal oxygenation. To
date, all of extracorporeal oxygenators available are
very strong additional stimuli. Furthermore, prolonged
extracorporeal oxygenation poses problems of quantitative
nature. Presently used extracorporeal circulatory assist
devices (such as the heart-lung machine for open heart
surgery) poses a *short, limited* challenge to the U.D.S.
followed by a long recovery period. Also, the presently
used "artificial kidneys" challenge the U.D.S. only for
a short periods separated by a long recovery intervals.
Artificial heart valves, small, well designed "artificial
organs" present an un-interrupted, but quantitatively
small challenge to the U.D.S.

In contrast, the long-term extracorporeal oxygenation
presents an uninterrupted strong stimulation to the

U.D.S. system. Extracorporeal oxygenation can thus only
be turned into a success provided that the stimulus,
the response, the interactive amplification of the U.D.S.
can be substantially depressed aiming at successful interference rather than further interactive amplification. To
this aim, more blood compatible biomaterials, better
hydrodynamic conditions and pharmacological intervention
have to be coordinated. The present difficulties encountered with the long-term extracorporeal membrane oxygenation are most likely related to the fact that none
of these goals have been met sufficiently to date. Easy
solutions to the problem in the future are not in sight,
but rather a pragmatic, stepwise approach with interdisciplinary efforts of engineering sciences, pharmacology and physiology.

The preceding attempts to focus on the general biological significance of the so-called blood trauma is largely based on the author's discussion remarks during the actual conference, as well as on the replies of the other participants. In the author's judgement, in the past the scientific community engaged in artificial organs research and application has neither acknowledged the physiology of the U.D.S., nor has the well established "interactive amplification" received the attention it deserves. While the central rôle of the Hageman Factor in the enzymology of three (or possibly four) plasmatic enzymes has generally been accepted, the rôle of cells, the multiple actions of mediators and the phylogenetic aspects of the U.D.S. as an archaic, but nevertheless fully operational partial function of normal human blood physiology has often been neglected. In patients subjected to artificial oxygenators the system is invariably activated (see textbooks of general and lung pathology). Possible ways of additional stimulation (especially by abnormal flow forces acting on the very fragile blood cells) will be demonstrated in the following chapters of this book.

On purpose, a proper citation of original literature was not included in the above introductory text. To allow an entry into the extremely complex material distributed in a scientific literature not familiar with most workers in the field of artificial organs, a highly selected list of comprehensive texts is given below which is by no means complete. Most of the statements made above are also born out by the prepared lectures and the discussion remarks of the participants of the symposion.

REFERENCES

1   BIGGS, Rosemary, (Ed), Human Blood Coagulation, Haemo-
    stasis and Thrombosis, second edition, Blackwell Scien-
    tific Publications, Oxford-London-Edinburgh-Melbourne,
    1972

2   COPLEY, Alfred L., S. WITTE, Editorial on Physiological
    Microthromboembolization as the primary Platelet Func-
    tion: Elimination of invaded particles from the circu-
    lation and its pathogenetic significance. In: Thrombosis
    Research, Pergamon Press, Inc., Vol. 8, pp. 251-262,
    1976

3   DEUTSCH, E., Blutgerinnung und Operation, Urban &
    Schwarzenberg, München 1973

4   KALEY, Gabor, Burton M. ALTURA, (Eds), Microcirculation,
    Vol. I, II and III, University Park Press, Baltimore,
    1978

5   MANNING, M.M. and R.J. TURNER, Comparative Immunobiolo-
    gy, Blakie, (Glasgow-London) 1976

6   MÄKELÄ, O., A. CROSS and T.U. KOSUNEN, (Eds), Cell In-
    teractions and Receptor Antibodies in: Immune Responses,
    London and New York, 1971

7   MEURET, G., Das Monozyten-Makrophagen-System in: Hand-
    buch der Inneren Medizin, 2. Band, Teil 3 (H. Begemann
    Ed.), Springer (Berlin, Heidelberg, New York), 1976

8   MÜLLER-EBERHARDT, H.J., Complement, Ann. Rev. Biochemis-
    try, 1975

9   SCHMID-SCHÖNBEIN, H., Physiologie des Blutes als Trans-
    port- und Abwehr-System, in: Arbeitsbuch der Physiolo-
    gie, K. Kramer u. E. Bassenge (Eds.), Urban und Schwar-
    zenberg (München), 1979 (in press)

10  WEISSMANN, G., Mediators of Inflammation, Plenum
    (New York-London), 1974

11  WILLIAMS, W.J., E. BEUTLER, A.J. ERSLEV and R.W. RUNDLES
    (Eds.), Hematology, (2nd Ed.), McGraw-Hill (New York),
    1977

12  ZWEIFACH, B.W., L. GRANT and R.T. McCLUSKEY, (Eds.),
    The inflammatory process, (2nd Ed.), Vol. I, II and III,
    Academic Press, New York, London, 1973

22

# 2. CONSIDERATIONS OF PLATELET FUNCTION MECHANISMS

G.V.R. Born, Department of Pharmacology, University of London King's College, Strand, London WC2R 2LS, UK.

Physiological haemostasis and pathological thrombosis are both initiated by platelet aggregation, and the involvement of platelets in both processes is more evident in arteries than in veins. Thrombosis in coronary arteries begins on sites damaged by atherosclerosis. Commonly a thrombus grows on an atherosclerotic plaque which has narrowed the lumen. With the blood pressure constant the blood flow is faster in the constricted lumen than elsewhere in the artery. Therefore, high flow and shear rates are no hindrance to thrombogenesis where the thrombus consists essentially of adhering and aggregating platelets. Indeed, the question arises whether the activation of platelets required for thrombus formation depends in some way on such abnormal haemodynamic conditions. When adequately anticoagulated blood is made to flow under conditions giving rise to flow separation or vortices, e.g., in artificial dialysers or oxygenators, platelets are deposited on the channel walls to form obstructive thrombi. Measurements of the haemodynamic forces required to activate platelets directly (Hellums & Brown, 1977) indicate that the flow abnormalities caused by atherosclerotic lesions in vivo cannot account for local activation of circulating platelets. On the other hand, there is considerable evidence for the indirect activation of platelets by the operation of haemodynamic forces on the red cells (see Born, 1977).

23

High collision frequencies between red cells and platelets do not by themselves cause the latter to aggregate. It seems that the activation of platelets by erythrocytes depends on their providing a chemical agent, presumably ADP (Gaarder, Hellem, Jonsen, Laland & Owren, 1961; Harrison & Mitchell, 1966). There are in principle three ways of inhibiting such effects of erythrocytes on platelets and so minimizing their contribution to atherosclerosis and preventing arterial thrombosis. First, by inhibiting the reactivity of the platelets themselves; secondly, by inhibiting the release of activating agents from the erythrocytes; and thirdly, by eliminating the activating agent in the plasma. The reactivity of platelets can be inhibited by a variety of agents, some of which are under trial as potential anti-thrombotic drugs. In support, it has been shown that inhibitory agents (adenosine without or with dipyridamole) can be used regionally to prevent platelet thrombi forming in artificial organs (Richardson, Galletti & Born, 1976). Recent experimental (Born, Bergquist & Arfors, 1976) and clinical (Zahavi & Schwartz : to be published) evidence suggests that the activation of platelets by erythrocytes may be diminishable by drugs. Chlorpromazine and similar drugs, in concentrations which stabilize the erythrocyte membrane against haemolysis but are too low to affect platelets directly, increase the 'bleeding time', both experimentally and clinically under conditions in which this time is determined by the reactivity of platelets. It has also been shown experimentally that platelet activation associated with the presence of erythrocytes can be prevented by the addition of an enzyme such as apyrase or the phosphoenolpyruvate kinase system which removes ADP (Harrison & Mitchell, 1966). On the basis of all this it has been proposed (Born, 1977) that in the course of non-laminar blood flow in the vicinity of atherosclerotic lesions, erythrocytes undergo reversible deformation through which, without being haemolytic or permanently damaging, the cells release enough ADP (probably together with other adenine nucleotides and other small molecules) to activate the accompanying platelets.

24

In the blood channels of artificial organs, thrombi tend to develop even when coagulation is prevented locally or systematically with heparin (1,2). Thrombi are undesirable because they may embolize and so endanger the patient and because they impede moving parts of the artificial organ and obstruct the flow of blood. Obstructive effects are particularly important when narrow passages are used in transport devices, e.g. in artificial kidneys, oxygenators, because thrombi increase resistance to flow (3) and decrease the areas available for the exchange functions.

Effects to minimize platelet thrombosis in artificial organs have so far been directed mainly towards optimizing choice of material, design of blood passages and assembly techniques. The introduction of silica-free silicone rubber coatings has improved oxygenator bypass circuits (4,5), but they are not suitable for devices with hydrophilic surfaces. A different approach towards preventing platelet thrombi is by inhibiting the adhesion and aggregation of circulating platelets. Such inhibition can be produced by various chemical agents including some established drugs, such as aspirin (6,7). Some of these agents are not suitable for systemic administration to patients because of rapid metabolism and/ or undesirable side effects. Such agents may, however, be appropriate for regional use in artificial organs, if it can be established that comparatively high effective concentrations can be limited to the blood passing through the organ and that concentrations in the general circulation are too low to induce side-effects.

METHODS

To test the possibilities that regional administration of inhibitors of platelet function can reduce thrombus formation in artificial organs, 3 factors in particular were considered. First, an artificial organ should be chosen which is standardized in manufacture, readily available, and has a strong tendency to thrombus formation when used with a particular animal species; secondly, the animal should be

25

large enough to allow tests to be carried out with a bypass
flow rate perhaps only 20 - 25 % of cardiac output (to
allow plenty of systemic recirculation of locally infused
drugs); and thirdly, the extracorporeal circuit should provide test and control organs in parallel to eliminate he-
matologic variability from animal to animal.

The test circuit is shown in Fig. 1. The animals were an-
esthetized sheep, with bypass from the carotid artery to
the superior vena cava. The bypass included 2 Cordis Dow
artifical kidneys (CDAK), which were perfused in parallel.

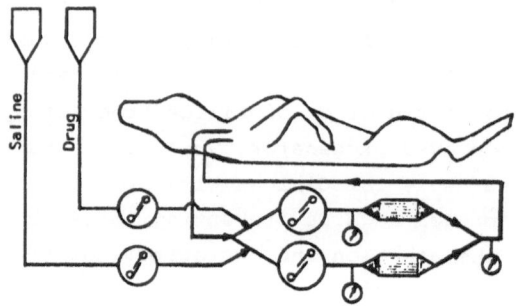

Fig. 1: Diagram of extracorporeal circuit. Blood drained from the
carotid artery is divided into 2 streams, each receiving its
infusate before being pumped through the artificial kidneys in
a 38°C bath. A common line returns blood to a venous cannula.
The triangles denote pressure measurement points.

Flow resistance of each unit was measured at flow rates of
200, 350, and 500 ml/min. The intubated, chloralose-an-
esthetized sheep had a Sarns cannula inserted, for drainage,
through which a catheter is advanced so as to measure arterial pressure. A short, flexible cannula (polyurethane
with wire-wound wall) was inserted for blood return. An
initial heparin dose of 5 mg/kg was administered.

Perfusion was started with blood flow in each kidney of
200 ml/min. If there were no counter-indications (big drop
in arterial pressure or big in flow resistance) within
1-2 mins the blood flow rate was raised to 350 ml/min, and
to 500 ml/min about one min following. The 2 infusion
pumps were started at the beginning of bypass and run at a
constant rate throughout. A saline drip was maintained to
the animal at 2-5 ml/min.
During bypass the pressure were monitored continuously.
If no thrombosis developed within the first hr, a drip of
banked sheep blood (ACD) of 1-2 ml/min was sometimes
commenced. Heparin was given in maintenance doses of
3 mg/kg/hr. Some experiments ran for 2 and most for 3 hrs.
The following problems sometimes arose during perfusion:
arterial cannula movement restricting blood drainage
(corrected by repositioning the cannula); fracture of an
infusion pump tube (irremediable); thrombi occluding
pressure-measuring catheters or ports (removed by flushing);
and massive thrombosis in the CDAKs, manifested by high inlet pressure which terminated the experiment.
In 2 runs, tritiated adenosine was added to the infusate
and blood samples were taken, after various times, from the
arterial outflow from the sheep and from the inlet to each
of the CDAKs.

## RESULTS

Thrombus formation during perfusion of a CDAK was indicated
by an increase in the resistance to flow measured by a rise
in pressure drop at constant blood flow rate.
Fig. 2 illustrates the variation in pressure drop as a
function of time for a CDAK, which developed considerable
thrombosis, together with the corresponding curve for a
CDAK, which was almost free of thrombi at the end of perfusion. It can be seen that the rise in $\Delta P$ was gradual,
though it can accelerate smoothly, and a 3 hr run is useful
in obtaining definitive changes in $\Delta P$.

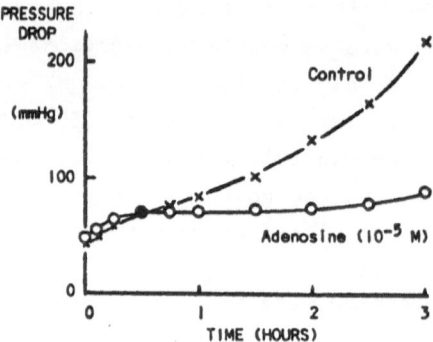

Fig. 2: Pressure drops measured in 2 kidneys perfused simultaneously
The control CDAK had saline infused; the other had adenosine.

Fig. 3 illustrates a typical variation of platelet count
and of HCT during perfusion. In most cases the platelet
count was reduced during perfusion compared with the count
immediately before bypass.

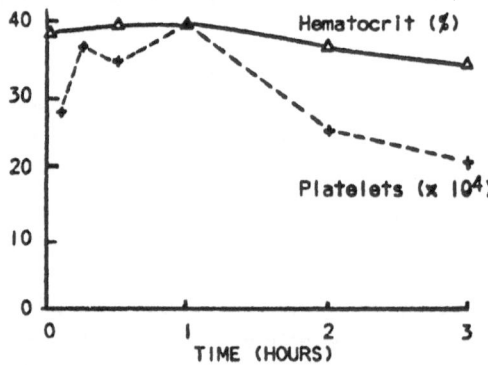

Fig. 3: The variation of HCT and of platelet count during a typical
experiment (the same as for the data shown in Fig. 2).

The drugs were adenosine ($10^{-5}$-$10^{-6}$ Mol/L), adenosine
($10^{-6}$ Mol/L) with persantin (dipyridamole) ($5 \cdot 10^{-6}$ Mol/L),
RA 233 ($10^{-7}$ - $10^{-5}$ Mol/L) and saline as control (concentrations are for blood, not for the infusate itself in
which they were 100 times greater).

Results are expressed as ratio of the pressure drop at the
end of perfusion to that at the beginning; the values of
this ratio for simultaneous test and control units are
plotted in Fig. 4.

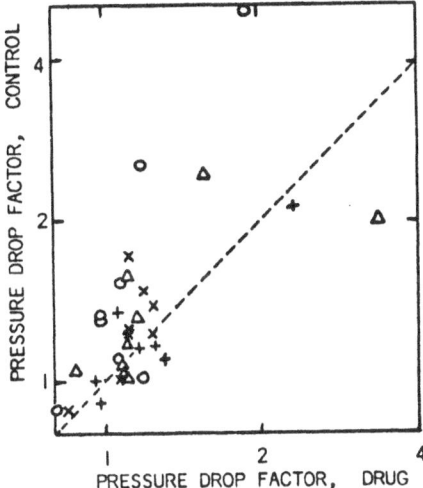

Fig. 4: Paired comparison between the pressure drop factors for drug
and control units, which were perfused simultaneously. The
pressure drop factor is the ratio of final pressure drop to
initial pressure drop, at 500 ml/min blood flow. Dashed line
is the line of identity: data points lying above it indicate
that use of the drug helps reduce the pressure drop factor.
$\Delta$, adenosine $10^{-6}$/M; 0, adenosine $10^{-5}$/M; x, adenosine $10^{-6}$/M
plus persantin $5 \times 10^{-6}$/M; +, RA 233, $10^{-7}$ - $10^{-5}$/M.

Different series are shown with different styles of points.
If the drugs have no effect the points should be scattered
in the figure on both sides of the line of equality of
pressure drop change (the dashed line). However, most
points are to one side of the line of equality, indicating
that the drugs diminished thrombus formation. The distribution of $\Delta P_f/\Delta P_i$ is decidedly not "normal". The mean
values (and standard deviations) for the rise in pressure
drop are: $1.38 \pm 0.7$ for $10^{-6}$ M adenosine local concentration, $1.40 \pm 0.5$ for concurrent controls; $1.11 \pm 0.12$ for
$10^{-6}$ M adenosine plus $5 \times 10^{-6}$ M dipyridamole, $1.26 \pm 0.26$
for controls; $1.29 \pm 0.5$ for RA 233, $1.26 \pm 0.4$ for con-

trols; 1.15 $\pm$ 0.3 for $10^{-5}$ M adenosine, 1.77 $\pm$ 1.25 for controls; and the average of all controls, 1.43 $\pm$ 0.7.

## DISCUSSION

The protocol. The CDAK units were appropriate for these tests but there was some variability in the resistance to flow between different units. It may help to run such experiments with units having matched flow resistance. Units with fewer capillaries but otherwise similar would permit the use of smaller animals or a smaller rate of blood flow per unit. With sheep and an appropriate array of pumps, several small test units could be run in parallel. This would permit a range of doses to be tested simultaneously or a statistically significant number of units to be tested more rapidly.

A typical run of 3 hrs provided a reasonable compromise between producing significant differences in thrombosis, indicated by changes in flow resistance and morphology, and some degree of adaptation by the animal to extracorporeal blood flow. If the purpose were changed, for example to obtaining information on the spatial distribution and microscopic morphology of platelets during the initial adhesion phase, the bypass time could be much shorter.

The flow rate of 500 ml/min for each CDAK provided a blood flow per unit membrane area typical of modern transport devices and intermediate between those for kidneys and lungs. This rate of flow exposed erythrocytes to high shear forces in such devices. Recent evidence (BORN, BERGQVIST and ARFORS) suggests that under such conditions ADP released from erythrocytes initiates platelet aggregation and that this effect may be prevented by drugs acting on the red cells. Changes in resistance to flow in the CDAK whether to blood or to saline, provides a measure of thrombosis. Examination of the morphological events provides information about the mode of thrombus formation in relation to flow pattern and materials and about the mechanism by

which drug acts locally to reduce thrombus formation. At
the price of the corresponding effort one could extend
this, similar to the work of Dutton and Edmunds (8), to
observe and measure embolus formation; to carry out simultaneous tests of platelet function; and so on.

## REFERENCES

1) Hill, J.D., O'Brien, T.G., and Murray, J.J.: Prolonged extracorporeal oxygenation for acute posttraumatic respiratory failure
   (Shock-lung syndrome). N. Engl. J. Med., 286:629, 1972.

2) Ward, B.D., Hood, A.G., and Hershgold, E.J.: Pathology and mechanics of membrane lung performance deterioration. Trans. Amer.
   Soc. Artif. Int. Organs, 21:206, 1975.

3) Richardson, P.D. and Galletti, P.M.: Gas transport and flow resistance as diagnostic tools of membrane oxygenator malfunction.
   Proc. 3rd Ann. N. Engl. Bioeng. Conf., Tufts U., 1975, p. 271.

4) Kolobow, T., Stool, E.W., Weathersby, P.D., Pierce, J., Hayano, F.,
   and Suandeau, J.: Superior blood compatibility of silicone rubber
   free of silica filler in the membrane lung. Trans. Amer. Soc.
   Artif. Int. Organs, 20A:35, 1974.

5) Zapol, W.M., Bloom, S., Carvalho, A., Wonders, T., Skoskiewicz,M.,
   Schneider, R., and Snider, M.: Improved platelet economy using
   filler-free silicone rubber in long term membrane lung perfusion.
   Trans. Amer. Soc. Artif. Int. Organs 21:587, 1975.

6) Born, G.V.R.: Platelet pharmacology in relation to thrombosis.
   Adv. Cardiol., 4:161, 1970.

7) Agarwal, K.C. and Parks, R.E., Jr.: Adenosine analogs and human
   Platelets: Effects on nucleotide pools and the aggregation phenomenon. Biochem. Pharmacol. 24:2239, 1975.

8) Dutton, R.C. and Edmunds, L.H.Jr.: Formation of platelet aggregate
   emboli in a prototype hollow fiber membrane oxygenator.
   J. Biomed. Mater. Res. 8:163, 1974.

DISCUSSION          Moderator: Born

Wildevuur:          I want to comment on the initial platelet  reac-
                    tion, Dr. Born mentioned. We have seen this speci-
                    fic phenomenon (1) regularly in our dog experi-
                    ments (see Fig.4 , page 227). In this circuit,
                    consisting of PVC-tubing and a roller pump, the
                    thrombocyte number decreases in a matter of mi-
                    nutes to 50 % of the initial value. This is a
                    momentary reaction which is partly reversible
                    and stabilization on the value of 90 % is ob-
                    served during the further period of perfusion
                    (shaded area). Additionally a typical secondary
                    dip can be seen on the first postoperative day.
                    This dip is most logically explained by an early
                    elimination by the RES of the platelets sublethal-
                    ly damaged during the perfusion (1). Our interest
                    has been focussed on the determination of the
                    causes of the initial dip (1, 2). Because extra-
                    corporeal circuits (ECC) are primed by various
                    solutions, experiments were designed to show
                    their effects on the circulating platelets. While
                    a blood volume of 500 ccm was withdrawn, the
                    same amount of various priming solutions was in-
                    fused. Dextran, as well as gelatine cause a se-
                    vere initial dip to about 20 %. These dogs were
                    otherwise treated in the same fashion as in our
                    previous experiments regarding anesthesia, hepa-
                    rin and protamine chloride administration. I
                    would like to draw your attention to the dip
                    following protamine administration, a rather se-
                    vere effect that needs more attention. Basically
                    the same effects of the priming solutions were
                    observed on the thrombocyte function (3). I be-
                    lieve that these experiments pinpoint the problem
                    of platelet aggregation in ECC, not only the
                    effect of the circuit proper but also the major
                    contribution which priming solutions may have.

32

REFERENCES:

1      J.C.F. de JONG, C.Th. SMIT SIBINGA and Ch.R.H. WILDEVUUR:
      Platelet Behaviour in Extracorporeal Circulation (ECC). In:
      Artificial Organs, p. 27 (eds. R.M. KENEDI, J.M. COURTNEY,
      J.D.S. GAYLOR and T. GILCHRIST), The Macmillan Press Ltd.,
      London, 1977.

2      J. WOLTJES, J.C.F. de JONG, H.J. ten DUIS and Ch.R.H. WILDEVUUR:
      The Priming of Extracorporeal Circuits: The Effect on Canine
      Blood Elements. Transfusion, in Press.

Birnbaum:          From the clinical standpoint I am interested in
the impressive drop of the level of the thrombo-
cytes right after the start of an extracorporeal
oxygenation. Dr. Born, could you please amplify
your statement concerning the initial thrombocyte
loss and its correlation with an activation of
complement?
A second question to Dr. Wildevuur: Did you
account for hemodilution effects in the interpretation of the platelet dip? In our measurements,
even after accounting for the hemodilution effect,
we still have a net loss of thrombocytes.

Born:          It is quite established that complement is activated quickly under these conditions. There is a
C-1-Q-receptor on human platelets and one or two
other receptors. The activation of complement
components in some way causes platelets to disappear temporarily from the circulation, perhaps
by trapping in lungs and elsewhere.

Birnbaum:          Complement component activation would mean that
there is a change of the $C_3'$ and the $C_4'$. So we
have to do with protein denaturation, I think.
We have measured the concentrations of $C_3'$ as well
as of $C_4'$ in man under extracorporeal circulation.
We could not see any change in the concentrations
of these two components of the complement system.

Certainly these measurements cannot answer the question whether there is an activation! But I wonder whether any activation during ECC is due to a protein effec, i.e. a proteolysis, or whether the thrombocytes cause the activation.

Born:             It is interesting that you can't find activation because other people have done so. As far as I know, there is no other explanation for the temporary disappearance of the platelets. I do know that granulocytes disappear in the same way and that too is due to complement activation.

Wildevuur:        Indeed, PMN's showed an identical initial dip as described for platelets (1). About the location of trapping of these blood elements MIELKE (2) described that the platelets are mainly trapped in the liver, at least in splenectomized dogs. When hemodilution is used platelet numbers have to be corrected by the changes in hematocrit to obtain the actual disappearance in numbers.

REFERENCES:

1      C. WILDEVUUR-van HAMERSVELD, J.C.F. de JONG, M.R. HALIE,
       C.Th. SMIT SIBINGA and Ch.R.H. WILDEVUUR: Hematologic Abnormali-
       ties in Extracorporeal Circuits (ECC). In: Clinical Aspects of
       Oxygenator Design, p. 197 (eds. Dawids and Engell), Elsevier/
       North Holland, Biomedical Press, Luxemburg, 1976
2      C.H. MIELKE, jr., M. de LEVAL, J.D. HILL, M.F. MACUR and
       F. GERBODE: Drug Influence on Platelet Loss during Extracorpo-
       real Circulation, J. Thorac. Cardiovasc. Surg. 66: 845, 1973.

Agostoni:         I have a comment on platelet behaviour during long-term extracorporeal circulation experiments in sheep. After an initial period of thrombocytopenia at the 4th and the 5th day there is an increase in the platelet number which is stable also in the next days Why do platelets increase after 4 or 5 days?

Born:             I have no obvious explanation. You said that the

34

counts remain low for such long time? Well, it is curious that there is then a sudden change. A new platelet population would have changed the situation gradually. This sudden change I cannot explain offhand.

Wildevuur:     I probably could give a suggestion to explain the increase in platelets on about day 4. The experiments described are long-term perfusions for 7 days in sheep, if I am correct. We have not done long-term perfusion and our model is the dog. However, in these 2 hours perfusion we do see a steep increase in platelet numbers around day four. They might implicate that the stimulation of the bone marrow by an ECC will become apparent in the circulating numbers around day four.

Born:          I agree, I have not thought of that. Thrombopoietin is controlled by a feedback mechanism. If the count is low for such a long time, there may be an overshoot of thrombopoietin, producing too many platelets from the megakariocytes.

Birnbaum:      I am still not quite satisfied in my understanding of this tremendous initial thrombocyte loss of more than 100 %. Do you have clinical experiments, which support the view that this thrombocyte loss is not due to hemodilution? We have thrombocyte losses in patients which are not due to hemodilution and which are far less pronounced.

Wildevuur:     The severe initial dip is most typical in dogs but has also been described for sheep. However, we have not seen this dip so typical in the human situation. This initial dip is clearly influenced by several factors, of which priming solutions have been mentioned earlier as being very important. We have looked back through all our dog experiments if we could consider the initial dip as a sensitive measure of hemocompatibility. However, because of the large standard

35

deviations we failed to prove it.

Born:                    I was recently in a research center in the States
                         where they do many bypass operations and they
                         almost invariably find that the platelet count
                         decreases much more than accountable for by hemo-
                         dilution.

Birnbaum:                We have also studied the thrombocyte loss in
                         clinical cases in two groups of patients.
                         One group with the bubble oxygenator and one
                         group with membrane oxygenator. We have calcula-

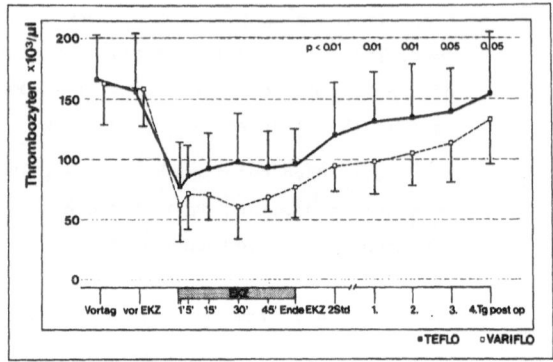

Fig. 1: Level of thrombocytes before, during and
after extracorporeal circulation (ECC) with two
different oxygenators for open heart surgery in
patients. (mean and std.dev., p = level of significance, n = 17 resp. 20)

ted exactly the thrombocyte loss by correcting
for the hemodiluting volume on basis of the hemoglobin concentration in the blood. We can see
that the value before extracorporeal circulation
starts at identical levels in the two groups. We
found   that the median of the losses during
extracorporeal circulation is much higher in the
group on a bubble oxygenator as compared with the
group on a membrane oxygenator. So we conclude
that the oxygenator or the extracorporeal circulatory system is responsible for the amount of
net thrombocyte loss.

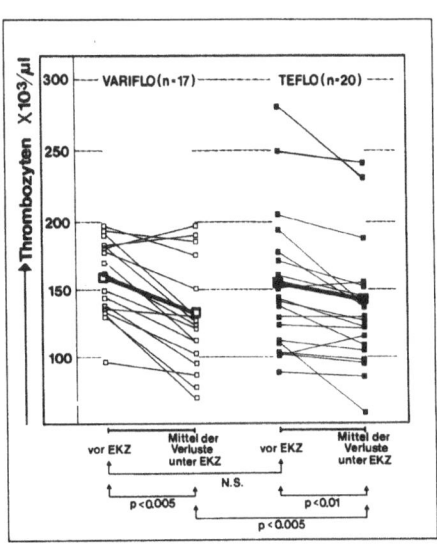

Fig. 2: Thrombocytes before ECC comparing the
mean of the counts during ECC (neclegting the
virtual loss by hemodilutional effects as caused
by the prime of heart lung machines).
(17 pts. with Variflo-Oxygenator, 20 pts. with
Teflo-membrane. Oxygenator; p = level of significance, n.s. = non significant).

Engell:     A decade ago, we learned that thrombocytes do
            not adhere to the intravascular wall surface, as
            following from the negative charge of the un-
            damaged endothelial cell. If that still holds
            true, and I suppose it does, can you possibly fit
            this into the present concept of platelet function?

Born:       First, a really crucial question is whether or
            not platelet adhere to the normal endothelium,
            for example in normal arteries or at least to
            endothelium which is minimally damaged, although
            no one knows what "minimally damaged" means. The
            reason for saying that is: There are now claims
            that the release of agents from platelets is
            essential in atherogenesis, e.g. the release of
            the smooth muscle stimulating factor. This hypo-

37

thesis implies that the edothelium must be sufficiently damaged in otherwise normal persons undergoing gradual atherosclerotic changes for the
platelets to adhere long enough to release this
factor; this has then to go on to the media and
stimulate smooth muscle cells, and so on. There
is now some evidence that platelets can adhere
to normal endothelium but only for *very short*
*periods of time.* Dr. Heino KORTENHAUS from Münster
and I are now looking at this very phenomenon *in*
*vivo* with quantitative methods. Concerning now
the other aspect as to whether platelets adhere
long enough to release this factor specifically
in atherogenetic situations, I think that it is
up to the people who are postulating this to
supply the corresponding proof. Surface charge
does come into this, but two neighboring negative
charges can be neutralized by calcium bridges. In
addition, there must be some highly specific
mechanism, because other cells, e.g. leucocytes,
do not adhere to the vessel wall.

Wenzel:    The drop of platelets in the dog and in human
beings goes parallel with a decrease of the mean
platelet volume. That is observed during extracorporeal circulation, and I think you have to
take into account that there are perhaps three
phases. First, there is hemodilution, you have a
drop in the platelet count but no change in the
mean platelet volume. When extracorporeal circulation is running, we have a decrease of the mean
platelet volume nad this is proportional to the
time of the perfusion. I will show details later
on. And then thirdly, you have again a drop, when
protamine is administered to neutralize heparin.
The last two phases are accompanied by a drop in
mean platelet volume and by an increase of the
number of very small platelets.

38

Schmid-Schönbein:    Coming back to the argument between Dr. Wildevuur
                     and Dr. Birnbaum, and to Dr. Born's presentation,
                     I would like to stress that while ADP is a very
                     potent activator of the platelets, which strongly
                     affects its metabolism, shape and therefore flow
                     behaviour, it is by no means the only platelet
                     stimulus. Instead, there are many unspecific sti-
                     muli. These unspecific stimuli also lead to a
                     shape change, albeit less pronounced. The follow-
                     ing figure (see Fig. 1, below    ), taken from the
                     very extensive work done by Dr. RIEGER (1) shows
                     the so-called "spontaneous platelet aggregation"
                     as tested in the "rheoaggregometer". The aggre-
                     gation is plotted as a function of time after

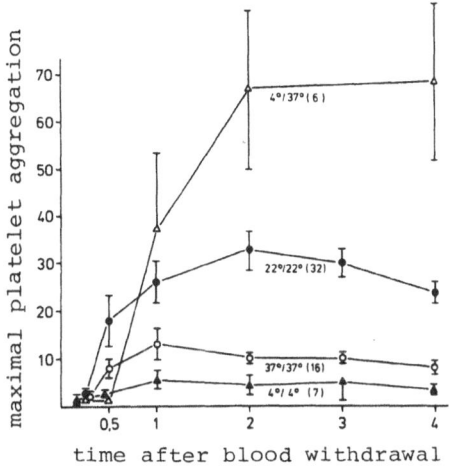

time after blood withdrawal

Fig. 1: Influence of temperature and time
elapsed after blood withdrawal on
"spontaneous" platelet activation

                     blood withdrawal, the aggregation measured in this
                     apparatus occurs without addition of so-called
                     aggregating agents. The machine is so designed
                     that the shear-rates are controlled. Therefore,
                     any encounter between aggregable platelets will

actually lead to a successful aggregate formation. Since the prevailing shear-stresses are relatively low, the formed aggregates will not be dispersed readily and their effect on light transmission can then be measured in the conventional way.

When we first used this machine, we thought we were measuring spontaneous or even "shear induced" platelet aggregation. Only later we found out, that this is not true, that we were rather caught in a trap that has been laid out by previous workers in the platelet field. I hope that Dr. Born will forgive me, but I would just like to remind you that if you read the platelet literature or even better talk to people who run platelet laboratories, you will notice that each laboratory has certain secret recipe concerning the preparation of platelet rich plasma for the actual platelet aggregating test. Most of these secrets include steps during which the platelets are allowed to cool or during which the $CO_2$ is allowed to evaporate. The resulting hypothermia or hypocapnia produces a very potent unspecific stimulus which can be seen to produce slight but significant changes in the platelet morphology (PIETSCH et al.). Most of the tests are done by first cooling the platelet and subsequent rewarming to $37^{o}C$ under which the actual test is executed. Dr. RIEGER's extensive work has finally brought an understanding of what is going on. During an isolated rise in pH, or during cooling to room temperature, "aggregability" increases quite substantial, "spontaneous" aggregation occurs provided the platelets collide under appropriate shear conditions. If both of these unspecific stimuli are avoided, no "spontenous" aggregation occurs, which, however, is very significant if the plate-

lets are first cooled and then subsequently rewarmed. The work of LIEPSCH and Dr. BREDDIN in
parallel with Dr. RIEGER's work, has provided
quantitative evidence that the "spontaneous"
aggregation we measure is in fact the consequence
of a spontaneous formation of pseudopodia, a finding we always also observe subjectively. We have
speculated earlier that such unspecific platelet
activation also occurs during extracorporeal circulation, for example during the oxygenator and
the early stages of the perfusion. This assumption
is born out by preliminary experiments done recently in our laboratory.

REFERENCE:

1    H. RIEGER: Zur Physiologie und Pathophysiologie der Blut-
     plättchen unter rheologischen Aspekten, Habilitationsschrift,
     Rheinisch-Westfälische Technische Hochschule Aachen, 1976

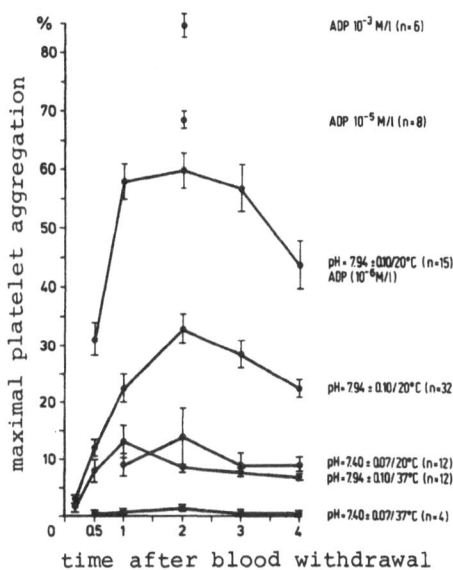

Fig. 2: Influence of temperature and pH on "spontaneous" platelet
aggregation (measured in a rheoaggregometer).
Note strong additive influence of two unspecific stimuli.
ADP effects ($10^{-3}$ and $10^{-5}$ Mol/L at 37$^{o}$C are shown for comparison
from (1)

The effective unspecific stimuli not only effect
the spontaneous aggregability of platelets but
likewise their response to the classical so-
called aggregating agents such as adenosin-diphos-
phate. The Figure, taken from Dr. RIEGER's work,
shows that for both response curves of adenosin-
diphosphate in citrated human platelet fresh
plasma can be shifted by two orders of magnitude
by these "unspecific stimuli". Taking into account
the time effect that was seen in Fig. 6, you will
notice that when PRP is prepared in the conventional way (in other words by allowing alkalosis
and hypothermia) the dose response curve is shifted to the left by a factor 100. If, on the other
hand, the pH is maintained, platelets are never
allowed to cool, the response to ADP in our aggregometer is drastically reduced over a very wide
range of ADP concentration. I believe that the
specific stimuli must be taken into account and
must have an important additional role in vivo
as well.

Born:                    This is very interesting. I would hesitate to use
the word unspecific and I would like to suggest
that you repeat these experiments in the presence
of apyrase or cratin-phosphokinase to remove any
ADP released during storage.

Schmid-Schönbein:        Thank you for your suggestion. We are well aware
that our results at $37^{\circ}C$ could be affected by
some kind of ADP-release; however, we are not
concerned about these as much as about the
"spontaneous" shape change (PIETSCH et al.) and
aggregability (RIEGER) found at room temperature
and room $pCO_2$. Under these conditions, a release
is much less likely. If we therefore find both
strongly enhanced aggregation without $^{14}C$-Sero-
tonin-release at $20^{\circ}C$, and also such a pronounced
shift of the dose response curve to ADP over the

42

whole range of concentrations we tend to take it as a "real" effect. This hypothesis is substantiated by recent clinical results in the field of platelet transfusion (2,3). Several groups have found that cooling of platelets prior to infusion leads to a very rapid drop in platelet count, whereas meticulous maintenance of isothermic conditions allows much longer survival. Under these conditions hypothermically stimulated "do their thing", i.e. induce hemostasis - by disappearing from the circulation ( 2 ). This concept from the field of platelet transfusion is important for our field as well.

REFERENCES:

1  PIETSCH, U., LIPPMANN, M., SCHARRER, I., BREDDIN, K.: Neue Befunde zur Wirkung von Acetylsalicylsäure. In Diabetische Angiopathien. Herausgeg. v. K. Alexander u. M. Cachovan, bei Verlag G. Witzstrock, Baden-Baden, (1977)
2  KATTLOVE, H.E., ALEXANDER, B.: The effect of cold on platelets I. Cold-induced platelet aggregation. Blood 38, 39 (1971)
3  VALLEJOS, C.S., FREIREICH, E.J., BRITTIN, G.M., DE JONGH, D.S.: Effect of platelets stored at 22°C for 24 h in patients with acute leukemia. Blood 42, 565 (1973)

Birnbaum:                May I add some information about the procedure in the clinic? We do normothermic perfusion, we warm up the prime of the extracorporeal machine and we regulate the $pCO_2$ to physiological ranges. Under these conditions were performed the platelet counts reported earlier. This might be the reason that the drop in thrombocytes in our patients is not as severe as in laboratory animals. We know from clinical experience (which might not be the value criterium for physiologists) that

normothermia does not cause so many complications
in the postoperative course.

Born: I want to throw one other complication into the
pot. It is now certain from work by GRYGLEWSKI
and MONCADA that the lungs produce continously a
prostacyclin as a circulating hormone. Now prostacyclin is the most potent inactivator of platelets
and may account for differences in the platelet
behaviour on the arterial and venous sides of the
circulation. The initial drop in platelet count
is presumably due to some stimulus which overcomes
any inhibitory effect of prostacyclin.

Van den Dungen: A comment on Dr. Born's remarks about the effec-
tiveness of the prostacyclin ($PGI_2$) and the
prostaglandin ($PGE_1$) to preserve platelets during
extracorporeal circulation. We used both platelet
inhibiting drugs during experiments in which dogs
underwent 2 hours of normothermic bubble oxygenator (Temptrol Q-110) perfusion nad were compared
to a control group (n = 6). $PGE_1$ (1-2 µg/kg/min,
n = 6) and $PGI_2$ (0.5-1 µg/kg/min, n = 6) were infused throughout the period of bypass into the
venous line. As compared to the control group
the platelet numbers (see Fig. 3, page 45 ) in
the $PGI_2$-treated group were significantly better
maintained throughout the period of bypass and up
to the second postoperative day, while the $PGE_1$-
treated group only at two hours after the end of
bypass and on the first postoperative day significantly higher numbers than in the control group
could be determined. The platelet function (see
Fig. 4; page 45 ) measured by the collagen - as
well as ADP - induced aggregation, was also one
or two hours after perfusion significantly better
preserved in the treated groups. The Borchgrevinck
bleeding time was in the treated groups only mo-
derately lengthened two hours after perfusion,
while in the control group the bleeding time was

longer than 15 minutes. The improvement in platelet function which can be achieved with these
drugs might be relevant because at a time when
optimal hemostasis is needed, the platelets are
shortly after clinical cardiopulmonary bypass,
almost completely refractory to aggregating agents.
However, the strong hypotensive side-effect of
these drugs might limit their application.

Fig. 3:

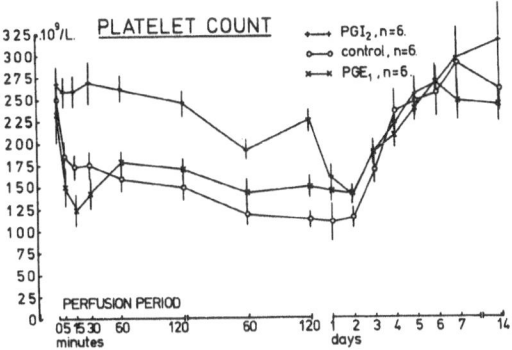

Fig. 4:

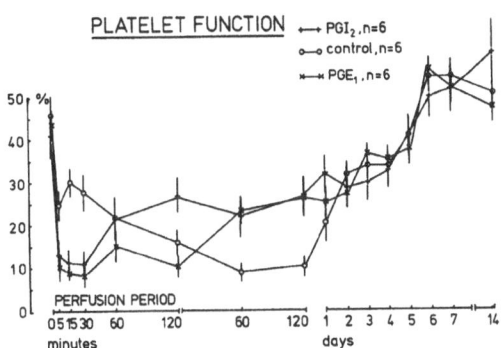

# 3. STIMULATION OF HUMAN PLATELETS UNDER THE INFLUENCE OF HIGH SHEAR STRESSES IN TUBE FLOW[1]

Forst, R.[2], Rieger, H., Schmid-Schönbein, H., Department of Physiology, Medical Faculty, RWTH Aachen, Melatener Straße 211, D-5100 Aachen, West Germany

## 1. INTRODUCTION

Thrombotic events in artificial organs (platelet deposition and fibrin formation) often manifest themselves in areas of retarded flow or stasis, "dead water zones" or areas of recirculation (RICHARDSON). However, there are exceptions to this, since platelet deposition is also seen in areas of high local flow. As a matter of fact, many forms of platelet deposition become the more pronounced the higher the local shear rate (FRIEDMAN, LEONARD, TURITTO). Furthermore, the possibility should be considered that the events (manifestation and triggering) of thrombosis do *not* take place at the same site. It has been argued (SCHMID-SCHÖNBEIN, 1977) that certain steps of the activation sequence for platelets might take place in the streaming blood - that activated platelets travel with the blood stream and become deposited in areas when wall structure and/or flow conditions favour the encounter with the wall or with thrombotic material already deposited there.

Lastly, there is even the possibility that high flow regimes not only *allow* but even *promote* the activation of platelets (or other components of the coagulation system).

---

1 Supported by Sonderforschungsbereich 109 (Projekt $C_2$) der Deutschen Forschungsgemeinschaft.

2 Experimental work done in partial fulfillment of a doctoral dissertation (D 82), Medical Faculty, RWTH Aachen.

Platelets are subjected to complicated tangential and normal forces when flowing, they rotate, become bent and they collide with other platelets (and/or with other blood elements) or with the wall in areas of disturbed flow. Physical forces are well-known to trigger "activity" of living cells, the best known example being the "myogenic activation" of smooth muscle by stretch (see Textbooks of Physiology, e.g. FOLKOW and NEIL). Physical contact (ZUCKER) or shear forces (RIEGER, GOLDSMITH et al.) have previously been shown to be essential for the completion of a "release reaction" triggered by chemical stimuli. The work of BROWN et al., HUNG et al. and ANDERSON have presented evidence of such "activation" following prolonged shearing of whole blood and platelet rich plasma.

The present work attempts to quantify possible platelet "activation" by *short* exposure times, such as they might occur in artificial organs. To this end, heparinized and citrated platelet rich plasma was perfused with varying wall shear stresses through stainless steel tubes of varying lengths.

47

## 2. METHODS AND MATERIALS

Heparinized human platelet rich plasma was perfused from
plastic syringes through steel canulae with internal diameters of 200 µm and a length of two to fifty cm (see
Fig. 1). The plastic piston of the syringes was driven by
a variable motor, which allowed to produce a constant
pressure and constant flow. The wall shear stresses were
computed under the assumption of a parabolic velocity
profile.

**PUMPELEMENT**

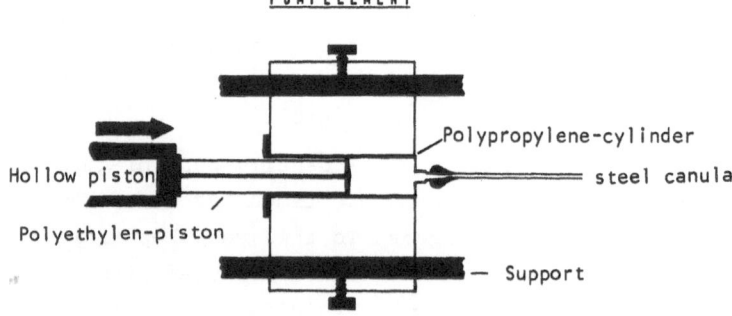

Fig. 1: Schematic sketch of the apparatus: mechanical support (1) of the polypropylene-cylinder (2). A
hollow piston (3) driven by the motor (not shown)
presses the polyethylene-plug. Flow of platelet
rich plasma through the stainless-steel-canula is
produced. The whole apparatus is maintained at
$37^{\circ}C$ (heating coil and air-ventilator) throughout
the experiment.

Platelet rich plasma was obtained from heparinized human
venous blood, and was loaded with $C^{14}$ Serotonin, as
described by MASSINI and LÜSCHER. Following complete $C^{14}$
Serotonin uptake, spontaneous release was inhibited by
Imipramine ($2 \cdot 10^{-6}$M/l ). Before and after the shearing exposure, the release of $C^{14}$ Serotonin was measured by
spinning down the platelets at high centrifugal force and
comparing the radioactivity  in the total to that of the
supernatant plasma sample. In additional experiments, we

determined the destruction of platelets by measuring LDH activity and the platelet factor III availability.

The rheological experiments were performed as follows: The Serotonin  labelled PRP was perfused once or several times through the apparatus. Before, during and after perfusing the temperature was maintained at $37^{\circ}$C throughout the experiment. We carefully avoided any cooling of the samples before or during the experiment.

## 3. RESULTS

Figure 2 shows the influence of wall shear stress and of the cumulative passage time. This is the calculated mean passage time for any single perfusion, multiplied by the number of perfusions. As can be seen $C^{14}$ Serotonin release was measured with a constant wall shear stress of 200 N/m$^2$. After a single passage, we found a small but not significant release (see Fig. 2). This small release is understandable, if one keeps in mind, that only a small fraction of the platelets are actually exposed to these shear stresses, since only a small fraction of the platelets is flowing near the vessel wall. In order to obtain information about the influence of passage time, we repeated the perfusions 5 and 10 times. For comparison, we used canulae with very different lengths, namely 20 and 500 mm. By appropriate control of the pump rate, we could obtain the same pressure gradient ($\Delta P/1$) but much shorter exposure times. In these experiments, we could also investigate the influence of the other parts of this setup, mostly a possible influence of the very steep stenosis, causing entrance effects, sudden accelerations etc. As indicated by the very small release even after 10 passages the apparatus per se does not produce a significant effect. Flow induced release is only found if the system contains a long tube, which produces a high shear stress for several hundred msec. This finding also suggested that besides the shear stress, the time of exposure is important for shear induced release. In all further experiments we therefore kept the cumulative passage time constant and varied the incident driving pressures by manipulation of the pump rate, producing wall shear stresses of 48.7, 100, 200 and 279.6 N/m$^2$.

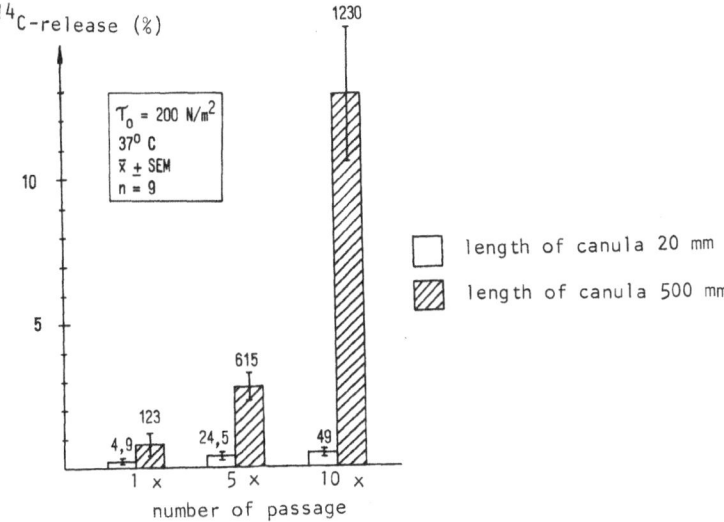

Fig. 2: Effect of the tube length and the number of passages on the percent release of $C^{14}$ Serotonin from platelet rich plasma subjected to flow (wall shear stress 200 $N/m^2$). The mean passage times (in milliseconds) of the platelets flowing through the tubes are given above the bars.

Fig. 3 shows the influence of the wall shear stress under the condition of 1230 msec cumulative mean passage time; there is a steady increase. The finite release at zero wall shear stress (unshared control) is not significant. At 279 $N/m^2$, we measured a release of 3.0 $\pm$ 0.5·$10^3$ CPM or 22 $\pm$ 2% of the total radio activity taken up as Serotonin by the platelets.

The shearing experiments provoked the release reaction but did not lead to a significant physical destruction of the platelets. As shown in Fig. 4, there was no significant change in the LDH activity in the supernatant of sheared platelet rich plasma. The dotted columns again show the increase in $C^{14}$ activity with increasing shear stresses, whereas the shaded columns show constancy of the LDH-activity in the plasma.

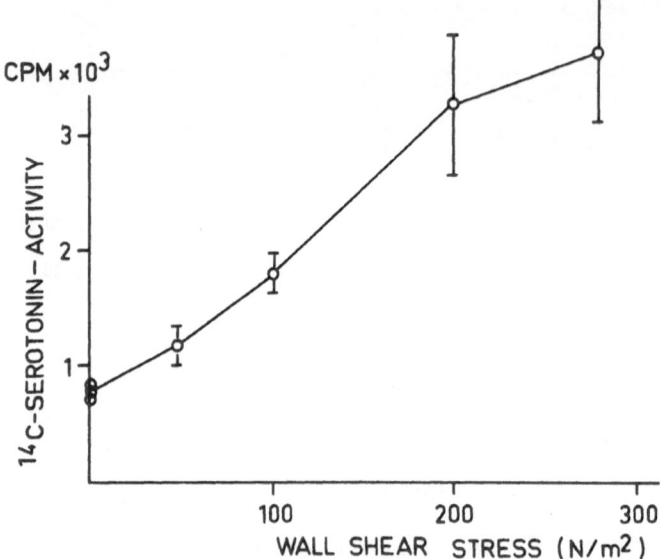

Fig. 3: Release of $C^{14}$ Serotonin ($\overline{X} \pm$ S.E.M.) during repeated shearing of human heparinized PRP as a
function of the wall shear stress. Cumulative
passage time 1.23 sec, i.e. the high values are
related to more frequent exposure.

In this set of experiments, both $C^{14}$ Serotonin and LDH
activity after shearing was always compared to the unsheared control to account for spontaneous loss of thrombocytes (which was not significant). The constant LDH
level of about 120 units/l in the control sample and in
the sheared samples in our experiments argues against any
significant platelet destruction in our experiments. Statistical evaluation shows, that in none of the three shear
stress stages there is any correlation between $C^{14}$ Sero-
tonin- and LDH release.

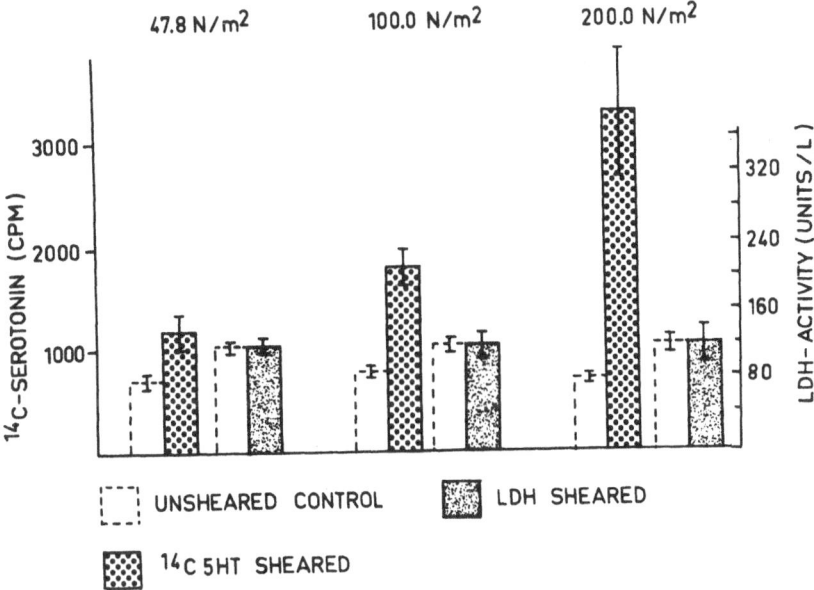

Fig. 4: Influence of wall shear stress on release of
C$^{14}$ Serotonin and LDH. Cumulative passage time
1.2 sec, 37$^{\circ}$C, heparinized human platelet rich
plasma.

As demonstrated in Fig. 5. phospholipids activating coagulation are made available during shear. To measure the
so-called "platelet factor III-activity", we simply took
the recalcification times with and without the addition
of caolin. Following shear exposure, we found a highly
significant reduction in recalcification times. The absolute difference to the unsheared controls is higher without caolin; the percent difference, however, roughly 40%
reduction in recalcification times is identical in both
tests. We also investigated the effect of the anticoagulant, keeping in mind, that heparin is the conventional
anticoagulant in artificial organs. Fig. 6 compares the
effect of sodium citrate alone to anticoagulation with heparin alone, left column, and to that of the addition of

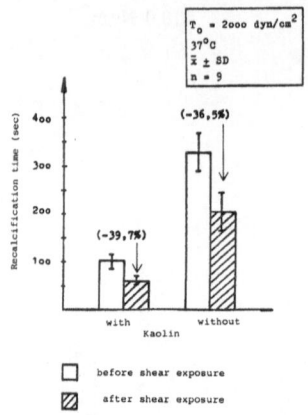

Fig. 5: Influence of shearing on recalcification time
of citrated human PRP. ReK = Recalcification
time with Kaolin, Re = recalcification time without Kaolin. Open columns: control, dashed columns:
PRP after shearing at 200 N/m$^2$.

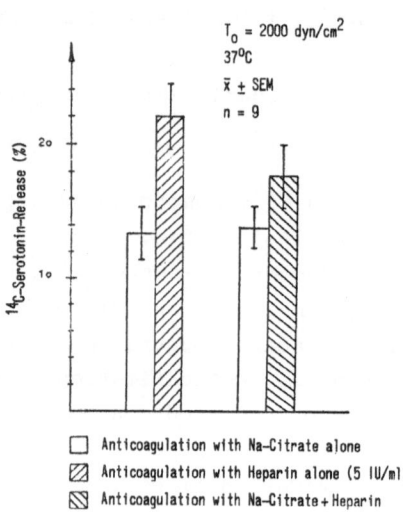

Fig. 6: C$^{14}$ Serotonin release in the presence of either
sodium citrate or heparin alone or of both of them.

heparin to previously citrated plasma (right column). In each case, the $C^{14}$ serotonin release is augmented, in absolute terms much more, when heparin is used as the sole anticoagulant. The difference between heparin alone and citrate alone is significant. We interpreted this as a result of the presence of calcium ions. The difference between citrate and citrate plus heparin is not significant.

## 4. DISCUSSION

The present data can be summarized as follows:
Exposure of platelets to shear stresses above 100 N/m$^2$
($\hat{=}$ 1000 dyn/cm$^2$) for time periods below 1000 msec induces
a release reaction (C$^{14}$ serotonin), makes available substantial amounts of platelet-factor 3   but does not lyse
the platelets. Unpublished experiments in our laboratory
have shown that these platelets after shear exposure in
the same apparatus also show significantly higher "spontaneous" aggregation when tested in a rheoaggregometer.

These results in principle agree with those obtained by
prolonged shear exposure in a rotational viscometer
(HELLUMS et al., COLANTUONI et al.); however, there are substantial differences in the interpretation of these results and ours. In our system, we did not destroy but
rather activate the platelets by inducing a classical
"viscous metamorphosis" by mechanical means.

(According to DAY and HOLMSEN) the release reaction is an
*active secretory, energy-dependent* process, which has been
regarded as a general biological response of the platelets
to a host of quite different stimuli and/or chemical
agents. Up to date mostly the *chemical stimulation* of the
viscous metamorphosis has been studied, easily triggered
off by reagents such as ADP, collagen and thrombin. We now
find that shear forces can also lead to a similar response;
the details of this mechanical activation awaits microrheological analysis. The result of this difficult task
notwithstanding, it must henceforth be accepted that even
stationary, laminar flow of PRP leading to wall shear
stresses in excess of 50 N/m$^2$ (500 dyn/cm$^2$) can trigger
significant platelet responses. A much more pronounced
effect, presumably at even lower shear forces, must be
expected under the much more adverse flow conditions ex-
perienced by platelets subjected to shear in whole blood
in non-stationary flow.

One of the most important open questions about shear activation of platelets concerns the activation time. In our experiments, the exposure time played a significant rôle, unfortunately, in tube flow experiments there is not only a distribution of shear rates and/or shear stresses across the tube radius, but also a distribution of passage times. In the region near the wall, where the *velocity* is *lowes t* and the passage time is highest, the *velocity gradient* and thence the shear stress is greatest. However, during each passage only a small fraction of the platelets is actually travelling in the marginal fluid layers experiencing the high shear. Therefore, the small release reaction found after a single passage (Fig. 2) is of substantial significance, as is the clear cut increase in release seen with rising wall shear stress but constant mean passage time (Fig. 3). The small, unsignificant release found with short tubes despite of identical wall shear stresses and identical repetitions argues against possible artefacts by the apparatus used - and at the same time it strongly underlines the significance of the exposure *time*. Among many possible explanations for this phenomenon we would like to envoke two possible mechanisms:

1. there might be a finite activation time for each individual platelet and
2. there might be a cascade activation via a primary mechanical release of trace amounts of serotonin, followed by secondary chemical activation via serotonin or other aggregating agents.

The release of platelet phospholipids capable of accelerating the coagulation sequence is another noteworthy finding. The stimulation of both the aggregability of the platelets and the reactivity of the plasmatic coagulation system by high shear forces may have a bearing on our understanding of thrombotic events in artificial organs, which occur despite "adequate" heparinization (FRIEDMAN, RICHARDSON, LINDSAY). The "classical" theory relates localized coagulation phenomena to an activation

of enzymatic events that takes place at the very site of
fibrin formation and/or platelet deposition. Such an event
would require a local stimulus ("thrombogenic surface")
and "stasis" (long term accumulation of coagulatory enzymes and of platelets). It was therefore logical to
attempt to make artificial surfaces "non-thrombogenic",
(to avoid "topical activation"); it was likewise logical
to design artificial organs in a manner avoiding "stasis".

The "classical" theory can now be extended and/or replaced
by the theory of shear activation. The present data lend
support to the assumption that the components of the coagulatory system become activated in the entire artificial
organ, especially in areas of high shear. According to this
view, only the site of manifestation of thrombotic phenomena is determined by the local conditions, especially in
areas of recirculation, stagnation point flow or "stasis".
More experimental work is needed to establish or discard
the value of this heterodox theory.

REFERENCES

1 RICHARDSON, P.D., P.M. GALLETTI: Correlation of effect
  of blood flow rate and design features on artificial
  lung performance. In: Physiological and Clinical Aspects
  of Oxygenator Design. S.G. Dawids and H.C. Engell (Eds.)
  Elsevier (Amsterdam, Oxford, New York) 1976, p. 29-44

2 FRIEDMAN, L.J., H. LIEM, E.F. GRABOWSKI, E.F. LEONARD,
  and C.W. McCORD: Inconsequentiality of surface properties for initial platelet adhesion. Trans.Am.Soc.Artif.
  Organs 16, 63 (1970)

3 LEONARD, E.F.: The role of flow in thrombogenesis.
  Bull. N.Y. Acad.Med. 48, 273-280 (1972)

4 TURITTO, V.T., E.F. LEONARD: Platelet adhesion to a
  spinning surface. Trans.Am.Soc.Artif.Organs 18, 348
  (1972)

5 SCHMID-SCHÖNBEIN, H.: Microrheology of Erythrocytes and
  Thrombocytes, Blood Viscosity and the Distribution of
  Blood Flow in the Microcirculation. Handbuch der allge-
  meinen Pathologie III/7 Mikrozirkulation. H. Meessen Ed.
  Springer-Verlag Berlin, Heidelberg, New York, 1977,
  p. 289-384

6 FOLKOW, B., E. NEIL: "Circulation". Oxford University
  Press, 1971

7 ZUCKER, M.B.: Proteolytic inhibitors, contact and other
  variables in the release reaction of human platelets.
  Thromb.Diath.Haemorrh. 28, 393 (1972)

8 RIEGER, H.: Zur Physiologie und Pathophysiologie der
  Blutplättchen unter rheologischen Aspekten. Habilita-
  tionsschrift RWTH Aachen, 1976

9 GOLDSMITH, H.L., J.C. MARLOW, and S.K. YU: The effect
  of oscillatory flow on the release reaction and aggregation of human platelets. Microvasc.Res. 11, 335-341
  (1976)

10 HUNG, T.C., R.M. HOCHMUTH, J.H. JOIST, and S.P. SUTERA: Shear-induced aggregation and lysis of platelets. Trans.Am.Soc.Artif.Intern. Organs 22, 285-291 (1976)

11 BROWN, C.H., L.B. LEVERETT, C.W. LEWIS, C.P. ALFREY jr. and J.D. HELLUMS: Morphological, biochemical and functional changes in human platelets subjected to shear stress. J.Lab.Clin.Med. 86, 462-471 (1975)

12 MASSINI, P., E.F. LÜSCHER: The induction of the release reaction in human blood platelets by close cell contact. Thromb.Diath.Haemorrh. 25, 13 (1971)

13 HELLUMS, J.D., and C.H. BROWN: Blood cell damage by mechanical forces. In: Cardiovascular Flow Dynamics and Measurements. N.H.C. Hwang, N.A. Normann (eds.), Baltimore, University Park Press, 1977, p. 799

14 COLANTUONI, G., J.D. HELLUMS, J.L. MOAKE, and C.P. ALFREY jr.: The response of human platelets to shear stress at short exposure times. Trans.Am.Soc. Artif.Intern.Organs 23, 626-630 (1977)

15 DAY, H.J., and HOLMSEN, H.: Concepts of the blood platelet release reaction. Series Hemat. 4, 1-99 (1971)

16 LINDSAY, R.M.:Platelets, foreign surfaces, and heparin. In: Physiological and Clinical Aspects of Oxygenator Design. S.G. Dawids and H.C. Engell (eds.) Elsevier (Amsterdam, Oxford, New York) 1976, p. 183-194

Moderator: Born

Born:            Thank you, Dr. Forst. The release reaction is a
                 rather late reaction. The classical release re-
                 action with thrombin appears in a few seconds.
                 That sounds very fast but in relation to what
                 happens in vivo in a few milliseconds this is
                 very slow. So my point is that you should con-
                 tinue to look for some criteria of platelet re-
                 activity which is more rapid.

Forst:           Thank you for this suggestion.

Born:            Your method may be the quickest way of showing
                 the release reaction but the emphasis has to be
                 on still faster events.

Williams:        I would just like to say that we have developed a
                 technique in Manchester, which does essentially
                 the same sort of thing that we have presented
                 here. We are looking at the same cells, and I am
                 interested in what we have heard so far about the
                 shear "activation" of platelets. We have de-
                 veloped a technique in Manchester where we have
                 produced shear-stresses which are generated inside
                 intact blood vessels without any need to anti-
                 coagulate the blood or remove it from the animal.
                 We can in fact produce thrombi and watch these
                 thrombi grow even after very short exposure times
                 of the platelets  (see page 63 , paper presented
                 at this symposium).

Born:            Activation within a few hundred milliseconds
                 sounds very fast, but in relation to our joint
                 results obtained in shearing red cells (see
                 page 322, paper presented by Dr. SCHMID-SCHÖNBEIN,
                 ROHLING-WINKEL et al. at this symposium) this is
                 a very slow business.

Schmid-Schönbein: This may well be true, however, Dr. Forst's results show that there is in fact a release after an extremely short exposure. Let us keep in mind, if he measures free serotonin in the plasma following shear exposure which affects only a small proportion of the platelets (namely those travelling in the marginal layers of his capillary). This indicates that something has happened to the platelets. We have simply taken a biochemically measurable indicator of such activation. We know, that other experimental set-ups are much better to measure the kinetics of this biological event. In other words, I am not at all convinced that our results are a good model of the real behaviour and I am willing to accept that a much shorter exposure of platelets to physical stimuli activates them.

Born: It is a very interesting story, indeed.

Williams: I would just like to re-make the point that these very same things that we demonstrated here can be shown in vivo, occurring after very short exposure times of some milliseconds. Shear-stresses of the order of 300-500 dyn/cm$^2$ induce the platelets to aggregate giving micro-thrombi, and it is not an effect of the vessel wall because the thrombi which embolize do not re-grow on the same site. Therefore, the endothelium was not damaged to a significant extent.

Born: Thank you. We will return to this point later (see page 322) when we talk about red cell interaction. There are many other interesting points raised by Dr. Forst to which we will also return later. I made no criticisms at all, I think these are beautiful results.

# 4.

THE INDUCTION OF INTRAVASCULAR THROMBI <u>IN VIVO</u> BY MEANS OF

LOCALISED HYDRODYNAMIC SHEAR STRESSES

A.R. Williams

Department of Medical Biophysics, University of Manchester, England.

## Abstract

A small object oscillating at ultrasonic frequencies while immersed in a liquid generates around itself a second order acoustic micro-streaming field. The hydrodynamic shear stresses produced within this shear field are similar both in magnitude and time of exposure to the maximum stresses produced in blood during turbulent flow or in flowing around the valves of the heart. A novel technique has been developed whereby a vibrating probe is applied to the intact wall of a mesenteric vessel in an anaesthetised mammal so that a portion of its undamaged endothelium is driven to oscillate at this same ultrasonic frequency (85 kHz). Acoustic microstreaming can be observed within the intact vessels and aggregates of platelets can be seen to build up within the flowing blood.

A motion-picture film was presented which showed that at very low displacement amplitudes one could observe intravascular microstreaming which disappeared as soon as the power supply to the transducer was turned off. No aggregates of platelets were visible if the maximum applied shear stresses were less than about 10 to 20 Newtons $m^{-2}$. When the applied shear stress exceeded about 25 $Nm^{-2}$ translucent aggregates of platelets (white thrombi) could be seen to build up within the centre of the microstreaming vortices. This indicates that the platelets were "activated" by the shear stress alone, and did not require contact with a "thrombogenic" surface. These platelet aggregates were seen to be exceptionally adhesive and attached themselves to any solid surface with which they came into contact. If the aggregates did not contact the vessel wall, they were embolised downstream when the ultrasonic probe was switched off; under these conditions there was frequently no growth of a platelet thrombus at the site of application of the probe indicating that the vascular endothelium had apparently not been damaged by the application of the

63

vibrating probe.

It was proposed that this technique could be used as an <u>in vivo</u> model system to evaluate the effects on platelet function of the various anticoagulants in common use, and any other pharmacologically active agents which modify the haemostatic system.

## Introduction

Blood is subjected to shear forces during flow. The applied shear stress ($\tau$) is usually expressed in units of Newtons per square meter ($Nm^{-2}$) or dynes $cm^{-2}$ and is the product of the suspension viscosity ($\eta$) times the velocity gradient (G) existing within it. Estimates of the velocity gradients which are established within the normal human circulation range from about 100 $s^{-1}$ in the great veins and 200 $s^{-1}$ in the aorta to about 600 $s^{-1}$ or more within the microcirculation. It has been proposed that even these relatively low velocity gradients may determine the survival time <u>in vivo</u> of certain blood proteins (e.g. fibrinogen: Charm and Wong, 1970) and perhaps also the blood cellular elements. However, strenuous exercise markedly increases these velocity gradients to the point where the erythrocytes are instantaneously disrupted and free haemoglobin may appear in the urine (e.g. march haemoglobinuria). These potentially dangerous shear forces may be approached under sedentary conditions if the blood flow becomes turbulent (e.g. in a post-stenotic dilatation or around an artificial heart valve which has been fitted incorrectly).

Unfortunately, it is difficult to characterise or exactly reproduce the complex flow fields which exist in turbulent situations. Cells in a turbulent suspension are alternately subjected to very high shear stresses (probably in excess of about 60 $Nm^{-2}$) for short times (of the order of milliseconds) followed by equally brief intervals of near stasis. This complex cyclic shear history may be duplicated in a more convenient and reproducible manner by an acoustic microstreaming field.

Acoustic microstreaming is the name given to the small-scale steady-state (second order) streaming pattern formed around a solid or gaseous body vibrating at a high frequency whilst immersed in a fluid (Nyborg, 1965). A graphical representation of the streaming pattern

64

around the hemispherical tip of a longitudinally vibrating cylinder is presented in Figure 1 (drawn from Holtzmark et al., 1954). Cells in suspension are accelerated towards the vibrating source and are subjected to high velocity gradients as they pass close by. The maximum velocity gradients developed by this device are given by:

$$G = 2\pi f \varepsilon_o^2 / a\delta$$

where f is the frequency of oscillation; $\varepsilon_o$ is the displacement amplitude; a is the radius of the vibrating source and $\delta$ is the boundary layer thickness which is equal to 2.7 μm for human plasma at a frequency of 85 kHz. The cells remain within this shear field for about a millisecond, and are subsequently decelerated as they enter the large streaming vortex.

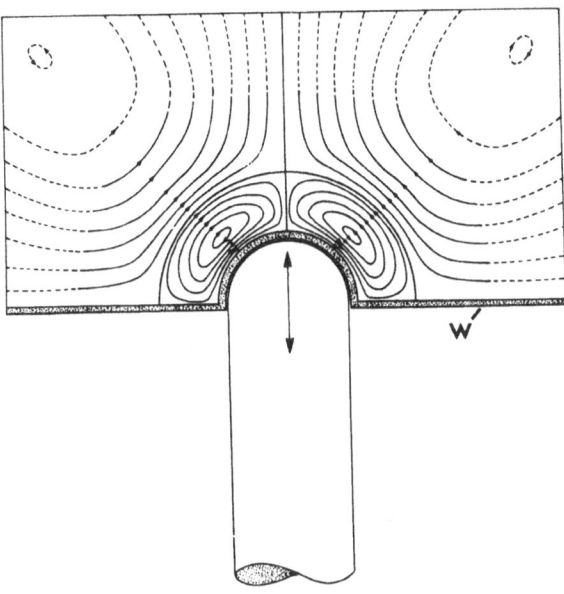

Figure 1. A graphical representation of the acoustic microstreaming pattern generated around the hemispherical tip of a longitudinally vibrating cylinder. W represents the wall of an intact blood vessel.

Thus, the amplitude of oscillation (and hence the magnitude of the applied shear stress) may be increased until a "threshold" point is exceeded and the suspended cells are damaged. Human erythrocytes in isotonic saline or in their own plasma are lysed when the applied shear stress exceeds about 160 $Nm^{-2}$* (Williams, 1971). However, human platelets are about ten times more fragile - this same oscillating wire system induces functional platelets in plasma to undergo the release at only about 14 $Nm^{-2}$ and ruptures the platelet outer membrane at stresses greater than about 89 $Nm^{-2}$ (Williams, 1974). These values are broadly in agreement with other workers (e.g. Brown et al., 1975) who showed that shear stresses of 5 to 10 $Nm^{-2}$ for 5 minutes caused the release of intracellular platelet components.

The main advantage of the acoustic microstreaming technique is that it may be used to subject platelets to controlled hydrodynamic shear stresses in an _in vivo_ situation without having to construct an elaborate by-pass circuit with its attendant problems of thromogenic surfaces. Williams (1977) has shown that a portion of the wall of an intact blood vessel can be driven to oscillate at an ultrasonic frequency by means of a vibrating metal probe or wire. The probe indents the wall of the vessel and contact is maintained by the animals own blood pressure (i.e. the situation is analagous to pushing one's finger into an air or water-filled balloon). When the probe is driven to oscillate, a hemispherical portion of the vessel wall moves with it and induces an acoustic microstreaming field within the flowing blood. When the amplitude of oscillation exceeded about 6 μm at 20 kHz, aggregates of platelets could be detected attached to the vessel wall even though the endothelium beneath them appeared to be undamaged (Williams, 1977). At even greater amplitudes (corresponding to shear stresses of the order of 100 $Nm^{-2}$) mixed thrombi were observed and all platelet aggregates were contracted and well

---

* It should be noted that the shear stress required to disrupt an erythrocyte depends upon the viscosity of the suspending medium (Morris and Williams, 1978). Consequently, the "critical shear stress" of 650 $Nm^{-2}$ required to disrupt human erythrocytes in a 31 centipoise medium using this same acoustic microstreaming technique (Williams, Hughes and Nyborg, 1970) is only valid for that particular value of suspending medium viscosity at 20 kHz.

permeated with fibrin.

The present article describes a modification of this in vivo technique whereby the microstreaming pattern is visually monitored throughout the time of sonication. This enables a direct estimate to be made of the "threshold" amplitude for the activation of platelets to aggregate in vivo; and enabled a motion-picture film to be made to record the effects of acoustic microstreaming on platelet function, as they occurred.

## Materials and Experimental Method

A cylindrical barium titanate/lead zirconate transducer (T) (3 cm long and 1.25 cm O.D.) resonant in its longitudinal mode at about 85 kHz was bonded with epoxy resin to a 4.3 cm long exponentially tapered (stepped) stainless steel velocity transformer (probe, P) (Figure 2). The tip of the probe was 52.5 μm in diameter and was ground so as to be approximately hemispherical (Figure 3). At 84.5 kHz the transducer/probe assembly was in resonance and the tip of the probe was a displacement antinode whose amplitude increased in a linear manner with increasing voltage supplied to the transducer.

A sinusoidal electrical signal was generated by means of a TG1800 oscillator (Green Industries Ltd.) and amplified by an EMI Model 240L-50dB power amplifier. A calibration curve was established so that any given peak to peak voltage across the transducer could be converted into the displacement amplitude at the probe tip (in μm).

Neonatal or young adult mice, rats, rabbits or guinea pigs were anaesthetised by means of gaseous Halothane or an intravenous or intraperitoneal injection of Nembutal (Pentobarbital) at a dosage of 60 mg/kg body weight. The ventral abdominal wall was incised and a portion of the small intestine pulled out so that part of its intact mesenteric circulation could be laid on a warm polished glass block, G (Figure 2). The animal rested on a transparent glass vessel (C) through which water was pumped at a temperature of $39^{\circ}$C.

The tip of the probe was positioned at the focus of a Leitz microscope to which was attached a Bolex 16 mm movie camera. The heated stage was raised and manoeuvred until the blood vessel to be treated made contact with the tip of the probe.

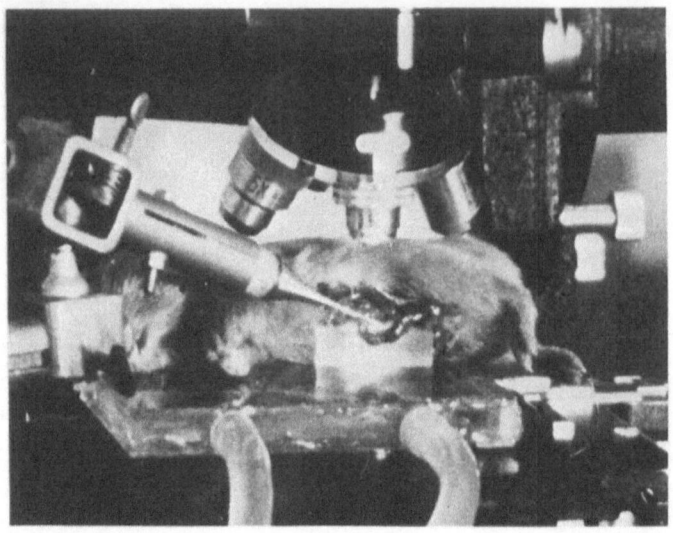

Figure 2. A frame from the 16 mm motion picture film showing the tapered probe (P) attached to the transducer (T). A portion of mesentry was exposed and placed on a glass block (G) which was kept warm by the transparent thermostated chamber, C.

A motion picture film was made at 10 to 20 frames per second to show the effects of hydrodynamic shear stresses generated by acoustic microstreaming on platelet function in vivo.

Results and Discussion

Figure 1 shows the predicted acoustic microstreaming pattern for a hemispherical solid or gaseous body oscillating in a longitudinal (or transverse) mode while immersed in a liquid (Holtzmark et al., 1954). The pattern consists of two small closed eddies situated immediately next to the oscillating interface, and two large scale eddies which bring fluid in towards the probe tip, subject it to shear, and then push it away. The small boundary layer thickness in blood plasma at 85 kHz (2.7 μm) means that the innermost eddies would not be readily apparent and so only the outer large scale vortices are visible under relatively low power (x 100) magnification (Figure 3).

68

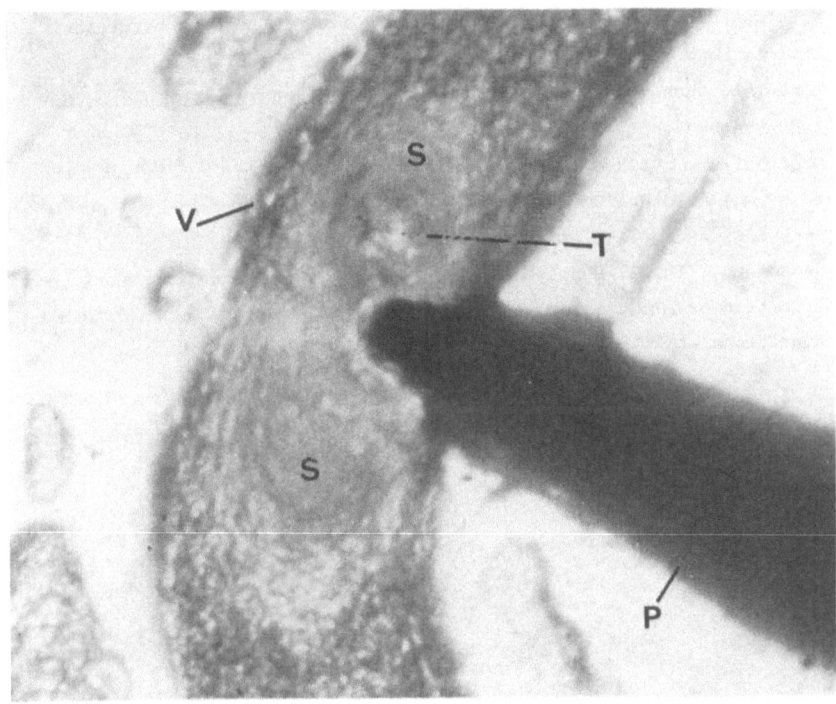

Figure 3. A frame from the 16 mm film showing the twin acoustic microstreaming vortices (S) within the intact blood vessel (V). The tip of the probe (P) indents the vessel from above. A gelatinous white thrombus of platelets (T) can be seen growing within one vortex.

The experimental arrangement is shown in Figure 2. The blood vessel to be treated was raised until it made contact with the probe tip. It was found that the size of the visible microstreaming eddies increased with the depth of indentation of the probe tip up to an indentation depth of about 20% of the vessel diameter; further indentation caused no detectable change. This effect was more noticeable with the lower frequency transversely oscillating wire assembly (Williams, 1977) than with the 85 kHz longitudinally oscillating probe and is presumably a reflection of the efficiency of coupling the vibrating source to the vessel wall.

At very low displacement amplitudes (less than about 1 μm which corresponds to a shear stress of about 16 $Nm^{-2}$) acoustic microstreaming could be seen to occur within the intact blood vessels, but there was no visible evidence of platelet aggregation or adhesion. However, electron microscopic examination of the site of these "sub-threshold" irradiations occasionally showed that damaged platelets (i.e. platelets whose plasma membrane had been torn and partially removed) had attached themselves to what appeared to be normal functioning endothelium. Figure 4 shows one such damaged platelet (P1) adhering to normal endothelium while another platelet (P2) has adhered itself to the damaged platelet and is beginning to form a minute mural aggregate. (N.B. For technical reasons this electron micrograph is of a portion of a mouse femoral vein irradiated under "sub-threshold" conditions at 20 kHz and not 85 kHz.)

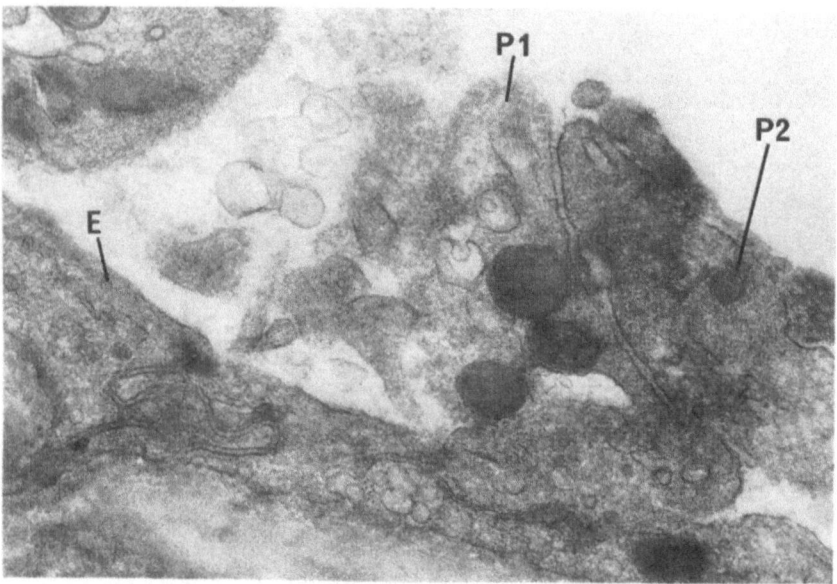

Figure 4. An electron micrograph showing the intact and apparently undamaged endothelium (E) to which has adhered a platelet (P1) which has suffered extensive rupture and removal of its plasma membrane and the loss of some intracellular organelles. Another platelet (P2) has adhered to this damaged platelet forming the nucleus of a minute mural aggregate.

Under the correct conditions of illumination, at displacement amplitudes greater than about 1 µm, one can observe the situation seen in Figure 3. Here, translucent spheres, which are large aggregates of platelets (containing white cells but few, if any, erythrocytes) can be seen to build up within the slowly rotating centre of the large micro-streaming vortices. This indicates that the platelets had been "damaged" or otherwise "activated" by the shear stresses to which they had been subjected while passing close to (but not in contact with) the endothelial surface. These "activated" platelets could then unite with other platelets to form an aggregate. The hydrodynamic conditions prevailing at the outflow from the high stress region result in three alternative routes for the "activated" platelets. Firstly, they could remain within the centre streamline and be carried around to re-enter the high stress region. Secondly, they could be deflected towards the centre of the vortex where they will spiral towards the centre and unite with the rapidly growing spherical aggregate (arrowed in Figure 3). Thirdly, they could be deflected away from the centre of the vortex. In this case they will leave the microstreaming pattern and be embolised downstream as a small platelet aggregate. It should be noted that numerous small platelet aggregates were detected when the blood downstream of a wire vibrating at 20 kHz was frozen <u>in situ</u> by means of iso-pentane cooled with liquid nitrogen (Williams, 1977). These same aggregates are visible as a "snowflake-like" appearance of the blood downstream of the vibrating 85 kHz probe.

The gelatinous roughly spherical aggregate of platelets found within the microstreaming vortex is extremely adhesive and will attach itself to any surface (including intact endothelium) with which it comes into contact. If the transducer is de-activated or if this large aggregate grows too big, it will leave its stable position and either attach itself to the vessel wall or be embolised downstream. It is important to note that there is frequently no visible growth of platelet aggregates at the site of irradiation after the probe has been switched off. This indicates that the endothelium has apparently not been damaged and therefore the platelets have been "activated" by shear stress alone and not by contact with a thrombogenic surface.

At displacement amplitudes of about 4 μm (corresponding to shear stresses of the order of 250 $Nm^{-2}$) the platelets are "activated" to such an extent that they unite together and can be seen to issue from

the rapidly rotating vortex as a continuous fluid stream. This
gelatinous stream is extremely adhesive, it attaches itself to the
vessel wall and "slithers" along it driven by the flowing blood.
After about 30 seconds the viscosity of this stream appears to
increase (possibly due to the formation of fibrin within the platelet
mass). In many cases this mass solidifies and blocks the vessel which
rapidly clots and then contracts showing that many of the platelets
forming the thrombus still retain an active thrombosthenin contractile
system.

## Conclusions

Platelets subjected to hydrodynamic shear stresses _in vivo_ are
"activated" and aggregate to give fluid adhesive masses which attach
themselves to any available surface, including undamaged endothelium.
A convenient method of generating these intravascular shear stresses is
by means of an acoustic microstreaming field which may be generated by
the application of an ultrasonically vibrating probe to the outside of
the intact blood vessel. It is proposed that this technique might be
of value as an _in vivo_ model system to evaluate the effects on platelet
function of the various anticoagulants in common use, and also any
other pharmacologically active agents which modify the haemostatic
system.

## Acknowledgements

I wish to thank the Bureau of Radiological Health, United States Food
and Drug Administration for the partial support of contract number
FDA 3177-75(J).

72

Brown, C.H., L.B. Leverett, C.W. Lewis, C.P. Alfrey Jr., J.D. Hellums. Morphological, biochemical and functional changes in human platelets subjected to shear stress. J. Lab. Clin. Med., 86 (1975).462.

Charm, S.E., B.L. Wong. Shear degradation of fibrinogen in the circulation. Science, 170 (1970) 466.

Holtzmark, J., I. Johnsen, T. Sikkeland, S. Skavlem. Boundary layer flow near a cylindrical obstacle in an oscillating, incompressible fluid. J. Acoust. Soc. Amer., 26 (1954) 26.

Morris, D.R., A.R. Williams. The effects of suspending medium viscosity on erythrocyte deformation and haemolysis in vitro. Biochim. Biophys. Acta, (1978) In press.

Nyborg, W.L. "Acoustic Streaming" in "Physical Acoustics" Vol. 2B. Ed. W.P. Mason. Academic Press, New York (1965).

Williams, A.R. Hydrodynamic disruption of human erythrocytes near a transversely oscillating wire. Rheol. Acta, 10 (1971) 67.
Williams, A.R. Release of Serotonin from human platelets by acoustic microstreaming. J. Acoust. Soc. Amer., 56 (1974) 1640.
Williams, A.R. Intravascular mural thrombi produced by acoustic microstreaming. Ultrasound in Medicine and Biology, 3 (1977) 191.
Williams, A.R., D.E. Hughes, W.L. Nyborg. Hemolysis near a transversely oscillating wire. Science, 169 (1970) 871.

DISCUSSION          Moderator: Williams

Müller-Mohnssen:          Did you determine the frequency for the lowest
                         energy producing a thrombus of a certain size?
                         Did you investigate the vessel wall morpholo-
                         gically after application of US? On nerve mem-
                         branes we found the strongest effect of sound-
                         waves also at 2 kilocycles, the frequency for
                         which the auditory threshold has a minimum.
                         Did you also apply audio sound frequencies?

Williams:                No, we did not investigate the effect of many
                         different frequencies because it is not the ra-
                         diated acoustic vibration which is causing
                         the microstreaming. It is the fact that you
                         have a solid probe actually in contact with
                         the vessel wall so that the wall itself is set
                         into oscillation. It does not really matter
                         very much what the frequency is. The frequency
                         of vibration just means, that the lower the
                         frequency the larger the microstreaming pattern.
                         It is exactly the same shape pattern, but has
                         a larger dimension. We wanted to keep the fre-
                         quencies in a region of about 20 to 80 KHz.
                         Because at lower frequencies the streaming
                         pattern is larger than the vessel. And so you
                         could not get a good streaming pattern within
                         it. When the frequency is higher than 85 KHz
                         it is difficult to generate and to produce a
                         good microstreaming pattern because the point
                         of the probe is so small that you begin to pe-
                         netrate through the wall. So we limited our-
                         selves to those frequencies. We did look at
                         the histological appearance of the vessel wall
                         at the point of contact and what we found was
                         that down at the very low subtreshold levels
                         of the order of about 100 $dyn/cm^2$ we see
                         nothing at the level of the light microscope.
                         Under the electronmicroscope we could see some

platelets attached to the vessel wall but the
endothelium looked normal. But the platelets
which were attached to it were damaged and what
we saw was that the platelets frequently had a
ruptured membrane. This damaged platelet membrane was perhaps responsible for them sticking
onto the wall. And so, the platelets that had
been damaged, were adherent to what appeared to
be normal endothelium. When we look at the film
you see that the platelet thrombus is built up
within the vortex of the streaming field. It
is not built up on the endothelium. So it is
just the shear stress which activates the platelets; the platelets then aggregate together,
and once they have aggregated they form a ge-
latinuous adhesive fluid mass which will adhere
to any surface. Once it has attached it flows
along the blood vessel wall because it is a
very fluid mass. But it is rapidly becoming
more viscous as fibrin is being formed within
it. If you look downstream at the emboli, you
sometimes see that these very adhesive large
platelet thrombi will harden as they go down
the vessel and so we get a region of normal
endothelium with a rigid mixture of fibrin and
platelet debris above it. This results in the
endothelium becoming anoxic. Frequently, the
rigid embolus contracts and this contracts the
whole vessel which blocks up.

Wurzinger:    When you looked at the electronmicroscopic pictures of the platelets did you also see membrane
damage in otherwise normally shaped platelets
with normal granular contents or were they all
shape-changed in that short exposure time?

Williams:     No, the platelets which were within the body of
the fluid blood were disc shaped and apparently
quite normal. The only platelets which we saw

which were atypical were those stuck onto the endothelium and those had broken membranes. The cells attached to the endothelium occasionally had what looked to be normal cells attached to these broken cells. In every case there would be a broken platelet on the endothelium and there was a normal looking platelet close by beginning to form an aggregate of platelets.

Wurzinger: What I meant is: the broken platelets, did they show normal tubular systems?

Williams: Yes, I could quite clearly see microtubules in them, dense bodies and mitochondria. It was just that the membrane had been torn and you could see where the membrane ended. The organelles were coming out and these were inflated and blown up because the osmotic strength of the plasma was not the same as that inside the cell and so all the organelles were exploded. But they could still be recognized as organelles and were found near the ruptured portion of the cell membrane.

Wurzinger: What about pseudopodia?

Williams: I saw no pseudopodia on these platelets. It just looked like a platelet which has been ripped open and stuck onto the endothelium.

Olijslager: Dr. Williams, we are impressed by this study but I think that your data will be different from the data other people have, for instance one we saw this morning. Could this be due to, I mention two things, the oscillating system that platelets are in an oscillating shear field, not laminar flow and second, is it possible that there are higher oscillations superimposed on your 85 KHz motion?

Williams: I will answer your second question first. The shear field itself is not oscillating motion

resulting from first order effects. The streaming pattern which you could see there was a
second order pattern. Look at that as a DC flow
where a given particle moves continuously within the flow field which is laminar. The maximum shear occurs in a narrow layer close to
the endothelium, and its scale is so small that
it remains laminar even at very high velocity
gradients. This is one of the few situations
I know of where one can get velocity gradients
of the order of $10^7$ sec$^{-1}$ and still have good
laminar flow conditions in the shearing zone.
So the shear field itself is not oscillating,
but the platelets are alternately subjected
to a high shear stress followed by a period
of low shear stress. It may get sheared hun-
dreds of times in the exposure period of several seconds. But we do not know what effect
this has as against a continuous laminar flow
shear field. But then again if you are going
to subject platelets to very high shear stresses
of the order of $10^4$ - $10^6$ dyn/cm$^2$, that implies
such high velocity gradients that you are almost certainly in turbulence using  any shear
system. In any case of turbulent flow you have
exactly the same situation of a high shear
stress for a short time, then it is off, then
it is on. And  so in may ways the time course of
exposure of the platelet to shear stress by the
oscillating wire is similar to turbulent flow,
but it is a more convenient and controllable
shear field.

Olijslager:      When you say that the platelets are in your vortex for one millisecond  or some milliseconds
in high shear stress region they come there
again and again. Don't you think that you perhaps should state that it is not one millisecond per platelet but that it is one second

for instance per platelet. And second, what do
you see at the tip of your probe
because there are no vortices there? It is
going up and down, so the fluid must come from
the sides again and again and then it is really
a pulsating flow.

Williams:       First of all, if the blood is still flowing
there is mixing within this vortex. Cells are
continuously coming into it, being retained in
it for a while as others are moving out and
being washed on down-stream. So there is a continuous mixing going on if the flow of blood
in the vessel is high enough. But once a cell
is in the high stress portion of the shear
field, close to the endothelium then it is in
a very intense laminar flow shear field. The
magnitude of these shear forces is comparable
to those encountered in turbulent flow or in
high speed flow through a jet. In the case
of jet flow, when it is actually passing through
that needle it is in a laminar flow system,
but once past the needle it is in a very complex turbulent shear field. In the case of the
oscillating wire it slowly goes from this
very intense  laminar shear field down to one
which is much more gentle, i.e. there is no
abrupt transition when the cells leave the
region of highest shear stress.

Fischer:        Mrs. Heidtmann called my attention to the fact
that you only used veins in your experiments.
Did you also try arteries with your ultrasound
method?

Williams:       Yes I did. The problem was for the most of the
animals I used the arteries were relatively
opaque, and so it was only in the case of neonatal mice or rats where the artery was sufficiently transparent. The vessels had to be re-

latively transparent before we could see the streaming patterns. It is exactly the same pattern we got, whether it was an artery or a vein, whether it was a rabbit or a mouse or a rat or a guinea pig.

Lambert:     Dr. Williams, may I ask you, have you done similar experiments in vitro to rule out the possibility that you trigger the extrinsic clotting system by this stimulation.

Williams:    Yes, I have done the control experiments in vitro. The slide I showed just before the film was in fact part of an in vitro series of experiments where I treated my own platelets in plasma. They form platelet aggregates first, and later generate film.
I also did the same thing with platelets suspended in saline. And I got exactly the same aggregation results from them. For any given drive frequency we got the same treshold aggregation whether the platelets were suspended in citrated plasma or in saline or if the platelets were in vivo in an animal.

# 5. SPECIES DIFFERENCES IN PLATELET AGGREGATION WITH SPECIAL REFERENCE TO HEPARIN AS ANTICOAGULANT

L.J. Wurzinger, W. Baldauf, E. Tobias, K. Mottaghy,
Department of Physiology, Medical Faculty, RWTH Aachen,
Melatener Straße 211, D-5100 Aachen, West Germany

## 1. INTRODUCTION

Thromboembolic events represent the most serious complications in the use of artificial internal organs (AIO), especially in those employed in the cardiovascular system
(FORBES and PRENTICE, 1978). It seems evident, that the
occurrence of thromboembolism is not only dependent upon
the primary process of a monolayered platelet adhesion
to foreign surfaces, but also on the further growth of
mural thrombi, caused by secondary platelet aggregation.
The growth of such mural thrombi is a conditio sine qua
non for the formation of emboli.

There is ample evidence showing that thrombus formation is
related to peculiar hydrodynamic conditions prevailing in
certain parts of AIO; regions of stagnant flow occur in
close proximity to regions of extremely high shear-rates.
Is has been shown (HELLUMS et al.) that high shear forces
in the order of magnitude of 100 $N/m^2$ can damage red blood
cells as well as platelets and thus cause the release of
so-called platelet aggregating substances (see papers
FORST et al. and SCHMID-SCHÖNBEIN et al.). Furthermore,
agents released from the damaged blood cells (e.g. ADP)
may subsequently accumulate in areas of stagnant flow, in
which convective transport is limited. If located behind
a constricted blood-conduit (stenosis or narrow channel)
these areas preferentially receive material coming from
upstream regions characterized by high shear-flow (BALDAUF

et al.). The biochemical consequences of shear damage to RBC or platelets in combination with these hydrodynamic conditions could well be a possible mechanism leading to shape-change and increased stickiness of platelets. Such "activated" platelets which, in other words, have undergone "viscous metamorphosis" would then more readily aggregate with already wall-adherent platelets.

There are pronounced species differences in tendency to thrombosis. Therefore, knowledge about the aggregability of platelets of different species is essential for testing AIO with regard to its potential hemocompatibility in man. In the literature there is only very limited information about species differences in platelet aggregability. Furthermore, practically all previous comparative studies were done with citrated PRP and using strong ADP stimulation in conventional aggregometers (SINAKOS and CAEN, McMILLAN and SIM; CALKINS et al.). Since heparin is used routinely as an anticoagulant in AIO we tested the so-called "spontaneous" and the ADP induced platelet aggregability under controlled viscometric flow in citrated as well as heparinized platelet rich plasma (PRP). However, in contrast to the high ADP concentrations used in conventional aggregometers (ranging from $10^{-6}$ to $10^{-4}$ Mol/l) we used much lower concentrations (from $10^{-8}$ to $10^{-6}$ Mol/l), as they might be expected to occur during haemolysis in AIO.

## 2. METHODS AND MATERIAL

For comparing the platelet aggregability of man, cattle, pigs, dogs, rabbits and sheep, we used the "rheoaggregometer", that was developed in our laboratory by KLOSE et al. By applying carefully selected, uniform shear-stresses to the entire sample, this technique allows to measure spontaneous PA which occurs when unspecifically stimulated platelets are colliding in viscometric flow. As we have shown earlier (RIEGER et al., 1977), platelets become activated by small unspecific stimuli such as cooling down to room-temperature or progressive drop in pH following evaporation of carbondioxyde. At least in human PRP these unspecific stimuli are sufficient to promote platelet aggregability to a degree that is quantatively measurable in our apparatus.

A PRP sample in a cone-plate-chamber is tangentially illuminated and the transmitted light is registered by a photoresistor, which is part of a Wheatstone-bridge. The PA was quantified by means of a calibration curve, obtained by diluting PRP with autologous platelet poor plasma. During each aggregation experiment the shear-rates in our cone-plate-device rose steadily within 12 minutes from 4.5 to 115 /second. The photometrically recorded changes in light transmission reflect the build-up of platelet aggregates until formation and break-down of platelet aggregates reach an equilibrium (Fig. 1 and 2).

Whole blood of the species under investigation was anticoagulated both with sodium-citrate 3.8 % (1 part citrate to 9 parts of blood) and with heparin (Liquemin$^R$, Hoffman-la-Roche) 7.5 units/ml respectively). Heparin was diluted 1 to 67 in phosphate-buffered isotonic saline (added one part to nine parts of blood to achieve the same dilution effect as with citrate-anticoagulation).

Platelet rich plasma was prepared by centrifugation of the whole blood specimens according to the following scheme: Dog: 500 g for 3 minutes; man: 500 g for 4 minutes;

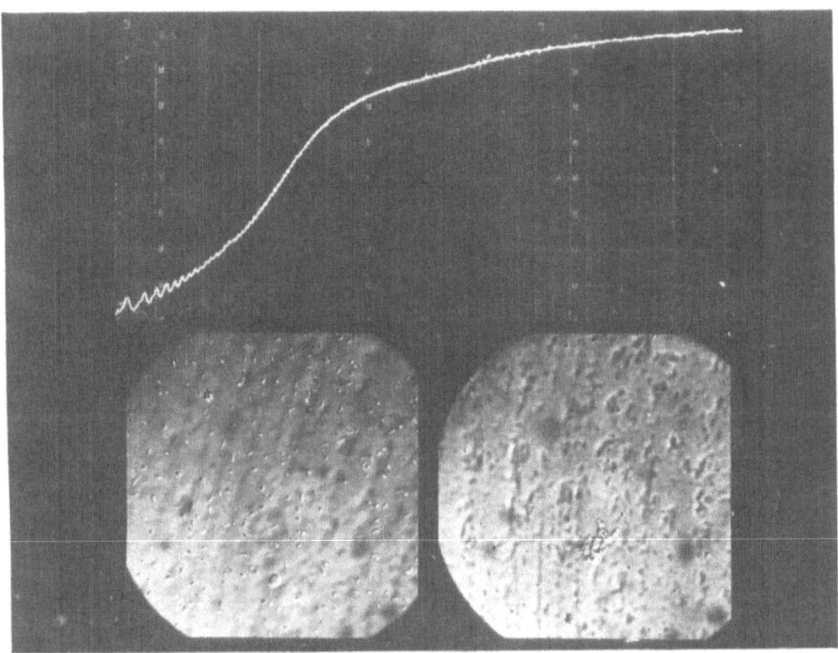

Fig. 1: Interference-contrast-micrographs showing citrated
porcine PRP before shearing (left pannel) and
after shearing (right pannel) with ADP $10^{-4}$ Mol/l.
A corresponding rheoaggregometer curve, amounting
to 64% PA is shown above. Note the drastic reduction of single platelets during the course of
PA.

rabbit: 800 g for 3 minutes; pig: 800 g for 4 minutes;
sheep: 800 g for 4 minutes; cattle: 800 g for 6 minutes.
The aggregation of platelets requires first activation
(leading to shape-change) and secondly adequate flow conditions for "successful" collision, resulting in formation
and not disruption of aggregates. Viscometric flow with
shear-rates of 30-50/second have been shown to be opti-
mally effective in this respect (KLOSE et al.). The application of this flow regime is probably responsible for the
great sensitivity of the "rheoaggregometer", which
allows to quantify not only spontaneous aggregability but
also the effect of comparatively low doses of activating
agents (e.g. ADP). Figures 1 and 2 showed typical aggrega-

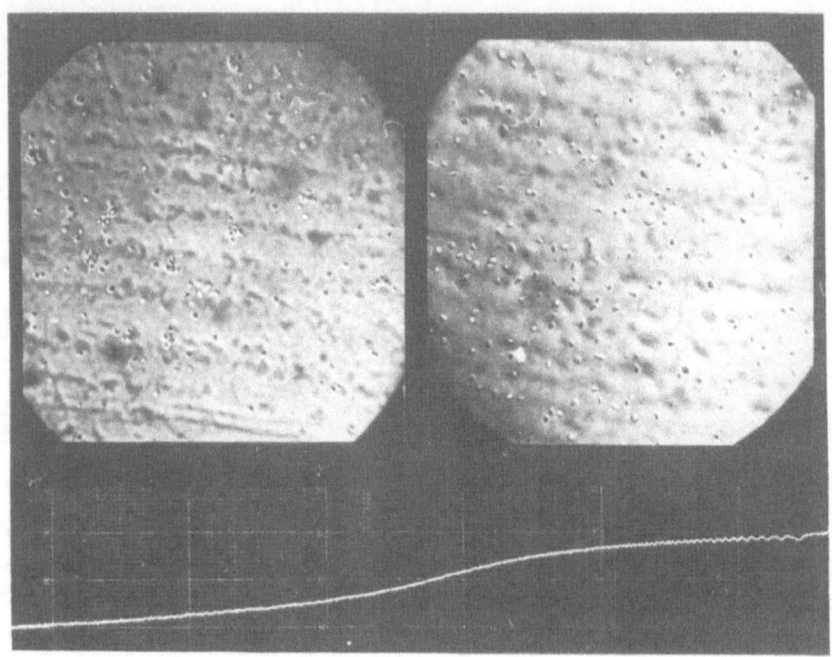

Fig. 2: Interference-contrast-micrographs showing citrated canine PRP before shearing (left pannel) and after shearing (right pannel) with ADP $10^{-7}$Mol/l. A corresponding rheoaggregometer curve shows 15% PA. Small and middle-sized aggregates have formed, reducing the number of single platelets.

tion curves obtained at rising shear-rates with strong ($10^{-4}$ Mol/l ADP) and weak ($10^{-7}$ Mol/l ADP) stimuli in PRP from a pig and a dog. The photomicrographs show individual platelets before, and platelet aggregates after the shearing experiments in the rheoaggregometer, individual platelets virtually absent after strong stimulation (see Fig. 1).

84

## 3. RESULTS

In citrated PRP of man the spontaneous aggregability increased during the time of storage under the conditions mentioned above, until it reaches a maximum 2 hours after blood withdrawal; later it falls gradually off.

When anticoagulated with citrate the PRP of all tested animal species without exception showed a very low spontaneous PA as compared to human citrated PRP (Figures 3 and 4).

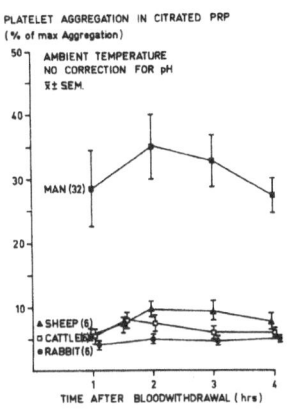 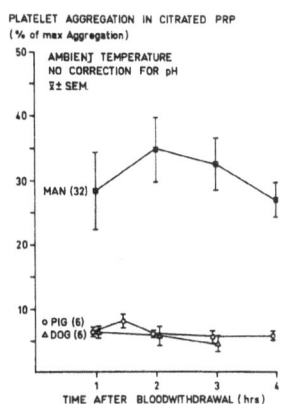

## Fig. 3 and Fig. 4:

Figures 3 and 4 show the extent of spontaneous PA (in percent of maximum possible PA) in dependence of storage time of platelet rich plasma under "room conditions". PRP from man, rabbit, sheep, cattle, pig and dog are compared under anticoagulation with citrate (1 : 9).

When testing PA in heparinized PRP (heparin concentration 7.5 units/ml) a distinctly different behaviour was found. Under these conditions canine platelets are so reactive that during blood-withdrawal and preparation already extensive spontaneous PA occurred in heparinized PRP. As a consequence of this, we were unable to prepare suitable

platelet suspensions and thus measurement was impossible
in heparinized canine PRP (Fig. 5).

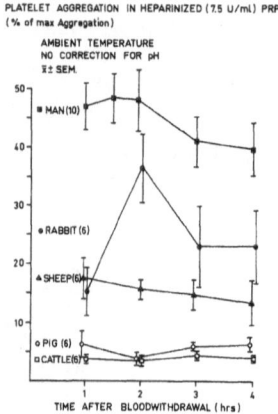

PLATELET AGGREGATION IN HEPARINIZED (7.5 U/mL) PRP
(% of max Aggregation)

AMBIENT TEMPERATURE
NO CORRECTION FOR pH
x̄ ± SEM.

TIME AFTER BLOODWITHDRAWAL ( hrs )

Fig. 5: Spontaneous PA in dependence of storage time of
PRP under "room conditions". PRP from man,
rabbit, sheep, pig and cattle are compared under
anticoagulation with heparin (7.5 units/ml).

Spontaneous aggregability in human heparinized PRP was
again more pronounced than that of any other species investigated. Spontaneous aggregability was higher in heparinized than in citrated PRP of man, of rabbits and also
of sheep, although the extent of the augmentation in heparin varies from species to species.

Only porcine and bovine platelets remain as "inactive" as
under citrate-anticoagulation. This behaviour corresponds
well to the pronounced differences in the platelet counts
in the PRP's of the respective animals, which consistently
occur despite the fact that citrated and heparinized PRP
were prepared under identical conditions in every case
(Fig. 6).

86

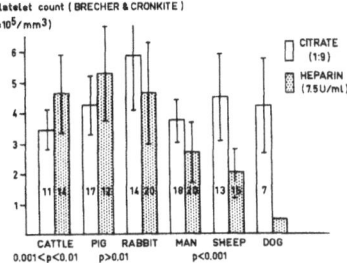

COMPARISON OF PLATELET COUNTS IN PRP FROM DIFFERENT SPECIES
WITH REGARDS TO THE ANTICOAGULANT USED ( MEAN VALUES ± S.D.)

Fig. 6: Comparison of platelet counts of the species investigated and the influence of the anticoagulant
used upon the platelet counts in PRP.

In those species (cattle and pigs), where we found no
difference in "spontaneous platelet aggregability" we
found no drop in platelet count in heparin, sometimes even
a few more platelets. In those species (man, rabbits and
sheep), where we noted a higher aggregability in heparin
we correspondingly found lower platelet counts in heparinized PRP. The difference was highly significant in PRP
from man and sheep. Canine heparinized PRP (right column)
consistently contained less than 100.000 platelets/$mm^3$.

Similar species differences were found in aggregability
following stimulation with rising doses of ADP. In response to $10^{-8}$ Mol/l ADP citrated human PRP again reacts
most strongly (Figures 7 and 8), the dose-response-curves
of the other species being shifted to the right by two or
three decades.

Bovine and porcine platelets again were least reactive,
they do not respond to ADP even in a concentration of
$10^{-6}$ Mol/l. The platelets of sheep, rabbits and dogs,
although more sensitive than cattle and pig, respond to a
threshold ADP concentration of $10^{-7}$ Mol/l, whereas human

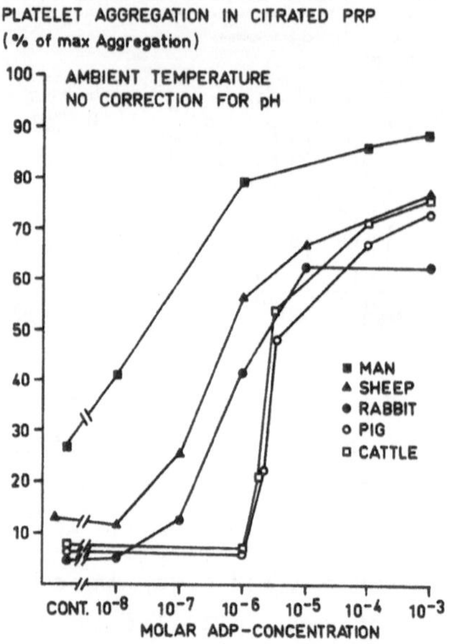

PLATELET AGGREGATION IN CITRATED PRP
( % of max Aggregation)

Fig. 7: PA in the rheoaggregometer as a function of molar ADP concentration in citrated PRP. Dose-response-curves for ADP in PRP of man, rabbit, sheep, cattle and pig.

platelets exhibit a significant increase in aggregability at $10^{-8}$ Mol/l under the conditions of $22^{\circ}C$ and mild alkalosis (pH 7.75 - 7.90).

The effect of the anticoagulant upon ADP-induced platelet aggregation is quite complex. In contrast to the more pronounced "spontaneous" aggregability, heparinized PRP from man, sheep and rabbits exhibited a significantly lower sensitivity towards ADP as aggregation-promoting stimulus than the citrated PRP of these species (Figures 9, 10, 11).

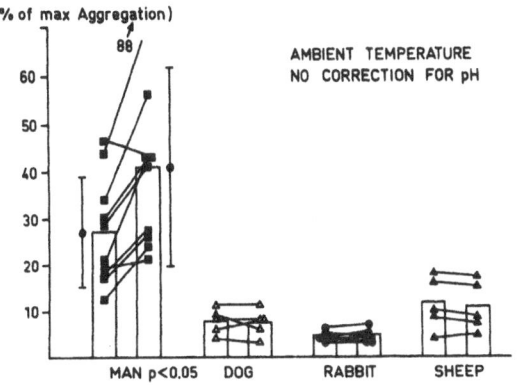

Fig. 8: Enhancement of platelet aggregability by small doses of ADP ($10^{-8}$ Mol/l). Comparison of citrated PRP from man, dog, rabbit and sheep.

89

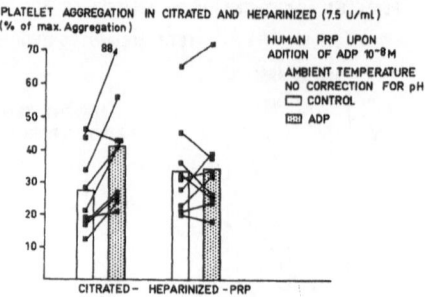

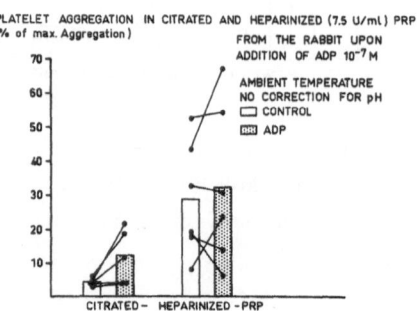

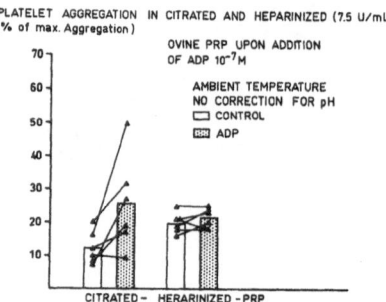

Figures 9, 10, 11: The effect of small, just aggregation-promoting, concentrations of ADP upon heparinized and citrated PRP from man, rabbit and sheep are compared.

90

The ADP response of bovine and porcine platelets, the spontaneous PA of which is not influenced by the use of citrate
or heparin  as anticoagulant is not significantly altered
by the choice of anticoagulant (Figures 12, 13).

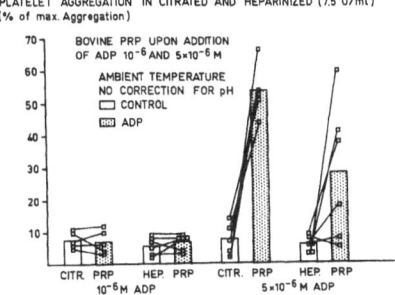

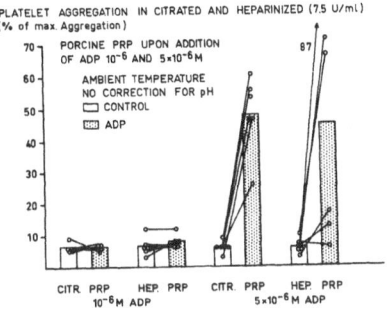

Figures 12, 13: The effect of small, just aggregation-
promoting and just inefficient concentrations upon heparinized and citrated PRP
from cattle and pig are compared.

# 4. DISCUSSION

The results presented clearly show significant species differences in the tendency of platelets to form aggregates either following unspecific stimuli such as a rise in pH - or exposure to low temperature - or following the specific activation by low doses of ADP. As discussed in detail elsewhere (SCHMID-SCHÖNBEIN, 1977) the process of aggregate formation depends both on platelet changes (shape-change or viscous metamorphosis) and adequate flow conditions for successful collision of "activated" platelets. In the conventional cuvette-aggregometers, the   flow conditions imposed by stirring rods are so complicated and non-uniform that they defy hydrodynamic definition. In the cone-plate-chamber used in the present experiments the flow conditions are characterized by uniform shear-rates which can be easily computed and/or altered. In this apparatus one can control the kinetics of platelet collision in uniform shear-flow, which is in principle identical to the natural prerequisit for aggregation. This means that the most optimal conditions for a successful collision between platelets can experimentally be determined in each case; "success" being defined as the formation of an aggregate. In order to save experimental time and material we chose to apply the same "shearing protocol" to all PRP samples, shear-rate increasing steadily from 4.5 - 115/sec within 12 minutes. While there are justified objections to the simultaneous change in shear-*rate* and shear-*time*, this procedure did allow to determine the range of 35-50/sec as an optimal velocity gradient for the aggregation of weakly stimulated platelets. This behaviour, originally established for human platelets, is now being confirmed for all species by the present results. Thus having established a sensitive method to detect "aggregability", we were able to detect (and corroborate  by microscopic inspection) significant aggregation in human platelet rich plasma, prepared by conventional methodology.

In keeping with the results of BREDDIN  we found that pla-

telet aggregability was very small immediately after
blood-withdrawal, increased during the first two hours,
reached a plateau and decreased after three to four hours.
Again in keeping with BREDDIN's results we found that the
time-dependent change in aggregability was paralleled by
"spontaneous", time-dependent "shape-changes", i.e., the
transformation of "smooth discs" to "spiny spheres" (PIETSCH
et al.). For citrated human PRP RIEGER found "spontaneous"
aggregability and shape-change depend on the experimental
conditions: they can be totally supressed if the evaporation of $CO_2$, usually occurring during storage of PRP
samples is avoided and if the temperature is meticulously
kept at $37^{O}C$. This applies within certain limits for the
platelets of cattle, pig and sheep too, which in a higher
percentage than human platelets retain their discoid
smooth shape during storage at room-temperature. Almost
no spontaneous aggregability was observed in citrated PRP
from dogs and rabbits (see Figures 3 and 4), despite the
fact that their platelets showed a tendency to undergo
shape-change comparable to human platelets. This seems con-
tradictory but under anticoagulation with heparin  (and
normal calcium-level), these species show a quite pronounced "spontaneous" aggregability. This makes evident,
that temperature and alkalosis indeed act as unspecific
stimuli to platelets, activating the metabolic events leading to a shape-change and thereby conditioning the platelets for "successful" collision in flow with the consequence of aggregate formation. "Spontaneous" aggregability
therefore results from the response of platelets to unspecific stimuli of cold and alkalosis, the  susceptability
to which is different in different species. Obviously, the
susceptability depends on such factors as calcium, heparin
and other factors that await elucidation.

In light of this interpretation, we conclude that when
heparin  is used as an anticoagulant the most susceptable
platelets in the blood samples of man, rabbit and sheep
become aggregated during blood sampling and preparation
of PRP. This fact is reflected by a systemically lower

platelet count in heparinized than in citrated PRP. Nevertheless, the higher concentration of ionized calcium or some platelet activating effect of heparin are obviously sufficient to render them more activated as shown in our test for "spontaneous" PA. In those species where decreased ADP sensitivity of heparinized platelets occurs despite finite "spontaneous" aggregability, heparin induced subliminal release-reaction could occur during storage, subsequently leading to partial refractoriness of the platelet exposed to its own ADP. EIKA has presented data suggesting that heparin per se can induce a release-reaction in platelets.

The results obtained have a number of practical consequences:

Firstly, we were able to show that the "aggregability" as tested in the rheoaggregometer was correlated to platelet adhesion and secondary aggregation in deposition experiments using glass models of various arteries (BALDAUF et al.).

Secondly, the aggregometer proved to be very helpful to monitor induced changes of platelet aggregability, such as they occur after addition of red cell hemolysate (see Fig. 14) in vitro and in artificial organs (WURZINGER and BLASBERG, unpublished observations). When testing the influence of artificial organs, i.e. bubble and membrane oxygenators a two-phase response was found. 15 minutes after commencement of extracorporeal circulation platelet reactivity was increased, 2 hours later it was decreased. More detailed analyses of these important changes in "spontaneous" aggregation are in progress.

Our results are understandable when we differentiate in the rheology of blood between flow conditions and flow properties of the media involved and resulting flow behaviour, in our case the presence or absence of platelet aggregation. There are differences in platelet properties between species which are modified in addition by the type of anticoagulant used. Whether or not activated platelets are deposited or aggregated greatly depends on flow con-

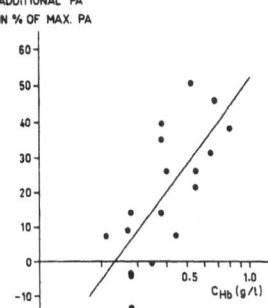

INCREASE IN SPONTANEOUS PLATELET
AGGREGATION (PA) UPON ADDITION OF RED
CELL HEMOLYSATE

ADDITIONAL PA
IN % OF MAX. PA

Fig. 14: Increase in spontaneous platelet aggregation (PA) upon addition of red cell hemolysate.


ditions. The pronounced species differences in platelet susceptability to specific and unspecific stimuli appear to be consequential in the selection of appropriate animal species for testing AIO.

95

REFERENCES

1   BALDAUF, W., WURZINGER, L.J., KINDER, J.: The Role of
    Stagnation Point Flow in the Formation of Platelet
    Thrombi on Glass Surfaces in Tubes with various Geo-
    metry. Path. Res. Pract. 163, 9, (1978)

2   BREDDIN, K., GRUN, H., KRZYWANEK, H.J., SCHREMMER, W.P.:
    Zur Messung der "spontanen" Thrombozytenaggregation,
    Plättchenaggregationstest III-Methodik. Klin.Wschr. 53,
    81, (1975)

3   CALKINS, J., LANE, K.P., LO SASSO, B., THURBER, L.E.:
    Comparative Study of Platelet Aggregation in Various
    Species., J. Med. 5, 292, (1974)

4   EIKA, C.: On the Mechanism of Platelet Aggregation
    Induced by Heparin, Protamine and Polybrene., Scand.
    J. Hemat. 9, 248 (1972)

5   EIKA, C.: Heparin-Induced Platelet Release and
    Refractory Platelets., Lancet, 1, 1343 (1972)

6   FORBES, CH.D. , PRENTICE, C.R.: Thrombus Formation and
    Artificial Surfaces, Brit. Med. Bull. 34, 201 (1978)

7   HELLUMS, J.D., BROWN, C.H.: Blood Cell Damage by
    Mechanical Forces, Chapter 20 in "Cardiovascular Dyna-
    mics and Measurements", (Eds. N.H.C. HWANG and
    N.D. NORMANN), University Park Press, Baltimore (1977)

8   KLOSE, H.J., RIEGER, H., SCHMID-SCHÖNBEIN, H.:
    A Rheological Method for the Quantification of Platelet
    Aggregation in Vitro and its Kinetics under Defined
    Flow Conditions, Thromb. Res. 7, 261 (1975)

9   KRATZER, M., KINDER, J.: Hydrodynamic Conditions at
    the Areas of Depositions in the Model of an Arterial
    Branching, Pflügers Arch. Europ. J. Physiol. 355,
    Suppl. R 39 (1975)

10  MACMILLAN, D.C., SIM, A.K.: A Comparative Study of
    Platelet Aggregation in Man and Laboratory Animals.
    Thromb. Diath. Haemorrh. 24, 385 (1970)

11  PIETSCH, U., LIPPMANN, M., SCHARRER, J., BREDDIN, K.:
    Neue Befunde zur Wirkung von Acetylsalizylsäure. Die
    Hemmwirkung auf den Formwandel der Thrombozyten und
    ihre Bedeutung für die Dosierung als Antithrombotikum,

in: Diabetische Angiopathien, Ed. by K. Alexander,
u. M. Cachovan, bei Verlag G. Witzstrock, Baden-Baden,
(1977)

12    RIEGER, H., WURZINGER, L., SCHMID-SCHÖNBEIN, H.:
Einfluß der Temperatur auf die scherinduzierte
Plättchenaggregation in vitro.Klin. Wschr. 55, 121
(1977)

13    SCHMID-SCHÖNBEIN, H.: Microrheology of Erythrocytes
and Thrombocytes, Blood Viscosity and the Distribution
of Blood Flow in the Microcirculation. In: Handbuch
der allgemeinen Pathologie III/7 Mikrozirkulation/
Microcirculation, Springer Verlag, Berlin, Heidelberg,
New York (1977)

14    SINAKOS, Z., CAEN, J.:.: Platelet Aggregation in
Mammalians (Human, Rat, Rabbit, Guinea-Pig, Horse,
Dog). A Comparative Study. Thromb. Diath. Haemorrh.
17, 99-111 (1967)

DISCUSSION           Moderator: Hemker

Fleming:

Have you ever tested the aggregation of platelets of animals in plasma in which the animal itself had been heparinized? It has been shown that heparin releases fatty acids from tissues. Can you make any comments on the effect of fatty acids on platelet reaction?

Wurzinger:

We tested platelet function in our heparinized rabbits during extracorporeal oxygenation but we could not find - as the number of experiments was too small - any significant differences between heparinization in vivo or heparinization in vitro after blood withdrawal. This work will go on.

Wildevuur:

Could I ask you which animals should be chosen as a model for our experimental work? Dog platelets are much more sensitive to damage, but I see these platelets behave differently from those of man. Therefore, you cannot transpose your results to the human clinical situation. However, if the dog platelets were behaving the same as the human platelets then I would like to use the dogs because our parameters for measurements are still very poor and if you have sensitive platelets you might quantitate differences between surface activity in the dog model which probably will not be seen in the human or any other species.

Wurzinger:

Well, if you are looking at reactivity of platelets to foreign surfaces the picture might change entirely. As Grabowsky (GRABOWSKI, E.F. et al., Trans. Am. Soc. Artif. Intern. Organs 23, 141 (1977)) has shown the surface reaction is dependent on the sort of polymer used, so that dog's platelets may even be less reactive than human platelets. We only tested platelet-platelet-interaction, but not what occurs, when a monolayered platelet deposit forms on a foreign polymer. From

the aggregation behaviour sheep platelets would
be most similar to human.

Schmid-Schönbein: These are experiments which only cover the aspect
of aggregation, but I think they have important
consequences for the artificial organs  work. One
could argue as follows:
If one designs a *new* instrument and wants not to
be bothered by thrombotic complications, one
should use cows, sheep or dogs. However, one
should not be surprised if later one runs into
thrombotic complication when working with other
species including man. Severe testing conditions
for blood compatibility are desirable. And here,
the dog is most probably a very good species. If
a new artificial organ is tolerated in terms of
platelet and/or coagulation in the dog, it will
probably be tolerated by man, also. Incidentally,
I would predict that there are species' differences as well in red cell suceptibility to trauma.

Wildevuur: I think this is a very important statement. If
that is true, we should use the dog model preferentially in the oxygenator field. Especially,
if we are looking for small differences between
various different configurations. But it is
essential to be sure that the platelet-reaction
in the dog is not basically different from that in
man, otherwise, one would probably have to look
for the sheep-model.

Wurzinger: Yes, I would agree to that. If one gets complications with the dog, one should try the sheep.

Wildevuur: I do not have problems with the dog. But the
question is, does it make sense to perform dog
experiments, if the result cannot indeed be trans-
posed to the human situation ? In other words:
if I see in dogs that we get definitely better results with a certain new material, would you say
that the same results will be obtained in man?

Do dog experiments have any relevance for the human blood compatibility?

Wurzinger:      No, not in the least! I cannot say anything about the platelet reactivity towards any material. Let me come back to Grabowsky's studies, in which he prepares the platelets from different animals and then determines their tendency to stick to various biopolymers. This could be called primary adhesion. And this is quite different from what I investigated, namely secondary aggregation. I agree, that the tendency of platelets is to stick to each other.

Wenzel:         I agree with Dr. Schmid-Schönbein and I think it is essential to decide which laboratory method one wants to chose for controlling blood-trauma in dogs. I think, for example, that dogs can be taken if one wants to test the platelet damage or erythrocyte damage by simple methods. For this purpose, you can use clinical routine methods. But, of course, you are only allowed to compare the results within one species, you cannot make any quantitative prediction concerning blood trauma in human beings. Thus, this leads to the important question which control methods should actually be used to study blood trauma in extracorporeal circulation.

Schmid-Schönbein:  We should definitely keep this problem in mind, because one of the prime aims and duties of the work of the concerted action is to propose standardized testing procedures.

# FLUID DYNAMIC ASPECTS OF THE BLOOD CELL-VESSEL WALL INTERACTION

Helmuth Müller-Mohnssen and Michael Kratzer

Abteilung für Physiologie der GSF, Ingolstädter Landstr. 1,
8042 Neuherberg

## 1. INTRODUCTION

From earlier investigations of spontaneous intraarterial
thrombosis accompanying atherosclerosis we have learned that
for thrombogenesis in medium sized arteries at least the
following three (pipe installation-)components of the organism are to be considered: 1. blood, 2. vessel wall and 3.
arterial flow (18). Further experimental research was con-
ducted to clarify whether the cause of atherosclerosis and
spontaneous thrombosis is due to certain properties, either
of the blood, or of the arterial vessel system or due to a
characteristic arterial flow pattern. In this paper we will
simplify these aspects to the terms: 1. blood factor, 2.wall
factor, 3. flow factor. The blood factor is advocated mainly by the internists and hematologists. Their conjections
about atherosclerotic alterations of arteries are drawn,
among others, from examinations of patient's blood specimens
as they do not look at the interior surfaces of the living
vessel. In contrast, the vessel wall and its pathologic alterations (wall factor) are well within the scope of experience of the pathologist who also takes notice of the
blood factor but tends not to include this factor in his
final analysis. Both, internists and pathologists
agree      in ignoring the flow factor. The latter is mainly
the domain of the medical engineer or the physiologist; each
of these specialists tends as a rule, to treat the entire
problem solely on the basis of the terms belonging to his
field (magic number, Baier).

If the problem is limited to atherosclerosis, it is not mandatory that etiological investigation merge the three magic numbers into the same visual field, because medical treatment is obviously only possible by changing the blood properties. Wall factor and flow factor did not seem to be a suitable site of curative intervention. On the other hand, this incompleteness of methodical approach may explain why no decision is yet possible as to whether atherosclerosis is primarily a disease of the blood or of the arterial vessel. In the area of extracorporeal circulation the mergance of the three magic numbers became demanding. In order to overcome thrombogenesis in extracorporeal circulation, the blood is not the only site of intervention. We can also optimize the wall, i.e. the compatibility with blood of the bio-materials used for the artificial vessel walls. To minimize the flow factor of thrombogenesis, we can optimize the shape of the vessels as well.

In order to determine the extent to which each of the three factors is involved in thrombogenesis within arterio-grafts and in extracorporeal circulation, model experiments were carried out. We used an experimental device in which the properties of blood components, wall-properties and flow velocity field could   easily be determined and standardized. Thrombogenesis observed in this system was described empirically by an equation consisting of three terms, which describe the three magic numbers. If two of the factors are kept constant (for instance  the flow and the properties of the wall), the thrombogenic power of the third (properties of blood components for instance) can be measured directly. The wall factor can be studied in the analogous way.

This system, therefore, may be applicable to test qualitatively the thrombogenic or antithrombogenic effect of changes in the blood factor produced by several agents (clotting inhibitors, surface protecting substances, lipids) or of the changes in wall factor (biomaterials). Because the accuracy of the method depends on the accuracy by which the flow factor is determined, more detailed studies about the influence of flow on thrombogenesis are necessary. Results of hydrodynamic experiments carried out with glass models of a rectangularly branched artery (the main predilection site of coronary thrombosis) had shown that the localization of deposits of platelets or RBC's corresponds to regions where stagnation point flow occurs.

In order to prove these results quantitatively, microthrombosis produced by a concentrically symmetrical stagnation point flow (14) was examined. Due to the symmetry, observations in only one plane (containing the symmetry axis) are sufficient to draw quantitative conclusions for the entire flow.

## 2. METHODS

In this paper only a brief description of the experimental device shall be given; see previous reports for further details (1, 2, 17).

### 2.1 FLOW SYSTEM

The rotationally symmetric stagnation point flow was produced by directing the flow from a straight inflow tube (diam = 3.45 mm) perpendicularly towards a cover glass. The cover glass with its mounting terminates a second tube (diam = 60 mm) mounted coaxial to the inflow tube and forms a chamber which collects the flow from the stagnation area, thus creating the back flow. In order to standardize the properties of the wall, the cover glass was renewed for every experiment and cleaned with King's water according to Dutton et al. (8); diam means the inner diameter of the tubes.

### 2.2 FLUIDS REPRESENTING BLOOD PROPERTIES

Bovine or human platelet rich plasma (PRP) was prepared from 500 ml fresh citrated blood by centrifugation (800 g during 10 min). The plasma was diluted with Parpas buffer pH 7,4 (Ponder 1970) in order to adjust the concentration to 50000 platelets per $mm^3$; bovine PRP was stimulated with $2.5 \times 10^{-6}$ M ADP. The viscosity of the diluted PRP was $\eta = 1.2$ cP ($37^{o}$C); Newtonian behaviour was observed in the range of shear rate between $1.7$ $s^{-1}$ and $1700$ $s^{-1}$. Suspensions of human and bovine erythrocytes with a concentration of RBC $50000$ $mm^{-3}$ were prepared by diluting whole blood with Parpas buffer solution.

### 2.3 MEASUREMENT OF FLOW PARAMETERS

The streamlines of the flow were recorded using a laser ultramicroscope anemometer (LUA; 10). The principle of LUA

measurement is as follows: light of a pulsating Argon
laser is focused in such a way that it illuminates a
0.1 mm thick layer of a longitudinal section of the moving
fluid in dark field mode. The light scattered by anyone
illuminated particle suspended within the fluid leaves a
bright track on the photographic plate, the intervals between the streaks being proportional to the velocity, and
the shape of the curve showing the pathways of the particles
(streaklines). From the velocity vector v measured in a
distance of $y = 50$ nm from the wall, the velocity gradient
near the wall $\dot{\gamma} = dv/dy$ and the wall shear stress
$\tau_w = \dot{\gamma} \cdot \eta$ (dyn $cm^{-2}$) was calculated assuming that the velocity profile between $y = 50$ μm and $y = 0$ μm $(v = 0)$ is
linear. Moreover, the velocity component perpendicular towards the wall $v_i$ was determined from v measured at a wall
distance of 100 μm.


2.4 MICROSCOPICAL OBSERVATION OF THE DEPOSITS

2.4.1 A reflective dark field microscope was used to measure the number of cells and the growth rate of deposits
adhering to the wall and to investigate the shape of monocellular and plycellular deposits qualitatively as well
(Ultropak, Leitz, Objective UO 52 W). Pictures were recorded by means of micro-photography and video-kinematography.

2.4.2 To study the interactivity between blood cells and
the surface of the coverglass, the distance of deposited
particles from the surface was measured by means of interference reflection microscopy (12). The technique employed
differed from that applied by CURTIS (7), insofar as we
illuminated the object with circular polarized light and
suppressed background intensity with crossed polarizors
(objective: Leitz, Immers. Kontrast. NPL oil 100/1. 30 A).
The system works as follows:

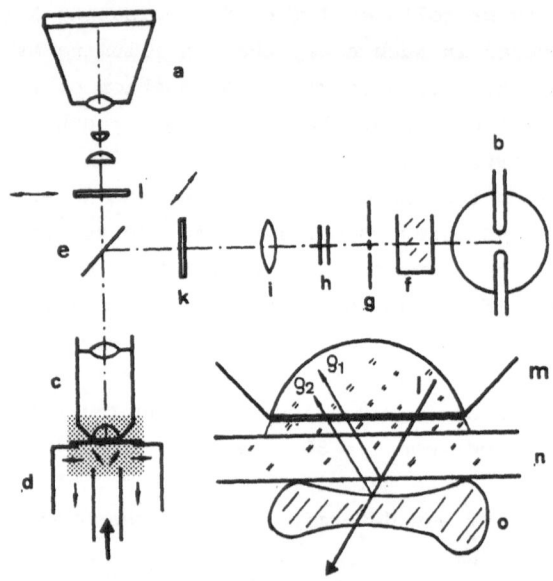

Fig. 1: Sketch of the reflecting interference microscope
        for the investigation of thrombogenesis in a
        stagnation point flow aggregometer: a) photogra-
        phic camera; b) Xenon arc lamp; c) immersion ob-
        jective; d) stagnation point flow chamber; diam of
        the outer tube forming the wall of the chamber re-
        duced by a factor 20 with respect to diam of the
        acial tube; e) half silvered mirror; f) heat re-
        flecting filter (water); g) central iris; h) 542 nm
        interference filter; i) collimating lenses;
        k) polarisator  l) analysator. Inset: magnification
        of the dotted section at the left; m) front lens
        with 1/4 λ plate; n) cover glass; o) Red blood cell
        (see text for further explanation)

The incident light beam I (see fig. 1 inset, solid line) is
reflected at the phase border glass/water and the border
water/cell. The reflected beams $\mathcal{S}_1$ and $\mathcal{S}_2$. In the case of
monochromatic light (λ=542nm) interference fringes can be
observed. The phase difference Γ between $\mathcal{S}_1$ and $\mathcal{S}_2$ was
estimated using the colour table of Michel-Lévy or measured
with the aid of a microdensitometer. These results allow
the calculation of the width d of the gap between the surfaces of the cell and the glass wall, if the value of the
refractive index of the gap material is known (termed as

$n_1$ provided a gap is present).

$$d = \frac{\Gamma - \frac{\lambda}{2}}{2 \cdot n_1} \cdot \cos \alpha$$

($\alpha = 45^\circ$ = angle of the incident beam in water; n refractive index of glass)

Estimates of the refractive index of the gap material and the cell plasma are possible on the basis of Fesnel's equations using the measured values of minimal ($\varphi_{min}$) and maximal reflectivity ($\varphi_{max}$) resp.; if absorption is neglected, the following equations are valid under the condition that the sequence of phase borders is $n > n_1$ and $n_1 < n_0$; $n_0$ stands for the refractive index of cell plasma provided a gap is present.

$$\varphi_{max} = \left[ \frac{n_1^2 - n_0 n}{n_1^2 + n_0 n} \right]^2 \qquad \varphi_{min} = \left[ \frac{n - n_0}{n + n_0} \right]^2 \qquad (1)$$

(if the gap is vanished as during viscous transformation $n_0$ terms the refractive index of extracellular solution – see 5.2; other equations, not mentioned here, are to be used to describe this case).

## 3. RESULTS, Monocellular deposits

In the first experiment the inflow was set at low flow rates. In figure 2, the upper photograph shows the pathways of RBC's under these conditions. The pathways of platelets are quite similar. In the axial flow, pathways appear which are directed perpendicularly towards the cover glass. In the other regions of the stagnation point flow the pathways of inflowing particles form a curvature of $90^{\circ}$ until they flow off nearly parallel to the cover glass. The curved pathways of the platelets are convergent with respect to each other and with respect to the wall surface. By microscopical observation of the cover glass in the direction of the tube axis, it could be established that the platelets touch the glass surface only in a region which corresponds exactly to the axial projection of the inflow tube opening on the cover glass. RBC's, however, touch the wall only in the central region of the stagnation area up to half of the tube diameter. In the diagrams (fig. 2) from top to bottom the dependence of the following values on the distance R from the center of the stagnation area are shown: a) $v_{\perp}$, $\dot{\gamma}$; b) number of particles $p_t$ which touch the wall; c) number of particles $p_d$ which adhere to the wall forming a monocellular deposit. The left column is valid for bovine platelets, the right column for bovine RBC's. In the vicinity of the wall where the streamlines of platelets are convergent, the numerical values of $v_{\perp}$ are found to be positive with a maximum near the center of the stagnation area. At the same time, the shear rate $\dot{\gamma}$ becomes zero and increases with increasing distance R. The stagnation point flow is thus characterized by positive values of $v_{\perp}$ indicating that particles gain an impulse toward the wall. $p_t$ (diagram b) was measured by means of reflective interference microscopy. A sudden retardation of the particle movement and the appearence of interference fringes indicate a collision of the particles with the wall. As shown by comparison of fig. 2 a and b (left) $p_t$ is nearly proportional to $v_{\perp}$. RBC contact $p_t$ with the wall, however, shows an exponential decrease to zero at $R = 0.4$ mm (2 b, right). Fig. 2 d demonstrates the radial distribution of platelets adhering to the wall and forming a monocellular deposit. Comparison of the maximal value of $p_d$ with that of $p_t$ shows that 10 % of the ADP-activated bovine platelets touching the wall eventually become fixed as a deposit ($2.5 \times 10^{-6}$ M ADP). Comparison of fig. 2 a with fig. 2 c shows that the location of platelet deposits corresponds to the overall region where $v_\perp > 0$, whereas RBC deposits only occur near the stagnation point (fig. 2 bottom at the right) By increasing the volume flow, not only $v_\perp$ but also $\dot{\gamma}$ and therefore $\tau_w$ are increased simultaneously. If $\tau_w$ exceeds a critical value $\tau_w^*$, the platelets, that are already deposited, are torn loose again, so that $\tau_w$ ($\dot{\gamma}$) is considered as a force that antagonize deposition. The values of $\tau_w^*$ are taken as a measure of the adhesive strength (adhesivity); for ADP-activated platelets $\tau_w^* \approx 60$ dyn cm$^{-2}$.

# 4. DISCUSSION OF THE MECHANISM UNDERLYING MONOCELLULAR DEPOSITION

## 4.1 TRANSPORT MECHANISM

In the region of stagnation point flow the pathways of particles are convergent if viewed at the plane normal to the wall and divergent in the plane parallel to the wall. According to the law of continuity, the fluid elements must undergo a deformation in such a way, that a cylindrical fluid element arriving at the center is deformed to a plate while moving tangentially to the wall in radial direction. If the distance of the streamlines from the wall becomes less than the radius of the particle $r_p$, mechanical contact with the wall occurs. On the basis of this approach the number of particles $p_t$ transported to the wall can be calculated:

$$p_t = C \cdot v_\perp^* \cdot t \qquad (2)$$

(C     concentration of blood particles, $v_\perp^*$     velocity component measured in a wall distance $r_p$; t time)
Assuming a linear velocity profile near the wall $v_\perp^*$ was calculated using the law of continuity:

$$v_\perp^* = \dot\gamma_1 \cdot r_p^2 \left(1 - \sqrt{\frac{\dot\gamma_1 \cdot R_1}{\dot\gamma_2 \cdot R_2}}\right) \cdot \frac{1}{R_2 - R_1} \qquad (3)$$

($\dot\gamma_1, \dot\gamma_2$ shear rate at a distance $R_1$ and $R_2$ resp. extrapolated to a difference $R_2 - R_1 < 1$ µm). Diagram fig. 2 b shows the calculated values for $r_p$ = 0.6 µm (crossed line). The curve of $p_t$     measured (solid line) fits quite well with the calculated curve. As shown by the diagram fig. 2 b (right) the transport mechanism for RBC's is quite different. Due to axial migration, net transport is diminished.

## 4.2 DEPOSITION MECHANISM

The mechanism of monocellular deposition can be illustrated by the following qualitative formula:

$$p_d = f(p_t) \cdot f(K_{pw}) \cdot f(v_\perp / v_\parallel) \qquad (4)$$

$f(v_\perp/v_{/\!/})$ allows for a force ($\sim v_\perp$) which presses particles towards the wall and a force ($\sim v_{/\!/}$) that shears off the particles. The term $f(k_{PW})$ describes molecular interactions which lead to adhesive bonding. For standardized hydrodynamic conditions, the adhesive factor $k_{PW}$ is defined by

$$P_d = P_t \cdot k_{PW} \qquad (5)$$

and can be compared with the respective adhesive factors measured by other methods (4, 11, 15). For ADP-activated ($2.5 \times 10^{-6}$ M) bovine platelets an adhesive factor $k_{PW} \approx 0.1$ was measured in the experiment described above (3.1). The adhesive strength of different surfaces (endothelia of living arteries, surfaces of arteriografts) can be tested in the same way as that of blood particles, provided that in this case besides the hydrodynamic conditions the properties of blood cells are standardized.

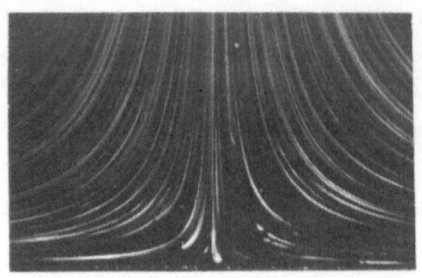

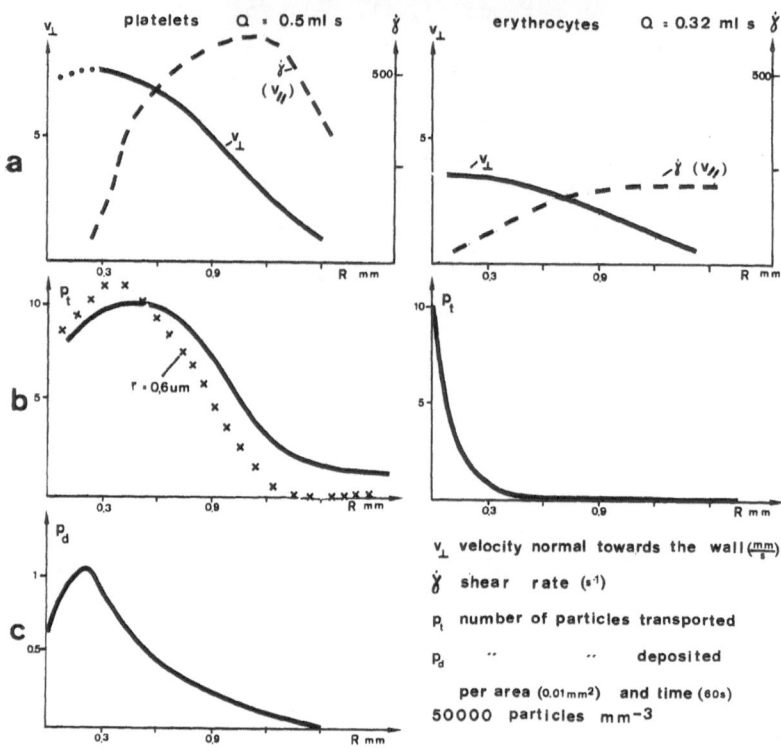

platelets  Q = 0.5 ml s

erythrocytes  Q = 0.32 ml s

$v_\perp$ velocity normal towards the wall $(\frac{mm}{s})$

$\dot\gamma$ shear rate (s$^{-1}$)

$P_t$ number of particles transported

$P_d$  "          "  deposited

per area (0.01mm²)  and time (60s)
50000 particles mm$^{-3}$

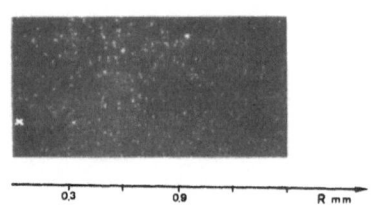

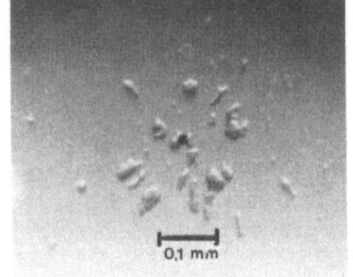

0,1 mm

Fig. 2  see text for explanation

## 5. INTERACTION OF BLOOD CELLS WITH THE GLASS WALL

As described in 3.1, stagnation point flow acts in decreasing the distance between the moving cells and the surface of the wall. If this distance becomes lower than a
certain minimal distance, $d_{min}$, adhesion between cell and
wall occur with a probability of 10 %. $d_{min}$ was measured
by means of interference reflection microscopy. The quo-
tient of $\tau_w^*$ and the distance to the wall represent the
strength of adhesive bonding.

### 5.1 HUMAN RED BLOOD CELLS

Fig. 3.5 and 4.5 show interference reflective micrographs of normal RBC's immediately after they had arrived
and adhered at the wall (12). The strength of adhesion is
low, i.e., they can be removed by a shear stress of $\tau_w^* =$
0.3 dyn cm$^{-2}$. From the margin to the center of the cell,
the following sequence of increasing interference colours
occurs: grey-blue, white, yellow, orange, red I.O. and blue
green II. O. near the center. The phase differences were
measured with the aid of a microdensitometer using monochromatic illumination (fig. 3.5); $d_{min}$ was estimated
assuming a constant refractive index of the gap matrix. The
gap attains its maximal width near the cell center, whereas the minimum width is at the margin (grey blue area)
corresponding to $d_{min} \approx 200$ Å. In a second experiment, thorn
apple shaped RBC's deposited at the wall were exposed to
shear stresses of increasing values and the morphological
changes recorded. In fig. 3.1, a thorn apple shaped RBC is
transported towards the wall at low flow rates ($\tau_w = 0.3$
dyn cm$^{-2}$). After adhesion, five points of black first order (I.O.) occur near the left margin, indicating that the
gap width is about zero, and that these points may be the
sites where the RBC anchors to the glass surface. In a second step, $\tau_w$ is increased to 3.4 dyn cm$^{-2}$ (fig. 3.2). The
cell body is shifted by about 5 μm in the direction of the
flow (indicated by arrow in 4.1). Because the RBC is fixed
to the glass wall by the anchoring points at the left margin, several strands of 5 μm length are formed tethering

the main body of the cell to the wall and preventing it
from being washed away. If the flow is stopped (fig. 3.3),
the cell moves back only about 2 μm. The remaining strands
and the deformed cell body show that the $\tau_w$-induced cell
deformation is not reversible. If the wall shear stress
exceeds $\tau_w^* = 7$ dyn cm$^{-2}$, the cell body is sheared off after
the membrane near the anchoring points is fragmented, as
shown by the residual strands (fig. 3.4 presents the cell
just before going adrift). These results, which correspond
to those of B l a c k s h e a r  (5), suggest, that fragmentation of RBC's and haemolysis may be induced by rather
small shear forces, if the cells come in close contact with
a surface of foreign material.

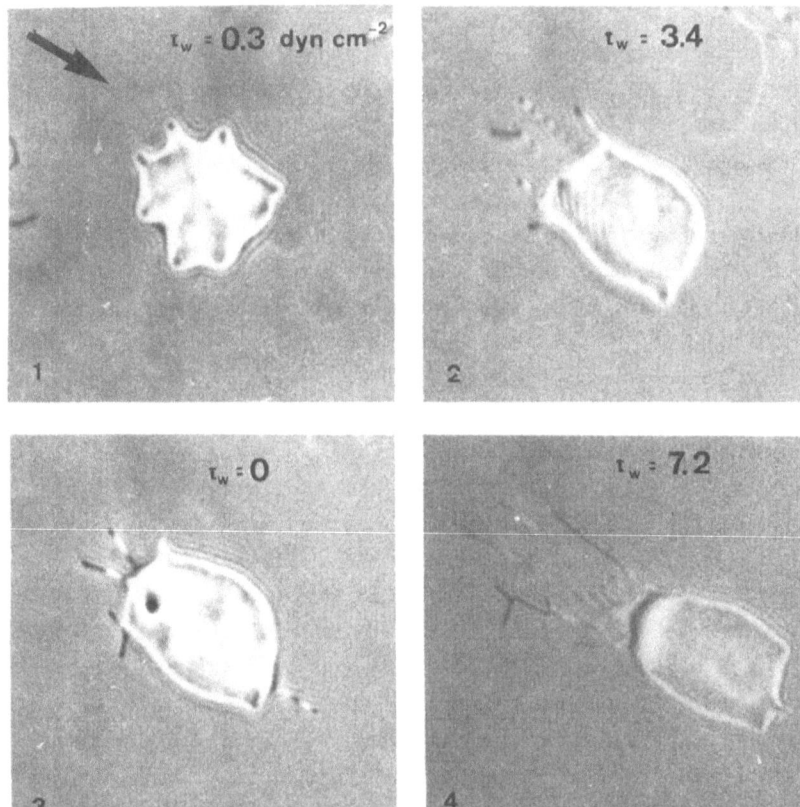

$\tau_w = 0.3 \ dyn \ cm^{-2}$

$\tau_w = 3.4$

$\tau_w = 0$

$\tau_w = 7.2$

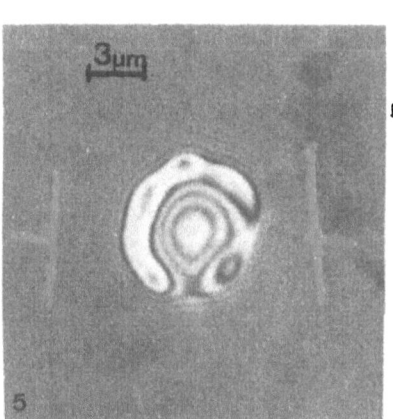

3µm

Fig. 3 Interference reflection micrographs (monochromatic illumination $\lambda$ = 542 nm); From
fig. 3.1 to 3.4 micrographs of the same
thorn apple formed RBC adhering at the wall.
The influence of different shear stresses $\tau_w$
(values indicated for each figure) on the
shape of RBC is shown. Fig. 3.5   normal
shaped RBC at $\tau_w$ = O for comparison.

115

## 5.2 HUMAN PLATELETS

Some characteristic morphological stages of platelet
deposition are demonstrated in fig, 4.1 ÷ 4.4 (12). Fig. 4.1
shows a platelet just arriving and settling down at the
glass surface. In the direction from the margin of the cell
to the center the following sequence of decreasing interference colours occurs: green blue II.O., red I.O., orange,
yellow, white I.O. In contrast to deposited RBC's, the gap
width of platelets attains its minimum value near the cell
center ($d \approx 600$ Å) and increases steadily toward the margin.
In the state represented by fig. 4.1 the $\tau_w^*$ is in the range
of 4.5 ($\pm$ 1.5) dyn cm$^{-2}$. 30 s after adhesion, the effects
of contact-stimulated excitation can be seen: the cell eva-
ginates pseudopods; at the same time the gap width in the
center of the cell is decreased to zero (interference colour
black I.O., see fig. 4.2 lower cell). Now the adhesion
strength increases to such a value that, under the conditions of our experiment, $\tau_w^*$ cannot be attained ($\tau_w^*$ > 20 dyn
cm$^{-2}$). Within the following 5 min the cell shape is transformed to a flat disc (viscous transformation; see fig. 4.3
and 4.4). As the distance of the gap is zero, the beam $\rho_1$
is reflected by the phase border glass/cell-front ($n/n_1$) and
the beam $\rho_2$ from the phase border cell-back/water ($n_1/n_c$). The
sequence of the phase borders in the direction of incident
light is now: $n$ > $n_1$, $n_1$ > $n_0$. No phase shift of 90° is
further superimposed on to the reflected beams. Therefore,
interference colours are complementary with respect to those
observed in the experiments described above. This could be
established by index matching (embedding the cell with a
medium of a nearly identical refractive index: silicone oil)
which causes the interference colours to disappear. The
thickness of the flat cells is measured to $d \approx 1000$ Å.

The tenfold higher values of $\tau_w^*$ for platelets than for
RBC's may be attributed to the more than tenfold higher
flow resistance of RBC's compared with that of platelets
(calculated regarding the different sizes of the cells). In

Fig. 4 Colour reproduction of reflective interference micrographs of deposited cells. From fig. 4.1 to
4.4 human platelets (no ADP-activation); 4.1 platelet immediately after having deposited (interference colour white I.O. corresponding to $d_{min} \approx 600$ Å). 4.2 other cells of the same proof 30 s after
deposition; appearence of black I.O. shows that $d_{min}$ is diminished to about zero. 4.3 same cells as
4.2 50 s after deposition; beginning of viscous transformation. 4.4 30 min final state of viscous
transformation (fried egg shape of platelets). 4.5 human RBC; $d_{min} \approx 200$ Å.

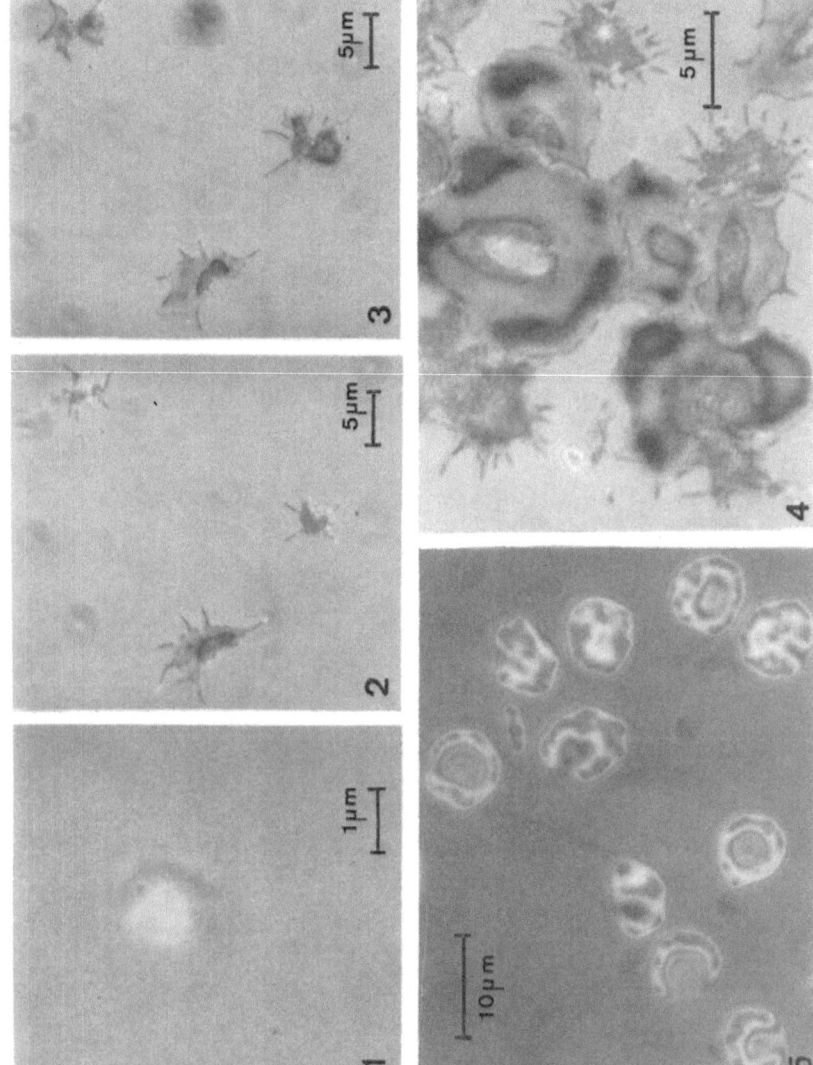

| d | RBC | | PLATELET | |
|---|---|---|---|---|
| $d_{min}/\text{Å}$ | 200 | 0 | 600 | 0 |
| $\tau_w^{\bullet}/\frac{dyn}{cm^2}$ | 0.3 | 7 fragmentation | 5 | >20 viscous transf. |
| $n_0(cell)$ | 1.48 | | 1.47 | |
| $n_1(gap)$ | 1.33 | | 1.36 | 1.38 cell |

Fig. 5: Relationship between the distance from the glass wall surface and the strength of adhesion: of normal human RBC, thorn apple RBC, human platelets in the earliest and in a later state of deposition (from left to right; fragmentation of RBC begins at $\tau_w^{*} = 1.5 \div 3.0$ dyn/cm². For the fragments is $\tau_w^{*} > 20$ dyn/cm²); $d/\tau_w$ represents the power of adhesive bonding.

the state in which they are sheared off, the $\tau_w$ which really strains the adhesive interface may attain comparable values for both cells, whereas the particle-wall distance d is different; d for platelets is greater by about a factor of three than it is for RBC's as intimated by the results of preliminary measurements (see fig. 5). The strength of platelet adhesive bonding to glass walls is thus remarkably greater for platelets, indicating a different bonding mechanism than for RBC's. The remarkably higher refractive index of the gap matrix suggests that a specific adhesive material is released by the platelets in the first phase of deposition thus supporting the assumption of different adhesion mechanisms.

## 6. RESULTS, Polycellular deposits

As described in 3. the platelets interact only with the surface of the glass wall; they do not adhere to other already deposited platelets if the velocity of stagnation point flow is small. Eq. (2) and the diagrams fig. 2 (left), therefore, describe the relationship between the hydrodynamic parameters and the p a r t i c l e - w a l l inter-action.

At higher velocities (where 60 dyn $cm^{-2}$ > $\tau_w$ > 2.3 dyn $cm^{-2}$) polycellular deposits occur. The pseudopodia of the monocellularly deposited platelets are elongated up to 30 μm and are trained parallel to the direction of the stream lines. Video-graphs show that those platelets already adhering to the vessel wall act as traps, entangling other passing platelets with their pseudopodia. Apposition happens only downstream from the point of the initial deposit in the direction of the flow, resulting in streak shaped polycellular deposits. They grow in the same region where

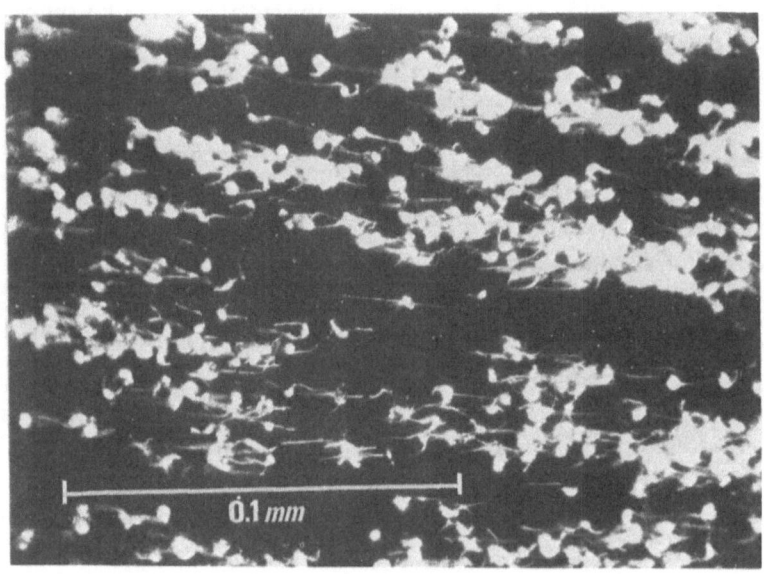

Fig. 6: Polycellular deposits of bovine platelets (re-flective dark field micrograph).

the single deposits appear ($v_\iota > 0$) but indicate p a r-
t i c l e - p a r t i c l e interaction predominantly.

To determine whether the observed particle-particle interaction at higher flow velocities is due to an increased
arrival rate of particles or whether it is due to an increased particle-particle adhesivity ($k_{pp}$), the following
experiment was carried out (3): The stagnation point flow
aggregometer was perfused by bovine PRP during 32 minutes
at low flow rates ($\tau_w = 0.7$ dyn cm$^{-2}$). Mainly monocellular
deposits of platelets occur (The adhesion rate of ADP activated platelets is constant only within the first 6 min
after activation. At t > 6 min a remarkable time-dependency
occurs. Therefore the freshly ADP-activated PRP was renewed
every 6 min, as indicated by arrows at the abszissa in fig.
7). The growth rate is small during the first 32 min (fig.
7). 32 min after onset of the flow, $\tau_w$ was increased to

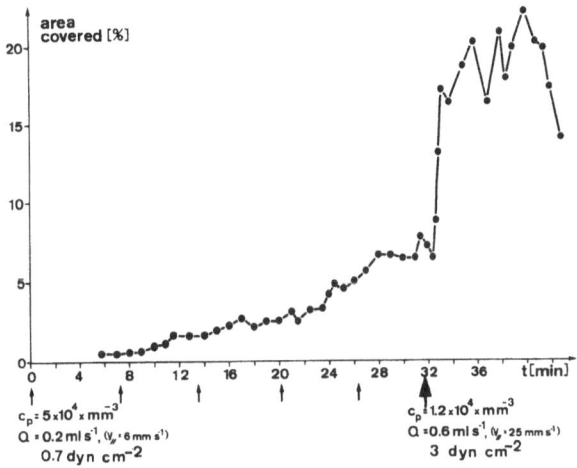

Fig. 7: Growth of deposits of bovine platelets in a stagnation point flow experiment. Different growth rate
of monocellular deposits ( t=0 ÷ 32 min) and polycellular deposits (t > 32 min). Polycellular deposition (induced by increasing $\tau_w$ from 0.7 dyn/cm$^2$
to 3.0 dyn/cm$^2$) is correlated with a sudden increase
of growth rate at the beginning (t=32) and disintegration (embolization) after 6 min (t=38). Growth
rate expressed in terms of change of surface area
covered by deposited platelets.

$\tau_w$ = 3 dyn cm$^{-2}$ (see heavy printed arrow in fig. 7). Although the arrival rate of platelets was held constant by reducing the concentration of platelets from $5 \cdot 10^4$ to $1.2 \cdot 10^4$ per mm$^3$, the growth rate of deposits increased remarkably.                As established by further experimental proof, the steep increase of growth rate appeared whenever $v_{/\!/}$ exceeded a critical value corresponding to $\tau_w$ = 2.3 dyn· cm$^{-2}$. The increase of growth rate can be attributed to hydrodynamically induced platelet-platelet adhesivity which is considered by introducing the empirical constant $k_{pp}$.

Whereas the deposition of monocellular deposits at the wall follows an exponential saturation curve (comparable to the charge curve of a capacitor), the growth of streak shaped deposits exhibits an exponential increment with time. Five minutes after onset of flow, the deposit growth is followed by embolization; the time course of which is also exponential (comparable to the curve describing the discharge curve of a capacitor). Only those platelets which originally had served as initiation points remain adhering to the wall. The rate constants of deposit integration and disintegration are different. The change of adhesive properties $k_{pp}$ (t) within a definite time indicates that platelet-platelet interaction is determined by biological processes. Whereas the first monocellular deposition may be explained sufficiently via physical mechanisms, streak-shaped deposition of platelets cannot be understood without taking these active biological processes into account (14). RBC's and inorganic particles also exhibit streak shape deposition but no disintegration could be observed, indicating that the mechanism of deposit formation is different from that of platelet-deposition.

According to these results, a close analogy exists to other mechanical adhesion processes. Stagnation point flow produces deposits by bringing the prospective adhering particles in contact with one another. This is achieved by overcoming the forces that antagonize such contact. The greater the compressing force which promotes bonding and the lower the shearing force which places a stress on the adhesive interface, the more stable is the resulting agglutination. The velocity field with its vector components $v_\perp$ and $v_{/\!/}$ determines the location of the deposit formation, whereas the deposit mass depends on the frequency of collision $p_t$ between the wall and the particles, as well as on the thrombogenic adhesive factor k ($k_{PW}$ and $k_{pp}$). If the rate of arrival and the rate of deposition ($p_t$ and $p_d$) are measured, the thrombogenic factor (k) of the blood elements or that of the natural or artificial wall can be determined quantitatively, provided that the unavoidable acting hydrodynamic forces are well known. Under laboratory conditions $v_\perp$ and $v_{/\!/}$ can be given experimentally as independent variables.

REFERENCES

1) Baldauf, W., L. Wurzinger and J. Kinder: The role of stagnation point flow in the formation of platelet thrombi on glass surfaces in tubes with various geometry. Path. Res. Pract. 163, 9-33 (1978)

2) Baldauf, W.: Behaviour of erythrocyte suspensions in flow through a branched tube. A study on the deposition hypothesis of atherogenesis. Beitr. Path. 160, 129-153 (1977)

3) Baldauf, W. and Kratzer, M.: Growth rates of platelet thrombi produced under definite flow conditions for stagnation point flow; in preparation

4) Begent, N. and G.V.R. Born: Growth rate in vivo of platelet thrombi, produced by Iontophoresis of ADP, as a function of mean blood flow velocity. Nature 227, 926-930 (1970)

5) Blackshear, jr., P.L., R.J., Forstrom, F.D. Dorman and G.O. Voss: Effect of flow on cells near walls. Fed. Proc. 30, 1600-1611 (1971)

6) Chien, S. and K.-M., Jan: Ultrastructural basis of mechanism of rouleaux formation. Micr. Vasc. Res. 5, 155-166 (1973)

7) Curtis, A.S.G.: The mechanism of adhesion of cells to glass. The J. of cell biol. 20, 199-215 (1964)

8) Dutton, R.C., R.E. Baier, R.L. Dedrick and R.L. Howman: Initial thrombus formation on foreign surfaces. Trans. Amer. Soc. Artif. Int. Organs 14, 57-62 (1968)

9) Goldsmith, H.L. and T. Karino: Platelets in a region of distrubed glow. Trans. Amer. Soc. Artif. Int. Organs 23, 632-638 (1977)

10) Kinder, J. and M. Kratzer: Geschwindigkeitsmessung im Inneren komplizierter Strömungen mit einem Lichtschnittverfahren. Biomded. Technik 20, 11-12 (1975)

11) Klose, H.I., H. Rieger and H. Schmid-Schönbein: A rheological method for the quantification of platelet aggregation (PA) in vitro and its kinetics under definded flow conditions. Thromb. Res. 7, 261-273 (1975)

12) Kratzer, M. and W. Baldauf: interferometric measurements of the distance between glass wall and adhering platelets or red blood cells at different strength of adhesion. Pflügers. Arch. ges. Physiol. 373, Suppl. R 58 (1978)

13) Leonard, E.F., E.F. Grabowski and V.T. Rutitto: The role of convection and diffusion on platelet adhesion and aggregation. Ann. New York Acad. of Science 201, 329-342 (1972)

14) Madras, P.N., W.A. Morton and M.E. Petschek: Dynamics of thrombus formation. Fed. Proc. 30, 1665-1676 (1971)

15) Marx, R. and S. Derlath: Über eine Methode zur vergleichenden quantitativen Bestimmung der Thrombozytenadhäsivität an blutfremden Oberflächen unter gleichzeitiger Erfassung der relativen Blutviskosität. Blut 3, 27 (1957)

16) Müller-Mohnssen, H.: Die Strömungsverhältnisse in den Koronararterien und ihre Bedeutung für die Manifestierung der Koronar Sklerose. In: Bad Oeynhausener Gespräche II (W. Lochner u. E. Witzleb, Hrgb.), Springer, Berlin, Göttingen, Heidelberg 179-196 (1958)

17) Müller-Mohnssen, H., M. Kratzer and W. Baldauf: Microthrombus formation in models of coronary arteries caused by stagnation point flow arising at the predilection sites of atherosclerosis and thrombosis. In: The role of fluid mechanics in Atherogenesis (R.M. Nerem and J.F. Cornhill, Eds.), Ohio State Univ., Ohio, p. 12 (1978)

18) Müller-Mohnssen, H.: Pathogenese der Koronarsklerose und Strömungsmechanik. Münchener Med. Wschr. 113, 604-616 (1971)

DISCUSSION          Moderator: Hemker

Schmid-Schönbein:          I would like to prompt a critical discussion about
                          the use of the word "dead water". In the eddies
                          and vortices you showed many dangerous things
                          happen which might kill organisms and human
                          beings. Thus, I think that these secondary flows
                          with the vortices and the stagnation flow, with
                          recirculation of activated blood-clotting factors
                          should not be called "dead water". Both from a
                          fluid-dynamic and a biological standpoint there is
                          a lot of action there. Could you please comment?

Müller-Mohnssen:          Dr. Schmid-Schönbein, I cannot oppose what you
                          said, but most of the people understand the mea-
                          ning of "dead water". In the presentation of
                          Dr. Naumann I heard: "dead water" and I cannot
                          find a better word. This is a region, where the
                          primary flow separates from the wall. One part of
                          the fluid no longer belongs to the far moving
                          fluid but becomes a part of the wall. This can be
                          seen on velocity profiles. Regions with the lar-
                          gest shear gradients, which were originally right
                          at the wall, are now located in the interior of
                          the tube, forming the boundary between dead water
                          and main flow. Within the dead water, the velocity
                          gradients are very low. The movements which can be
                          observed within the dead water are induced secon-
                          darily, the fluid behaves passively, in other
                          words: "dead". I find no other word, perhaps you
                          have one for it. - High kinetic energies are
                          necessary to form a dead water and high veloci-
                          ties can regularly be found in the areas surroun-
                          ding the dead water. This may be different bet-
                          ween dead water and stagnation flow. The forma-
                          tion of a circumscribed gangrenous area instead
                          of a progressive necrosis requires a certain vi-
                          tality of the organism. Excuse this non-scientific
                          but    illustrative analogy.

| | |
|---|---|
| Schmid-Schönbein: | Most people do understand, but there is still a considerable number of people who misunderstand this term. It implies to the non-fluid-dynamicist that there is stasis and this impression is positively wrong. There is no stasis, but rather stagnation point flow and also very rapid changes in shear rate. And, of course, the work of KARINO and GOLDSMITH (Microvascular Research, 1979, in press) will very nicely show how rapidly platelet aggregates can grow there. Dr. Lambert is here, and he can tell us what happens to the red cells. How would you like to call these flow-perturbations, Dr. Lambert? |
| Lambert: | In fact, a lot of things are going on in these "dead waters", e.g. red cells are migrating out of the centre of vortices. The separation area, as we could call it, is really very different from the main flow from which it is well separated by well defined separation streamlines ending in a stagnation point at the wall. |
| Schmid-Schönbein: | Can we agree to call them separated regions or simply vortices ("Wirbel" in German)? |
| Lambert: | I would not like to call them just vortices, because these are usually very well defined. But if you have a separation area, let's say behind a blunt body, there are not well defined vortices. Usually, there is a very complex motion which on the one hand cannot be called turbulence but which, on the other hand, I would not like to call plainly vortex, either. |
| Schmid-Schönbein: | This semantic difficulty has been the reason for much confusion in the medical literature. It is in fact complicating the communication between physicists and physicians. |
| Williams: | I would just say a slowly rotating vortex. This may be defined simply as a region which is bounded |

125

by a streamline of zero velocity.

Schmid-Schönbein: GOLDSMITH and his group have shown many rheological phenomena that occur in the vortices behind a stenosis. He has shown that the size of platelets, of red cells and of platelet aggregates has important consequences for the behaviour and the residence time of these species. A most important consequence of this is the progressive growth of platelet aggregates. This occurs primarily in the central region of low shear-stresses and there activated chemical species are also permanently trapped. The data of Dr. Müller-Mohnssen and Dr. Kratzer show that in very near proximity very high shear-stresses occur - and we are now beginning to realize that these are capable of activating the platelets directly or indirectly via a release of ADP from red cells. The boundary between the laminar flow and the ill-defined "dead water" is therefore certainly an area of high biological activity. I repeat my call for a more appropriate name for this type of flow perturbation. Maybe one can name it after a very famous fluid-dynamicist.

Williams: Dr. Müller-Mohnssen's group has in many ways duplicated some of shear exposure conditions I generate with my oscillating wire assembly. It might be of interest for you to know I see "activation" of platelets in the flow field, i.e. without contact with any solid surface. There "activated" platelets are extremely adhesive and will attach themselves to any surface with which they come into contact.

Müller-Mohnssen: I cannot answer directly but you said that you are excited about these high shear-stresses and this is really the fact. Very high shear-stresses also occur at the reflexion point, where the velocity profile changes from positive to negative.

126

But you can interpret it by saying that the
high shear-stress occurs now within the flowing
blood and not only near the wall. Motion occurs
here as a consequence of indirect acceleration
via inertial forces and not due to the pressure
gradient producing the primary flow.

Kratzer:                 We have a slide showing the velocity in the
                         dead water region (see Fig. 1).

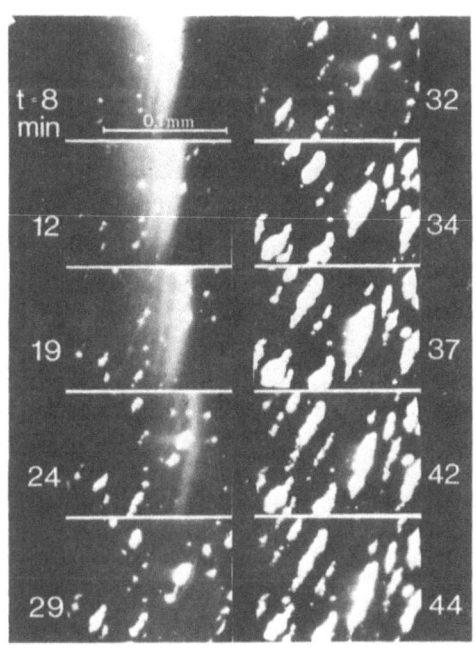

Tillmann:                Dr. Müller-Mohnssen, did you perform your studies
                         in pulsatile or in steady flow?

Müller-Mohnssen:         In steady flow.

Tillmann:                Would you expect any difference in your results
                         obtained in steady flow in rigid tubes and in
                         pulsatile flow in flexible boundaries? Do you
                         feel that you would get different results under
                         these different circumstances?

Müller-Mohnssen:         Thank you for your question which is very diffi-
                         cult to answer. We also investigated the effect of

pulsating flow, but so far only qualitatively. We are interested in the physico-mathematical treatment of our results in order to determine the cause and effect relationship between velocity field and deposition. Physical treatment of flow within geometrical complex regions is already a difficult task if the flow is stationary. Quantitative work on pulsating flow needs, moreover, the consideration of time-dependent properties (elasticity, visco-elasticity of the fluid, elasticity of the wall. Such tube investigations cannot start before we understand the deposition mechanism of particles at the wall under steady flow conditions. As far as we know today, deposition also takes place during pulsating flow; at the same sites as with stationary flow. The quantity of deposited cells is likely to depend also on amplitude and time course of the pulsations.

Feijen:
I remember from your presentation, you had values for $K_{pw}$ between 0.5 and 2 %. Is that due to different surfaces, standardization problems of surfaces or is it just a variation in the type of blood you are using? Can you comment on this?

Müller-Mohnssen:
First of all, we did not investigate the molecular basis of $K_{pw}$ and cannot explain quantitatively why the values of $K_{pw}$ are different for different samples. Only for some experiments with PRP, to which different concentrations of ADP were added, a correlation between the $K_{pw}$ and the ADP stimulation of platelets could be established qualitatively. In experiments using suspensions of RBC, the pH plays a predominant role in determining $K_{pw}$, the value of the $K_{pw}$ increasing with decreasing pH, thus, we may infer a correlation between $K_{pw}$ and the electrokinetic potential of the RBC. In most of the experiments we measured $K_{pw}$ as an empirical constant for which no detailed expla-

128

nation can be given. Investigation of the physico-chemical events underlying $K_{pw}$ (and also $K_{pp}$) will be started as soon as some fundamental problems - as standardization of particles and/or of the stagnation plane surface - will be solved so that the stagnation point aggregometer can be used in clinical laboratories. Values of $K_{pw}$ obtained from ward patients can be compared with a lot of other data. Provided a correlation will be found regularly between enhanced $K_{pw}$ and certain other findings, clinical investigations may lead to a better understanding of the events underlying pathological changes of particle-wall and particle-particle adhesivity as well as of thrombogenesis.

Wurzinger: We found that *human* platelets always adhere to glass which has been cleaned exactly as it has been done by Dr. Müller-Mohnssen. They are brought to adhesion to glass by Brownian motion only and subsequently undergo spreading. On the other hand, if you take fully ADP-activated bovine platelets, so strongly activated that they aggregate much more than human platelets do spontaneously,they do not adhere to glass although they interact among themselves. These activated bovine platelets need a velocity component normal to the glass wall which is considerably higher than that provided by the Brownian motion.

Schmid-Schönbein: There is more behind that information if I may say so. Dr. Wurzinger found that *bovine* platelets, which have not been stimulated chemically will never stick to glass, no matter how large the tangential or normal flow forces. Of course, human platelets do always stick to glass as we all know. This experiment has two messages: One is, the bovine platelets show (at least for this species) that even the very simple adhesion process is then dominated by both flow *properties*

129

(i.e. adhesivity) and by *flow conditions* (flow towards the wall). The resting bovine platelet is so inert, that even with the highest forces that will be induced in these experiments they cannot be brought to stick to glass. This can only be achieved first by activating them with a chemical stimulus and then providing an appropriate flow condition, namely a velocity component directed towards the wall. The second message suggests that in human platelets, which are spontaneously quite hyperreactive, both activation and motion to the wall happen simultaneously. Glass obviously acts as a "stimulus" and we probably just do not have an adequate method to detect the activation (e.g. shape change) quick enough. I would predict that if we had such a method we could probably see that adhesion in human platelets is also a two-stage process.

Kratzer:

I would like to come back to the question, which arose earlier, namely the wall shear-stress in a separated flow region. I measured the shear-stresses generated in the main branch of a T-shaped bifurcation flow. (KRATZER et al., Pflügers Arch. Europ. J. Physiol. 355, Suppl. R39 (1975)) which was a simplified model of a coronary artery. At a Reynold's number of 800 wall shear-stress decreases from 34 $dyn/cm^2$ at the entrance in the branch to lower values between 0 and 10 $dyn/cm^2$ within the separated region. Maximal values were observed at the apex of the bifurcation (150 $dyn/cm^2$). Shear-stress at the interface between fast flow (jet) and "dead water" was 30 $dyn/cm^2$.

Schmid-Schönbein:

There are important consequences that become obvious from the complex fluid dynamics of the stagnation point in non-stationary flow. There is not just a rapid local change in the shear-stress or shear-rate acting on the surface of

the cells near the wall, but also a sudden condensation of the fluid layers and therefore, an increase of the collision probability of suspended
particles with each other and with the wall. The
platelets and the red cells have a finite size
and the platelet size is by no means constant.
Irrespective of the unsettled question of volume
changes of platelets after activation, they become "extended" by any formation of pseudopodes.
Therefore, the local platelet concentration is
not constant. In a system containing platelets
we have to differentiate between the platelet concentration in a resting situation (either the number density or platelet volume per plasma volume)
and the "effective concentration". As shown by
KARINO and GOLDSMITH (Microvascular Research,
(1979), in press) in a flowing system we have
to consider a kind of "activity" in terms of a
collision probability. When flow produces a relative motion of blood-layers past each other, the
number of collision for any given shear-rate depends not simply on concentration as such but on
the hydrodynamically effective particle volume.
Normal, discoid or ellipsoid platelets are preferentially oriented in flow most of the time
and therefore their hydrodynamically effective
radius is equivalent to the minor axis of ellipsoid. Occasionally they flip over, and during
the rotation they have a larger radius. Thus, we
have sort of a time averaged  hydrodynamically
effective radius, and, of course, a hydrodynamically effective volume which is proportional to
the minor radius cubed. If two or three platelets are aggregated, their hydrodynamically
effective radius and consequently their effective
concentration is strongly increased in the case
of a small aggregate, especially since such a
body rotates always in a shear field. The forma-

tion of pseudopodia increases the hydrodynamically effective radius and the hydrodynamically effective volume by a factor which is proportional to the cube of the largest dimension of the platelets after activation. The effects of this are very pronounced, especially if averaged over extended times, since the normal discoid platelets are much better oriented in flow and rotate very seldomly whereas activated, shape-changed platelets rotate all the time (KRINGS and RIEGER, unpublished observation).

If one considers Dr. Kratzers and Dr. Karino's results together, one can envision a situation where shape-change results from any sort of mechanical or chemical stimulus that trigger the contractile proteins in platelets producing pseudopodia. Let us consider further, that this activation may be taking place upstreams in flow where high shear-stresses (ca. 500 dyn/cm$^2$) prevail and let us also consider that the formation of platelet aggregates may take place downstreams at a location where the flow-rates are lower and where the flow-lines are condensed. Under these conditions the "collision efficiency" will be drastically increased by cellular as well as by fluid dynamic forces. Needless to say that the probability of encountering platelets already deposited ("landing point" in Dr. Müller-Mohnssen's term) is likewise enhanced.

Kratzer:    I would like to show a little film, which was taken together with Dr. Baldauf. The film intends to demonstrate an increase of the probability of platelet aggregation caused by an increase of wall shear stress to values more than 2.3 dyn/cm$^2$. The main problem in illustrating such a dependence is to increase the wall shear stress without increa-

132

sing the arrival rate of platelets. Also one has
to compensate the time dependence of adhesivity
power of platelets after being activated with ADP
(2.5 M). Fig. 4 shows a micrograph of bovine platelet thrombi adhearing at a glass surface. Platelet deposits were induced by a stagnation point
flow. If the flow chamber is perfused with PRP
at low flow rates (0.7 $dyn/cm^2$) predominantly
monocellular deposits occure with a small growth
rate (Fig. 1, left side). If, however wall shear
stress is increased to 3 $dyn/cm^2$ (but reduced
concentration of platelets and thus constant
arrival rate) a much faster platelet thrombus
growth can be seen. The quantitative dependence
of thrombus growth and shear stress is shown
in the paper Müller-Mohnssen and Kratzer

# 7. THE ROLE OF SURFACES IN THE MECHANISM OF BLOOD COAGULATION

H.C.Hemker and G.Tans

Department of Biochemistry, Biomedical Centre, State University of Limburg. Maastricht, The Netherlands

## I. INTRODUCTION

Blood coagulation is brought about by a series of proenzyme - enzyme conversions. Except thrombin, the enzyme that converts fibrinogen into fibrin, the enzymes all serve to activate a specific proenzyme. The reaction sequence is therefore properly called a cascade (1) and has interesting amplifying properties (2). It can be represented as follows:

$$
\begin{array}{ll}
\overset{\overset{K}{\downarrow}}{XII} \longrightarrow XII_a & (1) \\[2pt]
\qquad \downarrow \\
\quad XI \longrightarrow XI_a & (2) \\[2pt]
\qquad\quad \downarrow \\
\quad\quad IX \overset{\downarrow}{\longrightarrow} IX_a \qquad VII_a \longleftarrow VII & (3\ a,\ b) \\[2pt]
\qquad\qquad \downarrow \qquad\qquad \downarrow \\
\quad\quad\quad X \longrightarrow X_a \longleftarrow X & (4) \\[2pt]
\qquad\qquad\qquad \downarrow \\
\quad\quad\quad\quad II \longrightarrow II_a & (5) \\[2pt]
\qquad\qquad\qquad\quad \downarrow \\
\quad\quad\quad\quad\quad I \longrightarrow Fibrin & (6)
\end{array}
$$

(see footnote on nomenclature and symbols).

Except for the last reaction, each of these reactions occurs at an interface. In these reactions not only the enzyme and the substrate interact but also a third type of protein, that we called paraenzyme (3) plays an important ,rate enhancing role.

In the reactions 1, 2, and possibly 3a, the surface can be provided by a variety of hydrophilic negatively charged solids (4). In the reactions 3b, 4, and 5 the surface is a negatively charged phospholipid surface (5). In all instances, the combination of adsorption

onto an interface and cooperation between enzyme and paraenzyme force-
fully augment the velocity of the reaction.We want to discuss what
mechanism can be held responsible for this effect.

First,we will shortly review what is known about the prothrombin activating reaction.On basis of that example we will discuss the interaction of coagulation proteins at interfaces in more general terms.

## II. THE ACTIVATION OF PROTHROMBIN (6)

Prothrombin is a proenzyme consisting of 582 aminoacids. Upon activation it is split at two sites:274 and 318 (bovine prothrombin).
Three polypeptide chains result: fragment 1-2, the $\alpha$-chain of thrombin and the $\beta$-chain of thrombin. The $\alpha$- and $\beta$-chains are linked
by an S-S bridge, together they form the active thrombin molecule.
Thrombin itself splits fragment 1-2 in fragment 1 and fragment 2 at
site 156.

In summary:

$$\text{prothrombin} \xrightarrow{E} \text{fragment 1-2 + prethrombin 2} \qquad (7)$$

$$\text{prothrombin 2} \xrightarrow{E} \text{thrombin} \qquad (8)$$

$$\text{fragment 1-2} \xrightarrow{\text{thrombin}} \text{fragment 1 + fragment 2} \qquad (9)$$

Thrombin can also attack prothrombin at the site
just as it does fragment 1-2. The resulting polypeptide is called
prethrombin 1. It can, in its turn be converted into thrombin in a
slow reaction

$$\text{prothrombin} \xrightarrow{\text{thrombin}} \text{fragment 1 + prethrombin 1} \qquad (10)$$

$$\text{prethrombin 1} \xrightarrow{E} \text{prethrombin 2 + fragment 2} \qquad (11)$$

$$\text{prethrombin 2} \xrightarrow{E} \text{thrombin} \qquad (12)$$

## III. PROTHROMBIN ACTIVATING ENZYMES

The enzyme capable to activate thrombin called E in the foregoing
paragraph under physiological circumstances is activated coagulation

factor X (factor $X_a$).Other proteolytic enzymes can split prothrombin and cause thrombin activity to arise; e.g. trypsin and several snake venoms (7 and references therein).The reaction scheme then may be different, meizo thrombin (i.e. thrombin cleft at place 318 only) can arise, thrombin may be broken down further etc. We will not discuss these enzymes further. It is interesting to note that proteolytic breakdown is not compulsory for prothrombin activation. In a highly specific reaction the staphylococcal exoprotein staphylocoagulase can form a stoichiometric complex with prothrombin in which no peptide bonds are cleft but that does have thrombin activity (8).

In the following,we restrict ourselves to the physiological activator factor $X_a$.

## IV. THE ACTION OF FACTOR $X_a$, FACTOR V AND PHOSPHOLIPID

Factor $X_a$ in free solution will convert prothrombin according to reactions 7 and 8.It has been known for several years that this reaction is accelerated manyfold by the presence of factor $V_a$, $Ca^{++}$ and phospholipids (9,10) and also that adsorption of the proteins onto the phospholipid surface is essential for this acceleration. In fact it is suggested by     binding as well as kinetic experiments that a molecule of factor $X_a$ adsorbed next to a molecule of factor $V_a$ on a phospholipid surface is the most active catalytic moiety (11-13).

Recent studies by Rosing and Tans (14) pointed out that addition of phospholipid caused the apparent $K_m$ of the prothrombin activation to rise 1000 fold. This means that the prothrombin concentration at which half maximal reaction velocity is observed drops 1000 times by the addition of phospholipid. The acceleration brought about by addition of factor V has a quite different basis. Here $k_{cat}$ is increased 250 fold whereas $K_m$ remains high. This means in popular terms that the time needed to activate a molecule of prothrombin is shortened by a factor 250.

The obvious question to be answered is also the question of interest to this symposion: how can interaction at an interface bring about these tremendous changes in katalytic properties?

## V. POSSIBLE INFLUENCES OF SURFACES

A global model of a protein molecule in solution is given in fig. 1.

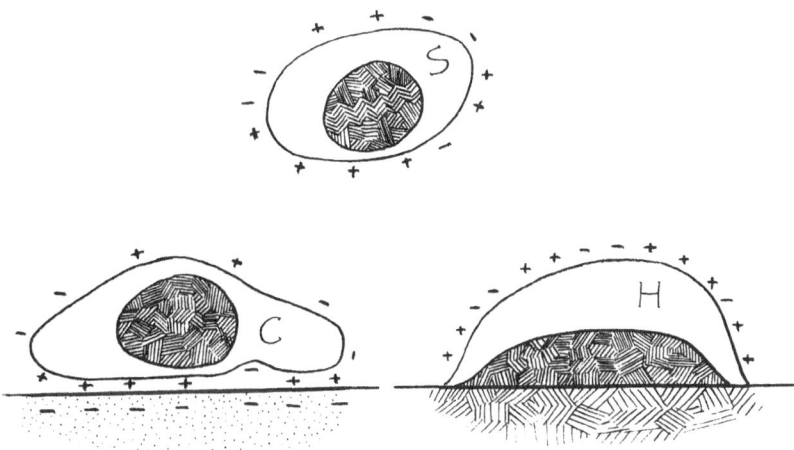

Fig. 1: Schematic representation of a protein in solution (S) and
adsorbed at a charged (C) and a hydrophobic (H) surface.
Hatched areas represent hydrophobic regions.

Usually the outside is formed by hydrophilic charged groups whereas
the more hydrophobic groups are sheltering from the surrounding
water in the inside of the molecule.
Positive and negative charges at the surface need not be evenly distributed. One part of the molecule can bear predominantly negative
charge whereas another part of the molecule is neutral or positively
charged.
Upon interaction with a charged interface the part of the molecule
bearing contrary charge will adhere to that interface. This can cause
the adsorbed molecules to be oriented in a more or less specific
way.Also the proteins can adsorb without gross conformational changes
because the charged groups are already present at the outside of
the molecule. On the other hand electrostatic forces are comparatively
strong so that formation of bonds can bring about deformation of the
molecule.

Hydrophobic interactions are weaker, but as the hydrophobic parts
of a protein molecule are not normally exposed at the surface interaction with a hydrophobic interface will tend to bring about gross
conformational changes. This is shown schematically in fig. 1 and
illustrated by the experiments of fig. 2.

137

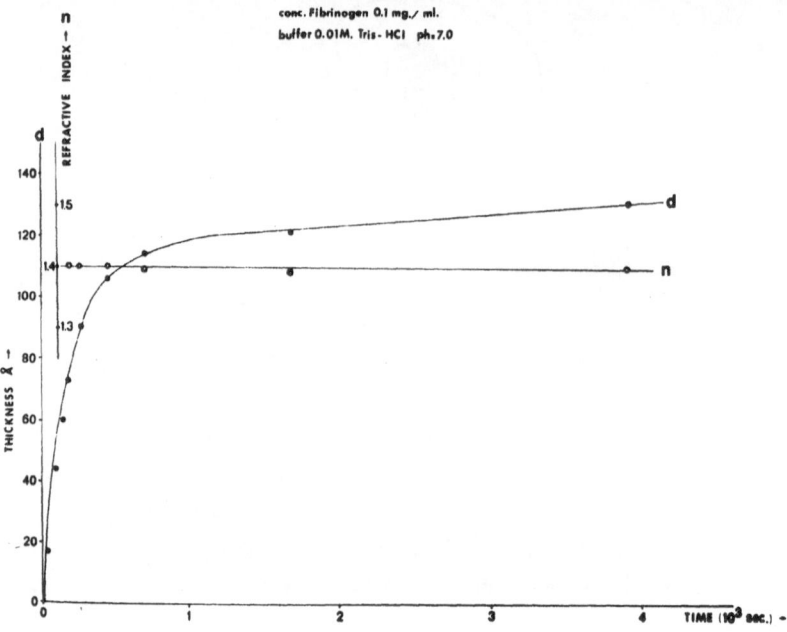

Fig. 2 a.

Figs. 2 a and 2 b.

a. Behaviour of thickness and refractive index as a function of time
   during the adsorption of fibrinogen (10 μg/ml) in 0.01 M Tris-HCl
   buffer pH 7.0 onto a chromium oxide (hydrophilic) surface.

b. Behaviour of thickness and refractive index as a function of time
   during adsorption of fibrinogen (10 μg/ml) in 0.01 M Tris-HCl
   buffer pH 7.0 onto chromium (hydrophobic) surfaces.

138

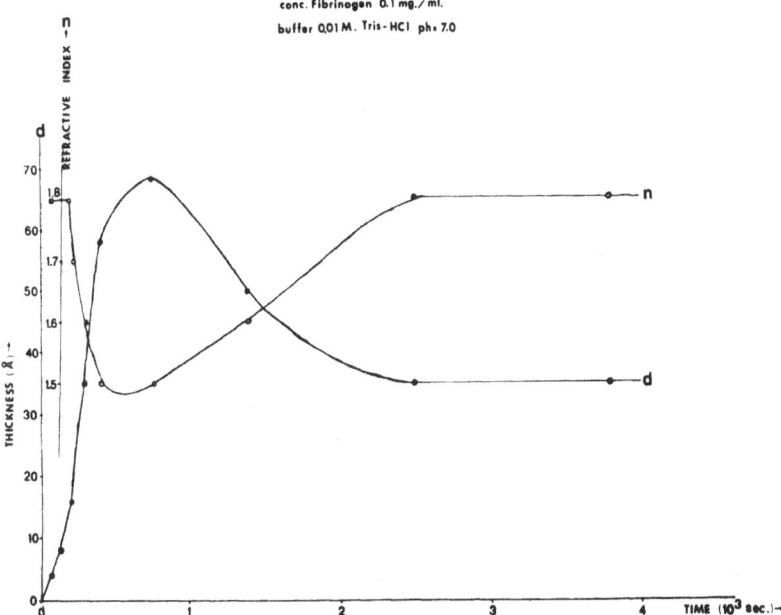

Adsorption of Fibrinogen on a chromium (hydrophobic) surface.

conc. Fibrinogen 0.1 mg./ ml.

buffer 0.01 M. Tris-HCl ph. 7.0

Fig. 2 b.

Adsorption will bring about concentration of selected proteins at the
surface, orientation of these proteins and conformational changes. Each
of these can cause an enhanced reactivity.

VI. REACTION RATES AT INTERFACES

Dealing in a quantitative manner with reaction rates involves
concentrations. Reactions at a surface can take place between two
molecules that are adsorbed or between an adsorbed and a free molecule. In the latter case the adsorbed molecule may be treated as a
molecule in solution with different properties. Modifications of the
reaction rates can occur because of orientation effects, conformational changes of the molecules and the presence of an unstirred layer
near the surface. Yet the reaction rate will be proportional to the
mean density of the reacting molecules per unit volume, i.e. the concentration.

When the reaction takes place between adsorbed molecules the density
per unit surface enters as a factor in the reaction rates rather

139

than the concentration.

The fundamental formula for any reaction rate constant:

$$k = Z.h.e^{-\alpha/RT}$$

where k = reaction constant, i.e. reaction velocity at unit amounts
of the reactants

Z = number of collisions per unit time

h = steric factor, proportion of the collision from which a
reaction may follow if the energetic conditions are favourable

$\alpha$ = activation energy

T = absolute temperature.

Three terms are influenced by adsorption of proteins on a surface.
We will treat each of them in the following paragraphs.
The collision frequency Z is related to two dimensional concentrations.
The steric factor h is influenced by orientation effects whereas the
energetic term can be influenced by conformational changes.

## VII. COLLISIONS AND CONCENTRATION AT A SURFACE (Z)

Concentration as such is a notion that cannot be used when the reactivity of adsorbed proteins is to be regarded. We have to go one step
back in the theory of reaction rates and realise that concentrations
determine rates because they determine the number of collisions per
unit time and because reaction rate is proportional to that number.

When molecules are adsorbed onto a surface the number of molecules
per unit volume no longer directly determines the number of collisions
but rather the number per unit surface.

In physical chemistry the number of collisions in solution between two
molecular species A and B is calculated as $Z_v = \pi . \sqrt{2}\ a.b.\bar{c}\ d^2 N$ (A)
where a, and b are the concentrations (e.g. mol per litre), c is the
mean velocity of the molecules and d is the diameter of the molecules,
assumed to be approximately equal. N is Avogadro's number. An analogous
derivation for molecules moving in a plane gives $Z_p = 2\sqrt{2}\ a^{*}.b\ \bar{c}^{*} dN$ (B)
Here $a^{*}$ is twodimensional concentration, i.e. moles per unit sur-
face, $\bar{c}^{*}$ is the mean lateral velocity. In coagulation the plane of adsorption is added as a suspension of phospholipid vesicles.

140

Dependant upon the type of preparation, i.e. size of vesicles and
nature of the phospholipids there will be a specific value S for the
surface added per mole of  phospholipid and the surface present will
be f.S. (f = concentration of phospholipid). When all A and B is adsorbed to the phospholipid water interface (upper limit possibility) a concentration a in solution means a concentration $\frac{a}{f.S.}$  in the plane of
the interface. Hence $Z_p$ in terms of bulk concentration  becomes

$A_p = 2. \frac{a.b.}{f.S} \bar{c}^* dN$. The ratio $R = Z_p/Z_v$  is the ratio of collision frequencies in absence or in presence of a surface.

$$R = 2/\pi .d^{-1} . \bar{c}^*/\bar{c} .f^{-1}s^{-1}$$

The proportion $\bar{c}^*/\bar{c}$  can be estimated from the diffusion constants
of proteins in free solution (D) and at a surface ($D^*$) as c is proportional to $\sqrt{D}$. It turns out to be between 0.2 and 0.01 (16-19).

S can be calculated to be about $2,5 .10^3$ $cm^2$ from the value of Avogadro's
number and a surface area of about 60 Å  for a phospholipid molecule in
an ordered layer. At phospholipid concentrations of 10 - 100  μM  R
can              be between $10^3$  and $10^4$ . Therefore enrichment of
the concentration of reacting molecules at the surface as such can be
held responsible for the catalytic effect of a phospholipid surface.

VIII. ORIENTATION AND STERIC EFFECTS (h)

Only a small part of the surface of a protein is occupied by its
reactive site. From the fact that pentapeptides can be relatively specific for a given coagulation factor (20,21) it can be inferred that
about the size of a pentapeptide will be a reasonable guess for the
size of the reactive locus on a clotting factor. This will be a surface
of some 50-100 $Å^2$. If we assume clotting factors II and X to be globular,
a radius of   about 40 Å corresponds to their molecular weight. This
means a surface of about 20000 Å. This means that about 2% of the surface is occupied by active or vulnerable sites so that in only 4 in $10^{-6}$
of the possible collisions these sites will meet. When the molecules
are non spherical this will hardly affect the size of the reactive
sites but the total surface will be larger than in a sphere and the
situation will be even less favourable.

Now when two proteins are adsorbed at a surface it is necessary for them to be reactive to retain a lateral mobility. Due to this mobility they can collide, but only at their broadest circumference. For being reactive in the adsorbed state the reactive sites of these molecules have to be located at that circumference. With the sizes quoted above, about 4% of the circumference will belong to the reactive site and the fraction of favourable collisions will be about $20 \times 10^{-4}$, i.e. about 50 times higher than with free molecules. When the molecules are not spherical but oblate they probably will adsorb with their long axis normal to the surface (22) and the circumference will be smaller than in a sphere. Hence the estimate of about 50 x obtained above must be regarded as a lower limit.

IX. CONFORMATIONAL CHANGE

Catalytic and vulnerable properties of proteins are completely dependent upon their tertiary structure. Adsorption anyhow will lead to                    distorsions. Hence, to hold conformational changes responsible for changes in catalytic properties is as easy as it is cheap. It will explain anything and is not easily put to an experimental test. In three cases it seems to be at the basis of fundamental phenomena though.

a. At present it is thought that factor XII adsorbs onto a surface and thereby becomes vulnerable to the action of kallikrein (23).

b. The interaction between prothrombin and staphylocoagulase gives rise to thrombin activity without changes in primary structure (24).

c. The adsorption of fibrinogen makes surfaces apt for adsorption of platelets, but denaturation (i.e. changes in tertiary structure) of fibrinogen (cf. fig. 2) brings about a change that prevents sticking of platelets.

It is hard to conceive that adsorption of proteins will to any marked extent strain vulnerable bonds and in that way cause bond breaking. For this to occur the number of degrees of freedom in a protein is too high. For that same reason it can be safely assumed that immobilization of a protein molecule although at first sight possibly equivalent to a drop in temperature will as such not necessarily decrease reaction rates. The cause for altered reactivity of adsorbed proteins rather is to be found in a favourable change in the tertiary structure and hence in the pattern of secundary binding sites between the reacting proteins.

## X. SPECIAL FEATURES OF THE PROTHROMBINASE COMPLEX

Thus far we discussed general ideas on interactions of proteins at interfaces on experience obtained with the prothrombinase complex. We are far from understanding completely the mechanistic role of proteins and phospholipids in this complex. Yet several features recently exposed in our lab may be as many examples of the behaviour of proteins at surfaces and merit attention.

a. Fluidity of the phospholipids

It has been suggested by Barton ( 25) and it has lately been demonstrated by Tans et al. (26) that the fluidity of the phospholipid is of prime importance in determining its efficacity as a support for the proteins. Mixtures of pure synthetic phospholipids are much more active at temperatures above the phase transition than below. The precise reason for this effect is still obscure. It may be related to the fact that factor V is bound to the surface by a hydrophobic bond and will be more mobile in a fluid membrane. The lateral mobility of factor II and $X_a$ that bind via electrostatic interactions to the interface may be dependent on the lateral mobility of the phospholipid to which they are bound.

b. Necessity of binding to the phospholipid

Factors II and X are vitamin K dependent. Vitamin K serves to carboxylate several glutamic acid residues in one region of these proteins. The $\gamma$-COOH-glutamic acid residues so created bind $Ca^{++}$ ions and via these ions bind to negatively charged phospholipid residues.

In vitamin K deficient men or cows the factors II and X (as well as VII and IX) are not carboxylated and circulate in their decarboxyforms. They can be isolated and serve as models for molecules that have all the features of the normal molecules but are unable to bind to    surfaces.When decarboxyfactor II is presented to a normal prothrombinase, it will be slowly converted but still appreciably quicker than without phospholipid (27). This indicates that bonds between factors V and/or $X_a$ and factor II contribute essentially to the function of the complex and maybe  also the

orienting effect of the phospholipids on the binding factors may play
a role.

The catalytic activity of decarboxyfactor $X_a$ towards normal prothrombin is not enhanced by the presence of factor V and phospholipid (22).

c. Fixation of intermediates

Decarboxyfactor $X_a$ and normal factor $X_a$ have an equal activity towards
small substrates (28). Towards prothrombin they both have a much smaller activity. With phospholipid and factor V the activity of normal
factor $X_a$, but not that of decarboxyfactor $X_a$, is brought to the
level of turnover of small substrates (14). This may mean that in the
normal complex the two bonds that have to be cleft in prothrombin are
attacked without the substrate dissociating from the enzyme whereas
factor $X_a$ in solution attacks one or the other of the bonds, then
looses the products and only seldomly finds them back to convert them
into thrombin. Schematically (E = enzyme, i.e. factor $X_a$ ($E_1$) or
complete prothrombin ($E_2$); P = product, i.e. prethrombin 2 ($P_1$) or
thrombin ($P_2$); S = substrate i.e. prothrombin) for complete prothrombin-
ase(i.e. at the surface):

$$S + E_2 \rightleftharpoons SE_2 \rightarrow P_1E_2 \rightarrow P_2E_2 \rightleftharpoons P_2 + E_2$$

for free factor $X_a$

$$S + E_1 \rightleftharpoons SE_1 \rightarrow E_1 + P_1$$

$$P_1 + E_1 \rightleftharpoons P_1E_1 \rightarrow E_1 + P_2$$

CONCLUSION

It is impossible at the moment to give a detailed account of the
precise mechanistic role of surfaces in the mechanism of blood
coagulation but the broad lines can be delineated. They can not
serve, however, as a general guideline for the design of non-
thrombogenic surfaces in artificial organs. There seems to be no other
way open in this field then first to screen for relatively harm-
less surfaces and then to study in detail thrombotic reactions occurring
at that surface to see if they may be specifically prevented.

It may be doubted, however, if coagulation as such plays a large role in the thrombogenicity of artificial surfaces. The specific requirements of a phospholipid surface will not be easily met by plastics etc.

On the other hand, there are surfaces that will hardly give any contact activation (steel, Teflon etc.) but that are not exquisitely non-thrombogenic. The first reactions of importance may be those of blood proteins and formed elements creating situations in which thrombin formation can start and, by its interaction with blood platelets, give rise to the self propagating interactions that end up in thrombi.

Footnote

The nomenclature of blood clotting factors is according to the recommendation of the International Committee on Hemostasis and Thrombosis. In schemes etc. a roman numeral indicates the corresponding factor. The subscript a indicates the activated factor.

REFERENCES

1. Macfarlane, R.G. An enzyme cascade in blood coagulation. Nature 202 (1964) 498-499

2. Hemker, H.C., P.W.Hemker. The kinetics of enzyme cascades. Proc. Roy.Soc. B. 173 (1969) 411-420

3. Hemker,H.C., H.L.L.Frank. Paratopic interaction, a mechanism in the generation of structure bound enzymatic activity. Experientia 33 (1977) 851-852

4. Nossel, H.L. (1969) The contact phase of blood coagulation. In Recent Advances in Blood Coagulation. Ed. L.Poller. Churchill, London, 60

5. Bangham, A.D.A. A correlation between surface charge and coagulant action of phospholipids. Nature 192 (1961) 1197-1198

6. Suttie, J.W., C.M.Jackson. Prothrombin structure, activation and biosynthesis. Physiol.Rev. 57 (1977) 1-70

7. Guillin, M.C., A.Bezeaud, D.Ménaché. The mechanism of activation of human prothrombin by an activator isolated from dispholidus typus venom. Biochim.Biophys.Acta 537 (1978) 160-168

8. Papahadjopoulos, D., C.Hougie, D.J.Hanahan. Influence of surface charge of phospholipids on their clot-promoting activity. Proc.Soc. Exptl.Biol.Med. 111 (1962) 412-416

9. Papahadjopoulos, D., D.J.Hanahan. Observations on the interaction of phospholipids and certain clotting factors in prothrombin activator formation. Biochim.Biophys.Acta 90 (1964) 436-439

10. Hemker,H.C., M.J.P.Kahn, P.P.Devilee. The adsorption of coagulation factors onto phospholipids; its role in the reaction mechanism of blood coagulation. Thrombos.Diathes.haemorrh. 24 (1970) 214-223

11. Jobin, F., M.P.Esnouf. Studies on the formation of the prothrombin converting complex. Biochem.J. 102 (1967) 666-674

12. Hemker, H.C., M.P.Esnouf, P.W.Hemker, A.C.W.Swart, R.G.Marfarlane. Kinetics of the formation of prothrombin converting activity in a purified system. Nature 215 (1967) 248-251

13. Barton, P.G., C.M.Jackson, D.J.Hanahan. Relationship between factor V and activated factor X in the generation of prothrombinase. Nature 214 (1967) 923-924

14. Rosing, J., G.Tans, J.W.P.Govers-Riemslag, R.F.A.Zwaal, H.C.Hemker The role of phospholipids and factor $V_a$ in the prothrombinase

complex. Submitted for publication.

15. Cuypers, P.A., W.Th.Hermens, H.C.Hemker. Ellipsometry as a tool to study protein films at liquid-solid interfaces. Anal.Bioch. 84 (1978) 56-67

16. Van Holde, K.E. Physical Biochemistry. Prentice-Hall, Int. London 1971

17. Edidin, M., Y.Zagyansky, T.J.Lardner. Measurement of membrane protein lateral diffusion in single cells. Science 191 (1976) 466-468

18. Poo, M.M., R.A.Cone. Lateral diffusion of rhodopsin in the photo-receptor membrane. Nature 247 (1974) 438-441

19. Smith, B.A., H.M.McConnell. Determination of molecular motion in membranes using periodic pattern photobleaching. Proc.Natl.Acad. Sci.USA 75 (1978) 2759-2763

20. All articles in Haemostasis 7 (1978) 61-183

21. I.Witt, Ed. New methods for the analysis of coagulation using chromogenic substrates. W. de Gruyter, Berlin, New York, 1979

22. Lindhout, M.J. Personal communication.

23. Bouma, B.M. Personal communication.

24. Hemker, H.C., B.M.Bas, A.D.Muller. Activation of a proenzyme by a stoichiometric reaction with another protein; the reaction between prothrombin and staphylocoagulase. Biochim.Biophys.Acta 379 (1975) 180-188

25. Barton, P., E.J.Findlay. The lipid phase separation model for prothrombin activation. In The significant platelet function tests in the evaluation of hemostatic and thrombosis tendencies. Day, H.J., M.B.Zucker and H.Holmsen, Eds. (1977) U.S. Natl.Inst.Health, Bethesda, Md. 461-470

26. Tans, G., H.v.Zutphen, P.Comfurius, H.C.Hemker, R.F.A.Zwaal. Lipid phase transitions and procoagulant activity. Accepted for publication in Eur.J. Biochem. 1979

27. Vermeer, C., J.W.P.Govers-Riemslag, B.A.M.Soute, M.J.Lindhout, J.Kop, H.C.Hemker. The role of blood clotting factor V in the conversion of prothrombin and a decarboxyprothrombin into thrombin. Biochim.Biophys.Acta 538 (1978) 521-533

28. Lindhout, M.J., B.H.M.Kop-Klaassen, H.C.Hemker. The effect of $\gamma$-carboxyglutamate residues on the enzymatic properties of the

147

activated blood clotting factor X. I. Activity towards synthetic substrates. Biochim.Biophys.Acta 533 (1978) 342-354.

Moderator: Wenzel

Wenzel:                   We have got now some basic knowledge on platelet
                          and cell damage during ECC and in addition, after
                          information on platelet and red cell damage
                          Dr. Hemker gave important facts on contact acti-
                          vation and plasmatic coagulation. This is a real
                          challenge for discussion in order to build up a
                          bridge between clinical and experimental facts.

                          So I would like to open now the discussion on this
                          paper. Are there questions?

Feijen:                   I would like to ask a question to Dr. Hemker about
                          the deposition of the phospholipids. When we have
                          coagulation of plasma in a tube we frequently ob-
                          serve that the thrombus or the clot is growing at
                          the surface. So can we imagine that we have the
                          active complex of $X_a$ on the surface with a
                          bridge of a phospholipid on it

                              or do we have only to look into the solution
                          for phospholipids? If phospholipids are present
                          on the surface, then I have a next question: Could
                          Dr. Hemker comment on the conformation of the
                          phospholipids on the surface and, more specifi-
                          cally, on the position of the phosphate groups?
                          Will you compare hydrophobic with hydrophilic
                          surfaces and in this way make prediction on the
                          influence of hydrophobicity of the surface on
                          *clotting times*?

Hemker:                   The water-air interface of course is well known
                          as a hydrophobic surface and phospholipids will
                          tend to float to that surface and orient with
                          their fatty acid tails upwards and their polar
                          heads downwards. So, in principle, I think, it is
                          very well possible that coagulation occurs at
                          that surface. But on the other hand, if you re-
                          move the lipopreteins very carefully from the

                                                                    149

plasma it will not clot at all. So I think that phospholipids present in the lipoproteins will by far outnumber the phospholipids at the plasma-air interface.

Feijen:          Still one question is not, I think, completely answered. When we have artificial hydrophilic surfaces I can imagine that the charged groups of phospholipids are more directed to the surface as compared with hydrophobic surfaces. And then the possibilities of attachement via calcium bridges to the glutamic acid residues of factor X will become less.

Hemker:          As far as I can see from our experiments with an ellipsometer in which we measure the deposit onto hydrophilic and hydrophobic interfaces from plasma or from protein solutions or from phospholipid solutions, it is very hard to get any phospholipids on to a surface. *I do not think* that the interaction of free phospholipid molecules with a hydrophilic or a hydrophobic surface will be of any importance at all in plasma because of the low concentrations of phospholipids present and the heavy competition with the abundant proteins.

Schmid-Schönbein:   This presentation is worth millions of any currency which will be saved if the people involved in designing non-thrombogenic polymer surfaces take notice of your work. I do not think that we can say at the moment that either platelets or fibrinogen which we measure at a specific surface site are actually originating there; and I think your approach to this whole area of coagulation enzymology, the investigation of physico-chemical interactions not only brings to light many biological phenomena of great significance, but will lead the problems bothering the design of biocompatible polymers into an entirely new perspective. And anybody who has read literature on biopolymers will know that this technology is conceptually in a crisis. Nobody knows whether or not fibrinogen, when it is coated on a surface has any advantage or disadvantage. Would you suggest that the formation of phospholipid fragments from destroyed cells, from leukocytes, red cells or most of all from platelets which are so easily destroyed, could act as an additional nucleus for the sequence of events that you have shown to produce active thrombin? Could thrombin, in turn, produce fibrinogen oligomers with low solubility which have a high tendency to attach themselves to any surface they can find, for example biopolymer surfaces? In other words, do you think that it is possible that the whole argument went wrong so far? Could it not be that the active deposition is already an end-stage rather than the beginning of fibrin-formation (which, of course, later triggers new deposition)?

Hemker:                          I think this might very well be possible and I had a question in that vein regarding your own presentation and that is: Do you know what happens to the erythrocyte ghosts and to the membranes that must arise during hemolysis? I am asking this because Zwaal from our laboratory has shown that both for platelets and erythrocytes the outside of the membrane in non-active as a support for coagulation reactions, whereas the inside is active. So when the ghosts turn inside out they set free something that would be measured as platelet factor- 3 -activity. And quantitatively more I think the platelets can do that. The platelets do have their own phospholipid flip-flop from inside-outside, but that must occur in a relatively late state of thrombus formation. I do know that platelet factor- 3 -release or availability has been shown in an early stage, but when you carefully correct for the amount of lysis of pla-

151

telets, then you will find that tiny amounts of lysis will already give rise to much apparent platelet factor- 3 -activity.

Schmid-Schönbein: To answer your question directly: No, we have not looked at the ghosts as yet but we will certainly do that. But I would like to report another little experiment which we do in the labcourse where coagulation is taught according to Dr. Hemker and we produce a very simple but very convincing experiment, by comparing the coagulation time in glass tubes of platelet-rich, platelet-poor and platelet-free plasma (the latter we filter carefully through millipore-filters). While the thrombin times and prothrombin times in these three systems are not significantly different, the recalcification times are so much different that a platelet-free plasma in glass will often not clot during two and a half hours. This shows that even the most aggressive surface without the presence of phospholipids is non-thrombogenic.

Feijen: Of course, it is in the later stages that the presence of phospholipids is important, but in the beginning, I think, we have the activation of factor XII and the point is that an aggressive surface can activate factor XII. Of course, in combination with the presence of phospholipids we see the final result in the formation of a thrombus. So I think we can distinguish between aggressive surfaces and non-aggressive surfaces also with respect to this phenomenon.

Schmid-Schönbein: Could we possibly concentrate a bit on contact activation and on the contact product? Is it essential in all types of coagulation? How can we explain the coagulation experiments in platelet-free plasma, where, as I would have guessed, a glass activation occurs but no coagulation in the absence of phospholipids? A "contact product" may

152

be a prestage, but it is by no means proved in
my opinion that the presence of contact products
must lead to coagulation.

Hemker: As you said, contact products can initiate coagulation. Of course, it will not initiate coagulation when you make impossible one of the lower
steps and whether it is physiologically important
I very much doubt, because anyhow the reactions
of the extrinsic pathway (that is factor VII and
phospholipids from damaged cells) are much quicker.

It is well-known for instance that leukocytes
do contain large amounts of tissue factor which
can bring about coagulation bypassing the activity of factor XII. Also, when factor XII does not
get a chance to start the coagulation reaction,
XIIa and XIa will be inactivated relatively quickly in the plasma.There is another aspect I should
like to stress. Rather than to prevent activation
of coagulation factors you should try to get a
kind of steady state in which a treshold of coagulation is just not surpassed. It may well be
impossible to prevent activation of coagulation
altogether. Clinicians very well know that because by adding heparin they do not prevent the
coagulation mechanism at all. They just increase
the removal of the activated products like thrombin and factor Xa or XIa.

Deggeler: I remember well, a patient lacking factor XII,
a Hageman-patient, is not known as a bleeder, but
can only be identified as such by coagulation
studies in vitro; perhaps Dr. Hemker can tell
more about it.

Hemker: This is completely true and I can even add to the
folklore at this point by saying that Mister Hageman himself died of a thrombosis.

Feijen: May I make one more comment? I think in the situations which we are looking at, we would like

153

to diminish the amount of heparin that we are using. Furthermore, we have availability of phospholipids and I think contact activation of factor XII will be an important factor for distinguishing between surfaces. I agree that factor XI can also be activated on platelet membranes, as we all know in the presence of ADP. So if we have damage to platelets we can have activation of the intrinsic coagulation mechanism without the interference of surfaces.

Hemker:

I just would like to add a brief remark and that is that the most interesting patients from the biochemical and physiological point of view may be dead. I have two examples. The most interesting subject concerning prevention of thrombosis at this moment is to get a clear insight in the antithrombotic properties of the blood. Now there are no complete deficiencies of antithrombin III known presumably because they die before they are born. The only patients we have are those with 50 % of antithrombin III. I always hesitate to answer questions of the kind of: "How is it that a factor XII deficiency does not bleed while a factor VIII deficiency does bleed", or "factor VII can be of no physiological significance at all". We actually should be aware of the fact that the amount of clotting factors we have circulating is in a tremendous excess. When you express the concentration in terms of times $K_m$ (that is maximal reaction velocity) we find $K_m$ at around 2 %. So we have a tremendous excess of clotting factors of around 50 $K_m$. We also determined the residual activity in a number of factor VII deficient patients and the $K_m$ in their plasma. Then you very clearly find two groups of factor VII deficient patients. First, those with a residual amount of about 2 % and a $K_m$ of around 1 %. These still have

154

an excess of factor VII. But there also is
another group, those with a $K_m$ of 2 % and a residual amount of $^1/2$ %. These are really deficient. Now these patients are very hard to find
and mostly very young. They come from families
with a high death rate of new borns because of
bleeding complications shortly after birth. We
must conclude that the population of patients we
are looking to in medical practice are only those
that survived with their handicap for some reason
that we very often do not know.

Wenzel:        Thank you very much: there is one more question.
You spoke of activities, but I think, we should
specify what kind of an activity we really mean.
Is it an activity in coagulation or is it an activity to split off a fibrinopeptide A or B or is
it an amidolytic activity or an esterolytic activity? Now my question to you is in detail: Is
there a difference of activities bound, e.g. to
proteins or streaming in the liquid?

                         The second question in
addition to that: if you have one system using one
signal (e.g. aminolytic) for measurements what
is the effect of physiological inhibitors on the
so measured activity?

Hemker:        To answer your last question first: There have
been experiments from Marciniak and from others
that show that as long as a coagulation factor is
adsorbed in an active complex it is immune to
the action of antithrombin III. Then you asked if
there is a difference in activity between ab-
sorbed factors and non-absorbed factors. There
is, of course, a big difference in the magnitude
of the activity, that will be clear to you. You
may also ask if there is a qualitative difference
towards different substrates and as far as our

experiments go we did not find that. I do know that it has been published that the activity of a factor adsorbed onto an artificial substrate might be higher but when you read this article carefully you may find out that there are trivial reasons to explain this finding. As far as I know absorption does not influence the properties of the active center of the enzyme.

Birnbaum: In our patients on extracorporeal circulation there are facts which I wonder how they could fit into your way of regarding the problem. It is a fact that protein solutions like albumin solutions, gammaglobulin solutions, even solutions with factor XII or fibrinogen show adhesion to all known material with the exception of the amicon material which obviously is a very exciting new material for extracorporeal devices. How can we understand this fact in the light of your views on thrombogenesis?

Hemker: I am not sure to give a very good answer to this. To quote Leo Vroman who studied proteins at interfaces quite a lot "any protein will get anywhere unless another protein will get there first". An interesting fact is that for some rare proteins like Hageman factor the adsorption is part of their physiological function, but we may doubt if the adsorption that we find onto any artificial or natural surface does serve any function. Plasma coats any surface with a layer of more or less denatured proteins. Those that get there will be the most abundant proteins like albumin, gammaglobulin and fibrinogen. After that there may be a reaction of some very specific system in the blood, like platelets that adhere to fibrin coated surfaces when the fibrin is in its native and not in its denatured form. So, after the coating with the proteins a specific,

156

more or less physiological phenomenon may start playing a role. You cannot prevent the proteins from acting physically and very quickly as soon as a surface is offered.

Schmid-Schönbein: Mayby , I can answer Dr. Birnbaum's questions. But I am not sure. I can vizualize how surgeons, experimentalists and bio-engineers studying artificial organs got together and saw a clot on a surface and they interpreted it by what was written in the physiology textbooks. They were "brain-washed" by a misquotation of a very famous medical dogma which says that stasis is a prerequisite for *all* coagulation. Virchow's trias is formulated as part of the paper on "Thrombose und Embolie". Now, if one reads Virchow's original paper it becomes evident that Virchow clearly excluded from his pathogenetic theory all thrombotic event which take place in arteries. In other words, thrombotic events that occur in the presence of flow. Despite of Virchow's warning, the medical public is "brain-washed" into the idea that a clot found on the wall has been formed there, and that stasis was the fluid-dynamic condition that caused it. I have not found any direct evidence that the majority of clots one finds in artificial organs (including artificial oxygenators) are actually originating at the site where they are found.

Feijen: If we adsorb for instance fibrinogen on hydrophobic surfaces and compare this with fibrinogen on hydrophilic surfaces the same fibrinogen may have a different conformation and may interact in different ways with platelets and other cells. This experiment has not been done in the moment. We have some evidence that on hydrophilic surfaces the adsorption is more reversible, so this might be an indication for minor conformational changes.

157

Hemker:      I will not go into too many technical details of
our experiments with the ellipsometer. The ellipsometer is an apparatus in which you can determine the thickness and refractive index of very
thin layers down to the Angstrom range. So with
this instrument you can see what mono-molecular
layers are adsorbed onto surfaces from various
solutions. I completely agree with Dr. Feijen
when he says that the adsorption is not only
determined by the species of molecules. It also
depends upon the kind of interaction. When in one
experiment you adsorb fibrinogen onto a hydrophilic surface, you see that it will grow until
a mono-molecular layer is adsorbed with the
thickness of a fibrinogen molecule and a refractive index that remains constant and equal to
the refractive index of a hydrated protein molecule. When you do the same experiments with a
hydrophobic surface you will see that the thickness of the layer will grow and then decrease
again, to a value which is smaller than the diameter of the hydrated fibrinogen molecule whereas the refractive index goes up. This means that
on a hydrophobic surface the molecule is dehydra-
ted and spreads out, whereas on a hydrophilic
surface it is more or less in the configuration
it also has in solution. This may serve to illus-
trate that fibrinogen or any other molecule that
adsorbes may change its physical and chemical
properties. Now from experiments of Vroman it is
known that platelets will stick to native fibrinogen and not to transformed fibrinogen.

158

# 8. Blood trauma and Hypercoagulability produced by extracorporeal circulation

E. Wenzel, I. Volkmer, E. Laux, H.G. Limbach, M. Mierendorf, M.Müller, E. Saavedra, H. Monadjemi, O. Thetter, M. Morgenstern, G. Dhom, U. Rietkötter, B. Otte, G. Harbauer, L. Svendsen, H. Holzhüter, B. Angelkort

Department for Clinical Haemostaseology and Transfusion Medicine, Department for Cardiac and Vascular Surgery and Department for Surgical Research , FB 4/3, Inst.for Pathology, FB 3/4, Inst. for Med. Biology, University of the Saarland, Homburg-Saar, and II. Med. Department, Technical Highschool Aachen.

## 1. Introduction

Vinazzer (1969) and Deutsch (1973) have established that various degrees of disseminated intravascular coagulation and fibrinolysis syndrom (DICFS, Bowie 1971) occur during surgical interventions. In addition to these operative stresses, the blood is traumatised, when it comes into contact with blood foreign surfaces (Salzmann 1971). Moreover, when extracorporeal circulation is used (Bachmann 1975), the flow also has a traumatizing effect on the blood (Salzmann 1971). Therefore the hemostatic and metabolic equilibrium of patients is especially stressed during open heart surgery (Gans 1967).

In particular, we will outline our findings which have indicated hypercoagulability and damages occuring in human and in canine blood corpuscles during extracorporeal circulation. Prof. Dr. Schmidt-Schönbein who has done a very nice job in organizing this work-shop, requested that I also inform you of the results of the in vitro experiments completed earlier, when we used an enclosed devise for artificial blood circulation, a so called "Hydropulsator". This work was done in Aachen in cooperation with the Aerodyn. Institute of the TH (Prof. Dr. Nauman, Dr. Lambert and Prof. Dr. Kramer . S.C. Kramer,1973).

## 2. Methods and special in vitro experiments

### 2.1. Blood coagulation tests, hematological investigations, biochemical methods

Principle, method, interpretation etc. (s. table 1).

### 2.2.1. Platelet counts and volume distribution of platelets

Platelet counts were figured by a model ZB1 Coulter Counter

159

Table 1:

Blood coagulation tests, hematological investigations and
biochemical methods

| | |
|---|---|
| Prothrombin time, PTT,<br>Fibrinogen, Bleeding time etc. | Vinazzer, H.: Gerinnungsstörungen<br>in der Praxis. G. Fischer, Stuttg.<br>1972 |
| Recalcification time<br>0.02 M Calcium chloride | Owen, CA J. et al.<br>Amer.J.Clin.Path.25,1417,1955 |
| Thrombin T./Reptilase-/<br>Thrombincoagulase T. | Wenzel, E. et al.<br>DMW 99, 746, 1974 |
| Fibrin or Fibrinogen<br>Split Products | Mayo Clinic Laborat., Manual of<br>Hemostasis. Sounders Philadelphia-<br>London-Toronto 1971 |
| Stypven time PL-F 3 | Mac Farlane, Brit.J.Hemat.7,496,<br>1961 |
| Platelet factor 4 | Deutsch, E. et al., TDH 1, 397,<br>1957 modif. |
| Hemoglobin in Plasma (1)<br>LDH (2)<br>Glucose-6 P-D | 1. Meyer-Berthenrath (1975 )<br>2. G. Ceriotti*<br>3. W. Schröter*<br><br>*s. Clinical Biochemistry.<br>Principle and Methods.<br>H. Curtius, M. Roth.<br>De Gruyter Berlin 1974 |

Fig. 1: Coulter Counter Channelyser Computer equipment for measuring
the volume distribution of platelets (printout s.fig.3).

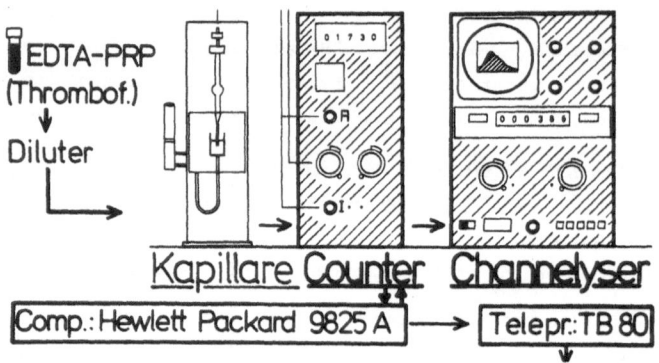

fitted with a 50 μ orifice tube. Isoton (Coulter Electronics Ltd.) was used as the diluting fluid and was dispensed from a Zepette to produce minimal agitation. Platelet rich plasma was centrifuged in a Thrombofuge (Coulter Electronics Ltd.)(s.fig.1) The best settings were found to be gain trim 10,matching switch 3, aperture 1/2, amplification 1/4, window 100, base channel threshold 0. The ZB1 Coulter was hooked up to a Channelyser (s.fig.1) and a Hewlett Packard computer (9825). Example for the outprint of data and normal values s.fig.2,3.

### 2.2.2. Studies on aggregation and adhesion of platelets using the Coulter Counter Channelyser equipment

0.5 ml citrated platelet rich plasma which was rotated in an ELVI aggregometer, Collagen was added to a final concentration in plasma of 0.25 μg/ml. The volume distribution of the unaggregated recirculating thrombocytes was measured. Corresponding to the decrease in platelet count and to the increase in transmission (Wenzel 1978), the plotted graphs indicate an extreme shift of mean platelet volume from 7.5 $\mu^3$ to approximately 3.5 $\mu^3$. The spontaneous aggregability of platelets using the method of Breddin (s.fig.4) was measured in the same way.

### 2.3. Amidolytic measurement of serin proteases using chromogenic substrates

Substrates, principle and methods s. tables 2,3,4.

### 2.4. The effect of extracorporeal circulation on platelets from experiments performed on the dog

In 12 dogs (X = 25 kg, S = 3.7 kg; 500 mg Trapanal i.v., Halothan 0.8 - 1.2 vol.%, laughing gas-oxygen mixture 2:1, heart-lung-machine, Weißhaar, München, using a Rygg-Kyvsgaard-Bubble-Oxygenator), extracorporeal circulation lasted for 120'. The dog was heparinized (3 mg/kg/bodyweight, 15 mg Heparin/500 ml Oxygenator volume and 1/3 of the initial dosis/h). The Oxygenator was filled with Ringer lactate and 5 % Glucose. The operation was performed in milde Hypothermia (30° body temperature). 90 minutes after the extracorporeal circulation was started, the animal was rewarmed. 30 minutes later, the heart-lung-machine was stopped, and Protamin chloride was administered in doses equivalent to the doses of Heparin (1 mg Heparin = 1 mg Protamin chloride). 60 minutes later,

161

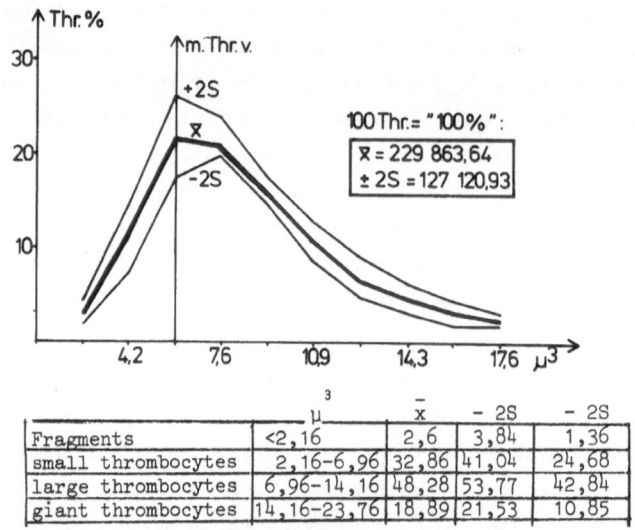

| $\mu^3$ | | $\bar{x}$ | $-2S$ | $-2S$ |
|---|---|---|---|---|
| Fragments | <2,16 | 2,6 | 3,84 | 1,36 |
| small thrombocytes | 2,16-6,96 | 32,86 | 41,04 | 24,68 |
| large thrombocytes | 6,96-14,16 | 48,28 | 53,77 | 42,84 |
| giant thrombocytes | 14,16-23,76 | 18,89 | 21,53 | 10,85 |

<u>Fig. 2:</u> Normal values for volume distribution (out of 177 volunteers, 43 were eliminated because of significant abnormal volume distribution caused by fat-liver). Studies of the stability of a 'thrombotrol' specimen (precision of the method controlled on 16 different days, s. left side of the fig.).

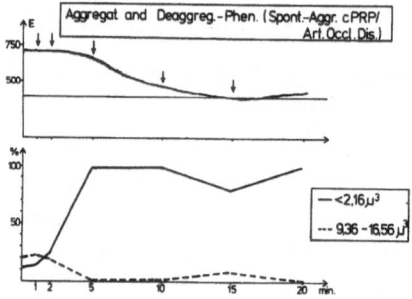

<u>Fig. 4:</u> Aggregation **and** deaggregation phenomenon in a spontaneous aggregating plasma from a patient with arterial occlusive disease. Above the increase in transmission is demonstrated, the graph below demonstrates the increase of small particles during aggregation and their decrease during deaggregation phenomenon.

162

Thrombocyte-Laboratory
Division of Clinical Hematology
University of Homburg/Saar


Determination of volume distribution of the thrombocytes in the
sample gave the following results:

Thrombocyte count:           225000
Sum of particles counted:    32285

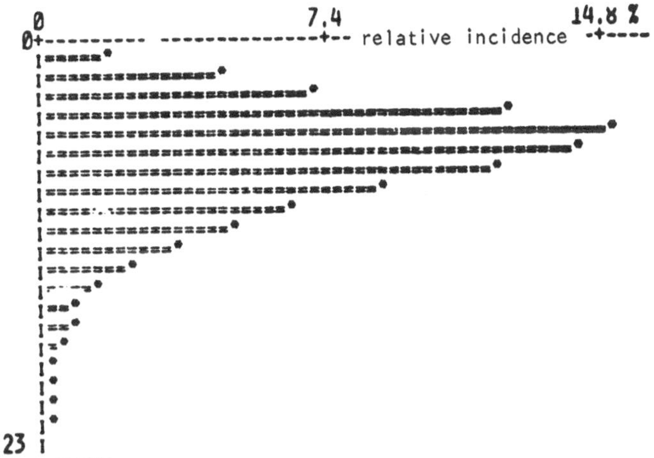

```
    0                7.4                        14.8 %
  0+--------- --------------+-- relative incidence -+----
   |=====•
   |=============•
   |==================•
   |==========================•
   |=================================•
   |==============================•
   |=======================•
   |===========•
   |=======•
   |=======•
   |==•
   |==•
   |=•
   |•
   |•
   |•
 23|•
```
Size CBMUE

| Mean Size | Normal value | % value | absolute value |
|-----------|-------------|---------|----------------|
| 2.16  | 2.6  | 6.9  | 2232.0 |
| 4.56  | 11.9 | 19.6 | 6316.0 |
| 6.96  | 21.8 | 28.9 | 9323.0 |
| 9.36  | 21.5 | 21.0 | 6795.0 |
| 11.76 | 16.2 | 11.8 | 3797.0 |
| 14.16 | 10.6 | 6.0  | 1944.0 |
| 16.56 | 6.7  | 2.7  | 882.0  |
| 18.36 | 4.4  | 1.6  | 532.0  |
| 21.36 | 2.9  | 0.9  | 302.0  |
| 23.76 | 1.9  | 0.5  | 162.0  |

| Evaluation Fragments | Small thromboc. | large thromboc. | Giant thromboc. |
|----------------------|------------------|------------------|------------------|
| 6.9 %  | 48.4 % | 38.8 % | 5.8 %  |
| NORM.:2.6 % | 32.9 % | 48.3 % | 15.9 % |

PEAK-channel                  :             22.0
REL. incidence in peak channel              3.1

Fig. 3: English translation of a computer print out for thrombocyte
        volumetry

| SYNTH. SUBSTRATE | ACTIVITY IN PLASMA | ACTIVITY OF PLASMA INHIBITORS |
|---|---|---|
| CHROMOZYM-TH BOEHRINGER | IIA | ANTITHROMBIN-III ▲ |
| 2224 KABI | XA | |
| S 2444 KABI | UK-LIKE | ANTI-UK (PLATELETS) |
| UK - PENTA * | | |
| PL - PENTA * | PLASM.-LIKE | ANTIPLASMIN ▲ |
| K - PENTA * | "KALLIKR."+ KONTACT-LIKE | - |
| TRY-PENTA * | TRYPSIN-LIKE | ANTITRYPSIN ▲ |

\* PENTAPHARM (SVENDSEN)  ▲ controlled by means of immunological measurem.of A-III/α₂Macro/α₁Antithr.

Tab. 2: Chromogenic substrates and their specificity for measuring serinproteases and their physiological inhibitors (see also tab. 3 and 4).

| SENSITIVITY AGAINST | SYNTHET. PEPTIDES |
|---|---|
| F.II(IIA) | TOS-GLY-PRO-ARG-PNA |
| F X(X A) | Bz-ILE-GLU-GLY-ARG-PNA |
| PLASM.AKTIV. | PYRO-GLU-GLY-ARG-PNA |
| PLASMIN | TOS-GLY-PRO-LYS-PNA |
| KALLIKREIN | Bz-PRO-PHE-ARG-PNA |
| TRYPSIN | H-D-VAL-GLY-ARG-PNA |

Tab. 3: Chemical structure and sequence of amino-acids in the chromo-genic substrates as used for measuring serin-proteases (see tab. 2) and their physiological inhibitors (see tab. 3). Typical differences in the sequence of amino-acids are underlined.

Tab. 4: Test system used to measure the biological functions of inhibitors of serin proteases in the plasma

| Inhibitors: Stand enzyme activity and substrate used for measurement | Principle of Method | Procedure (Kinetic measurement: 5 min., 405 nm) | I U |
|---|---|---|---|
| Antithrombin<br>15 NIH Thrombin<br>ROCHE<br>Substrate:<br>Chr.TH-Boehringer | AT-III + Hep ⟶<br>[AT-III · Hep] [AT-III · Hep]<br>+ Thrombin (excess) ⟶<br>[AT-III · Hep · Thrombin]<br>+ Thrombin | Sample A:<br>0.9 ml Plasm.dilut.(1:2.5)<br>+ 0.1 ml Thrombin(15 NIH)<br>Incubation:<br>5 min.,15 min.,30 min./37°C<br>2 ml buffer+0.25ml sample A<br>+ 0.25 ml substrate | $\frac{\Delta Ext.2260}{117.5}$ = mU Thr. ml<br>% of resid.thromb.activ.at<br>15 min. and at 30 min.<br>(5 min.: 100 %) |
| Antiplasmin<br>1.25 CU Plasmin KABI<br>(in 25 % Glycerol + ATU<br>Hirudin/ml)/<br>Substrate:<br>Chr.Pl-Svendsen | Plasma + Plasmin (excess) ⟶<br>[Plasma · Plasmin] + Plasmin | Plasma sample:<br>0.1 ml Plasmadilut.(1:20)<br>0.020ml Plasminsolut.(1.25CU)<br>90 sec. incubation/37°<br>1.7 ml buffer/0.2 ml substr. | $\frac{\Delta E\ Plin - \Delta E\ Pla \cdot V \cdot 20}{t \cdot V \cdot 10.4}$<br>= CU/ml Plasma<br>Blank:<br>buffer instead of plasma |
| Antitrypsin<br>8 mU Trypsin(Schwein)<br>MERCK<br>Substrate:<br>Chr.Try-Svendsen | Plasma + Trypsin (excess) ⟶<br>[Plasma · Trypsin] + Trypsin | Plasma sample:<br>1.7ml buffer,0.1ml Tryp.sol.<br>0.01 ml Plasmasolut.<br>4 min. incubation/37°<br>0.2 ml substrate | $\frac{\Delta E\ Try - \Delta E\ Pla \cdot t \cdot V \cdot 20}{10 \cdot 4 \cdot d \cdot V}$<br>= mU/ml Plasma<br>Blank:<br>buffer instead of plasma |
| Anti-UK in Platelets<br>500 E UK/ml MEDAC<br>Substrate:<br>Chr.-UK-Svendsen | Plasma + Urokinase (excess) ⟶<br>[Plasma · Urokinase] + Urokinase | Plasma sample:<br>1.6 ml buffer,0.2ml Plasma<br>(500 E UK/ml)<br>5 min. incubation/37°<br>0.2 ml substrate | $\frac{\Delta E\ UK - \Delta E\ Plasma \cdot V}{t \cdot V \cdot 10}$<br>= UKE/ml Plasma<br>Blank:<br>buffer instead of plasma |

165

| | N | | S |
|---|---|---|---|
| Hematocrit "0" | 24 | $\bar{x} = 43$ % | 3.34 % |
| Hematocrit "2-7" | 65 | $\bar{x} = 23-28$ % | 3.13 - 6.41 % |
| pO$_2$ arterial bl. | 81 | $\bar{x} = 168$ % | 52 % |
| " | 7 | $\bar{x} = 219$ % | 150 % |
| SO$_2$ arterial bl. | 91 | $\bar{x} = 96$ % | 4 % |
| SO$_2$ venous bl. | 91 | $\bar{x} = 75$ % | 10.5 % |
| " | | $\bar{x} = 52$ % | 11.3 % |
| pH | 91 | $\bar{x} = 7.40$ | 0.09 |
| pCO$_2$ ("4/5") | 18 | $\bar{x} = 34.0$ | 5.4 |
| " | 17 | $\bar{x} = 37.0$ | 6.5 |
| pCO$_2$ ("6/7") | 19 | $\bar{x} = 33.0$ | 7.8 |
| " | 18 | $\bar{x} = 48.0$ | 8.6 |
| Bicarbonate (H CO$_3$) ("4/5") | 18 | $\bar{x} = 22.0$ | 1,87 |
| | 17 | $\bar{x} = 22.8$ | 3.34 |
| Bicarbonate (H CO$_3$) ("6/7") | 19 | $\bar{x} = 21.6$ | 1.80 |
| | 18 | $\bar{x} = 28.1$ | 4.13 |
| Syst. RR (mmHg) | 91 | $\bar{x} = 169$ | 27.1 |
| | | $\bar{x} = 85$ | 27.2 |
| Diast. RR (mmHg) | 91 | $\bar{x} = 128$ | 27.3 |
| | | $\bar{x} = 85$ | 24.9 |
| Z.V.PR (mmHg) | 91 | $\bar{x} = 7.6$ | 5.5 |

Table 5:

Blood gases, blood pressure etc. in 12 dogs during open heart
operation and extracorporeal circulation. The findings indicate
the limits of standardization of this experiment. The indices
0 - 7 indicate the time, when the controls were performed,
before (0-2), during (3-5) and after extracorporeal circulation
(6-7), when no significant changes were observed; all the results
were summarized.

# Hydropulsator - Apparatus
## (Kaminski - Kramer)

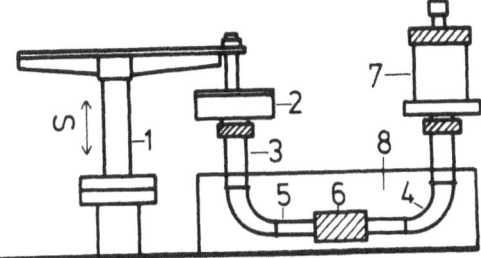

1 Control-Column   5 Measur. Line
2 Membr. Pump      6 Stenosis
3 Ascend. Pipe     7 Container
4  "       "       8 37°C-Bath

Fig. 5: Technical details characterizing the Hydropulsator:

1. Type of movement                        Sinusoscillation

   Frequency                               0.6 Hz

   Length of time of pulsation             0.833 sec.

   Increase in Pressure                    3,000 mm W.S./sec.
   (with a narrowness of 8,6 mm)

   Blood volume in one tube                125 ml

   Circulated volume per test              42 ml

   Diameter of suction pipe (pump)         25 mm

   Diameter of measureline                 14 mm

   Tides                                   85 mm

2. Influence of Stenoses

| | B1 | B2 | B3 | B4 | |
|---|---|---|---|---|---|
| Coefficient of resistance | 0 | 9 | 62 | 340 | |
| Influence of time | A1 | A2 | A3 | A4 | A5 | A6 |

| | | | | | |
|---|---|---|---|---|---|
| Number of pulsations | 50 | 1.000 | 3.000 | 5.000 | 10.000 | 15.000 |

3. Coefficient of resistance ( $\Psi$ ) $= (1 - \frac{A_1}{A_2 \cdot \alpha})^2$

   $A_1$ : Diameter of measureline

   $A_2$ : Diameter of stenoses

   $\alpha$ : "Strahlkontraktionszahl" (relationship between diameter
        of stenoses and rate of flow).

the animal was sacrificed, and several organs were taken for microscopic studies. During the experiment, several parameters of bloodgases were controlled and found to be constant (s.table 5).

2.5. Explanation of the device used to measure bloodtraumatization
     (Hydropulsator, Kaminski-Kramer)

The diagrammatic representation (fig.5) demonstrates the principle of the machine. The technical details can be seen on the graph (s.fig.5).

3. Results

In cooperation with the department of Cardiac and Vascular Surg., we studied 32 patients undergoing open heart surgery for congenital and acquired cardiac lesions and measured these parameters (fig. 6). 16 patients out of the total number had prolonged perfusions averaging from 45 - 147 min. Extracorporeal circulation caused a 15 % to 16 % decline in platelet count and a decrease of 10 - 30 % in concentrations of fibrinogen. Particularly the percentage changes between preoperative and postoperative count of platelets larger than 4.8 $\mu^3$ correlated with the time of bypass ( fig.6). Moreover in 15 of the 16 patients undergoing perfusion lasting more than 1 hour, the clottability of the fibrinogen was intraoperatively and postoperatively found to be reduced. The reduction of clottability was measured by the increasing length of time of thrombincoagulase in parallel to the decreasing concentration of fibrinogen ( fig.6). The kinetics of platelet change in the patients and coagulation parameters intraoperatively have already been described in detail in another publication. Electromicroscopic studies on platelet (fig.7,8) during surgery were done by Prof. Dr. Morgenstern. The platelets show considerable size heterogeneity and microcytoses (fig.7,8). A low concentration of dense granules,especially in comparison to the number of mitochondria are observed. This correlates well with our results on the decrease of mean platelet volume. Additional morphometric studies are still in their preliminary stages (Eckstein 1979).

During the first 48 postoperative minutes, the percentage of smaller platelets increased significantly in 10 patients out of a total of 21 ( fig.9 ) who had undergone prolonged bypasses (longer than 56 min.). Also during the first 60 postoperative minutes, the mean

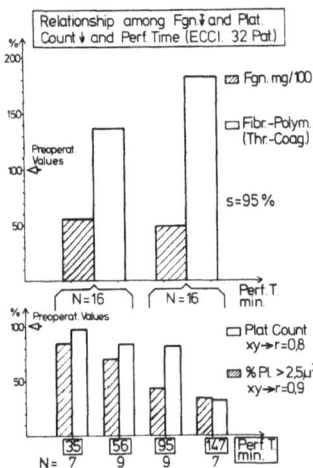

**Fig. 6:** Above the decrease of fibrinogen concentration and the disturbance of clottability (Thrombincoagulase time) and the perfusion time during extracorporeal circulation is demonstrated.
The columns below express the relationship among decreasing
numbers of big platelets ($> 2.5\ \mu^3$) and the decrease of platelet count and the perfusion time (mean) of the different
groups of patients (N = 7; 9; 9; 7; total: 32).

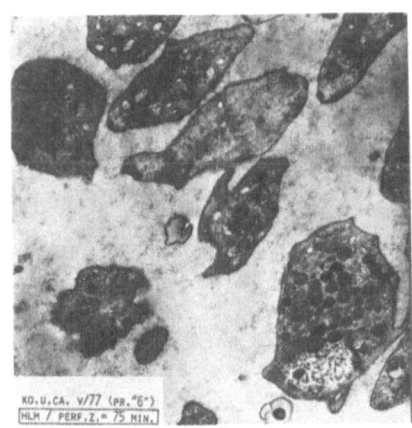

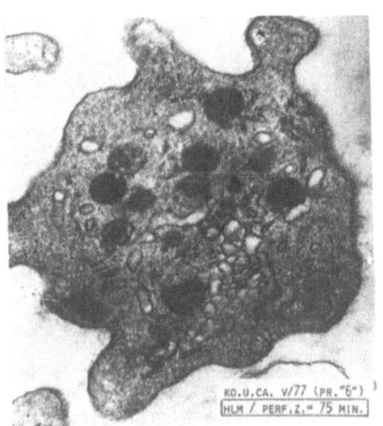

**Fig. 7:**

Electron microscopic studies on platelets during extracorporeal circulation (75 min.). The platelet show
considerable size heterogenity and
microcytoses.

**Fig. 8:**

Electron microscopic studies on
platelets during ECC (75 min.):
A low concentration of dense
granules, especial in comparison to the number of mitochondria was observed.

of the platelet count was found to be significantly below 80,000/
mm$^3$. Parallel to this, the percentages of small thrombocytes
($\leqslant$ 2.5 $\mu^3$) were significantly higher than the control group consisting of 11 patients who had postoperatively by mean of platelet
count higher than 80,000/mm$^3$. The graph shows in this group of patients up to the first 48 postoperative hours a gradual increase in
smaller thrombocytes (s.fig.9 ). In comparison with the control
group consisting of patients who had postoperatively higher percentages of larger platelets and the mean over 80,000 platelets/mm$^3$.
This could mean that altered platelets are stored intraoperatively
in the organs of the patients and begin to recirculate postoperatively.(see also Friedman 1970, 1971; Brown 1975).
In 11 patients, the biological function of Antithrombin, Antiplasmin, Antitrypsin was studied ( fig.10). During extracorporeal circulation and the first 6 postoperative hours, factor II$^A_3$ -X$^A_3$ Plasmin,
Kallikrein and Trypsin were measured. Significant activities of
factor II$^A$and -X$^A$were found postoperatively, but not during ECC,
when Heparin was administered. Kallikrein activities were found
intraoperatively. Decreased activity of Urokinase-like Plasminogen
activator in the plasma were observed postoperatively up to 6 hours.
No spontaneous Trypsin-like activities could be measured.(Table 6).
By means of immunological measurements, a slight increase of concentration of $\alpha_2$-macroglobulin and $\alpha_1$-antitrypsin was found and,
concentrations of Antithrombin III remained constant   (fig.10).
These findings were in definite contrast to the results of photometrically evaluated Antithrombin-III-function. The capacity of plasma to inactivate Thrombin,decreased in parallel to the inhibitory
activities of Antitrypsin. Antiplasmin remained constant.
This suggest that:
a) the disturbed reaction of Antithrombin III could be caused by
the continuous activation of factor II and -X during extracorporeal
circulation. Therefore, when heparin was postoperatively neutralized by Protamin injection, a significant increase in the activity
of these serinproteases was observed.(see also Büttner 1975).
b) The concentration of physiological inhibitors increases when
fresh blood mixes with the damaged blood during operations.

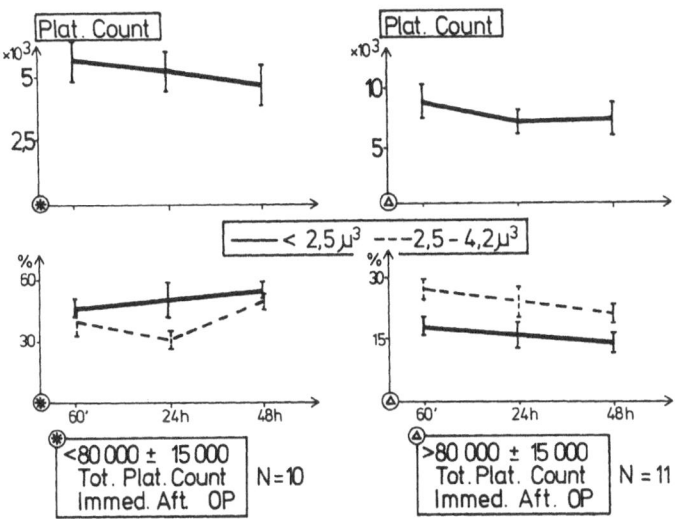

Fig. 9: Percentages of small thrombocytes (> 2.5 μ³) in patients who had postoperatively a mean of platelet count higher (lower) than 80,000/mm³. A significant higher increase in smaller thrombocytes was found in the group consisting of patients who had postoperatively a mean of platelet count lower than 80,000/mm³.

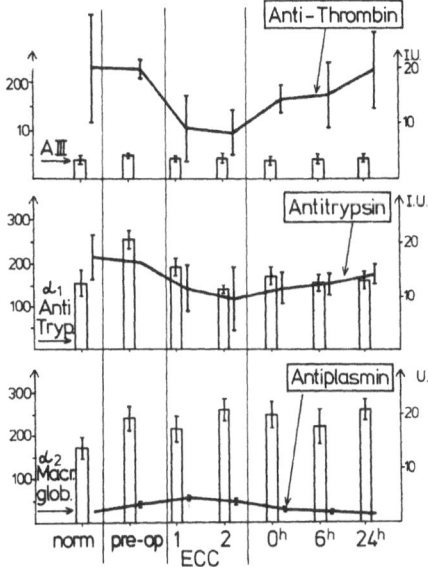

Fig.10: Effect of ECC on Antithrombin III, Antitrypsin and Anti-plasmin. Comparison of immunological concentration (columns mg/100 ml, left ordinate) and encymatic activity (1.U., right ordinate)

171

| Amidol.M. | Pre-/Intra.OP | 0 h | 6 h | 24 h |
|---|---|---|---|---|
| F II A | < 0.002 ΔE/min. | 0.02+0.01 | <0.002 | ΔE/min. |
| F X A | | 4.2 +1,2 | 1.3+0.4 | <0.002 |
| Pl.activ. | 0.8 ± 0.25 | 0.02+0.15 | 0.3+0.2 | 0.8+0.4 |
| Plasmin | < 0.05 CU. | | | |
| +Pl.ogen | 9.7+0.2 →16.1+1.2 | 16.8+1.6 | 15.4+2 | 13.6+2 |
| Kallikrein | 0.06ΔE/M.+0.023 | 0.5ΔE/M.+0.05 | <0.0008 ΔE/min. | |
| +MANCINI | Trypsine-like act.: < 0.002 Δ E | | | |

Tab.6 : Activities of factor IIa, factor Xa, plasmin and plasmin-
activator (PLAKTIV). As evaluated by photometrical measurement, using chromogenic substrates (see tab. 2 and 4).
Significant activities of factor IIa and Xa were only found
postoperatively, free Callicrein-like activities were found
intraoperatively. The (Urokinase-like) plasminogen-activator
decreased postoperatively up to 6 hours.

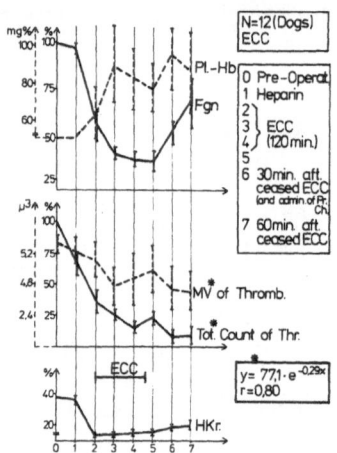

Fig. 11: Relationship among plasma hemoglobin (Pl-HB) concentration of
clottable fibrinogen (fgn) and the mean volume of thrombocytes (MV) as well as the total count of thrombocytes during
extracorporeal circulation in the dog. The relationship between the decrease of platelet count (or the decrease of mean
platelet volume) and the duration of ECC can be expressed
mathematically in relation to the perfusion time.

In order to gain better evidence on the effects of extracorporeal circulation, we operated on 12 dogs using the Bubble Oxygenator for 120 min. (fig.11) under well standardized operative conditions. This procedure is described in detail in 2.4.(Tab.5). As demonstrated before in precise correlation with the duration of extracorporeal circulation, the mean volume of thrombocytes and the total count of platelets decreased. Immediately after sternotomy, when hemodilution was performed and the extracorporeal circulation was primed, the count of platelets decreased, while on the other hand the mean platelet volume remained unaltered. When the extracorporeal circulation was started, the mean platelet volume decreased significantly parallel to the increasing amount of plasmahemoglobin, the decreasing of the concentration of fibrinogen and the dropping of total counts of platelets. The relationship between the decrease of platelet count or the decrease of mean platelet volume and the duration of extracorporeal circulation can be expressed mathematically by a logarithmical function of platelet count in relation to the perfusion time (fig.11). No correlation between the described parameters and the amount of hemodilution was found. When Protaminchloride was administered and the extracorporeal circulation was stopped, platelet count and mean platelet volume again decreased markedly (see also Eika 1972; Encke 1972).

The increase of very small thrombocytes ($< 2.5$ $u^3$) as well as the decrease in the percentage of thrombocytes larger than 4.8 $\mu^3$ during extracorporeal circulation caused the decrease in the mean volume of circulating platelets. Deaggregating drugs like Lysin-Acetylsalicylsäure or Benzyclan significantly protect platelets from changing during extracorporeal circulation, but does not influence the aggregation phenomenon induced by Protaminchloride (fig.12). The increase of small platelets during ECC is less significant, when Acetylsalicylic acid or Benzyclat are administered preoperatively and are infused continuously during extracorporeal circulation (fig.12). The percentage of large platelets didn't change in the group of dogs treated with the drugs mentioned above. After the dogs were perfused for 120 min. and then postoperatively observed for 60 minutes, they were sacrificed and, several organs were taken for microscopic studies. No microembolism or platelet aggregates were found in the examined sections. A significant lower

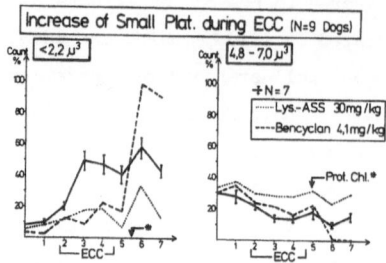

Fig. 12: Deaggregating drugs like Lysin-Acetylsalicylsäure or Benzyclan protect platelets significantly from damage during
extracorporeal circulation, but does not influence the aggregation phenomenon induced by Protaminchloride as indicated
by the differences in the increase of small thrombocytes
( $<$ 2.2 u$^3$) or by the decrease of large thrombocytes
( 4.8 - 7.0 u$^3$).

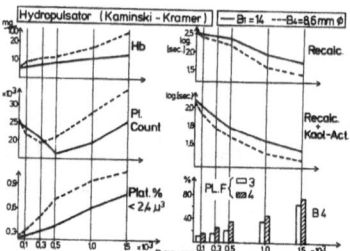

Fig. 13: Effect of standardized pulsations in a 'Hydropulsator' (see
fig. 5) on 250 ml of ACD-anticoagulated human blood. When a
narrow stenosis is used (B$^4$ = 8.6 mm Ø, plotted line), the
recalcification time is significantly shorter. Relationship
among plasma hemoglobin (Hb), platelet count, percentage of
small platelets (PLAT.% $<$ 2.4 $\mu^3$), the recalcification time
and the Caolin-activ. recalcific. time as well as the platelet factor 3 and platelet factor 4 release and the number
of pump procedures is demonstrated.

| FILTER* | A-III↑ | % PL.RET. | $\mu^3$ | |
|---|---|---|---|---|
| SURFACE(SW) | s! | 22,0 | > 4,8 | INTACT PLATEL. |
| SIEVE(MF10) | - | 14,25 | - | |
| SIEVE+SURF. | - | 7,0 | - | |
| SURFACE(SW) | s! | 36 | > 4,8 | ALTERED |
| SIEVE(MF10) | s! | 43,5 | > 9,36 | |
| SIEVE+SURF. | s! | 25 | > 4,8 | |

\* i.compar.with a stand.-filter
s (= 95 %) student-test.

Tab. 7: A significant effect (S = 95 %) of different filter types
(surface filter, Seaf filter and combined seaf- and surface-
filter on the retention rate of intact platelets (above) and
altered platelets and on the activation of Antithrombin III.
A significant rise in Antithrombin III activity was observed,
when altered blood had passed through the filters. Especially large thrombocytes are stored in the different filter
types.

174

number of extravasal erythrocytes as well as extravasal proteins
were observed in the lung of the dogs treated with ASS or Benzyclan.
The heart-lung-machine provides filters on the arterial line. The
incidence of neurological complications for the following cardiac
pulmonary bypass was significantly reduced, when Dacron-wool-fil-
ters were used (Bachmann 1975). This could explain the microscopical findings which were in definite contrast to the changes of platelets and of fibrinogen noted in our experiments. In vitro we studied the effect of several filter types on platelet retention using
ACD-anticoagulated human blood (tab.7). One part was fresh and
unaltered and the other one had been stored at 25°C for 21 days.
Using a constant low filtration pressure, 500 ml of ACD-blood were
sieved through a Swank filter. The retention rate increased significantly, when stored ACD-blood was used and increased in parallel
with the volume of thrombocytes passing through the filter. Retention rates not higher than 43.5 % were measured. A significant rise
in Antithrombin-III-activity was observed in the plasma after having passed through the filters and coagulation parameters remained
unchanged (tab.7). Especially no significant changes in the concentration of platelet factor 3 and 4 were observed in the ACD-
plasma (see also Ferbers 1958; Vinazzer 1972).
The amount of released platelet factors 3 and 4 was studied in a
"Hydropulsator" built at the Aerodynamic Institute in Aachen
(fig.5). An U-shaped plexiglass tube was filled with 250 ml of
ACD-anticoagulated human blood. A standardized pulsation was simulated by a membrane pump and, stenosis was inserted into the tube.
Recalcification time of the citrated plasma decreased in correlation with the duration of the pumping of the blood (fig.13). When
there is a narrow stenosis, recalcification time is shorter. The
phenomenon is caused by contact activation and by release of factor
3 from platelets. The amount of liberated factor 3 correlates with
the decrease of mean platelet volume as well as with the increase
of particles smaller than 2.5 $\mu^3$. In parallel to the liberation of
platelet factor 3, increasing amounts of platelet factor 4 were
measured in the ACD-plasma. The amount of released platelet factor4
was strong enough to equal 0.1 USP Heparin per ml of plasma, when
a narrow stenosis was used and the duration of pumping lasted
10.000 pulsations. In correlation to the increasing number of small

175

platelets and the decreasing number of the total platelet count, the concentrations of plasma hemoglobin increased (fig.13).

4. <u>Summary</u>:

4.1. During open-heart-operations (in 64 patients), the percentage of small thrombocytes ( $<$ 2.4 $\mu^3$) increases and platelet count decreases. In patients undergoing perfusion lasting more than 1 h, the clottability of the fibrinogene was intraoperatively and postoperatively found to be reduced. This parameters correlate quite well with the perfusion time of ECC. During the first 48 hours, a constant postoperative increase in small platelets is observed in only those patients with significant low (postoperative) values in their platelet count. The findings indicate a correlation between the perfusion time during the extracorporeal circulation and the degree of blood damage. (see also Wenzel 1977).

4.2. The biological function of Antithrombin and Antitrypsin decreases during extracorporeal circulation, but protein concentration of Antithrombin III as well as the protein concentration of $\alpha$-2-Antitrypsin does not decrease. Serin proteases (factor IIa, factor Xa, Callicrein) in particular were measured and found to be active up to 12 hours postoperatively. These results indicate a state of hypercoagulability, starting intraoperatively and increasing immediately, when the extracorporeal circulation ends, that means when heparin is neutralized by Protamin chloride.

4.3. The platelet damage was studied in the dog (N = 12) that underwent an open heart operation. No blood transfusions were performed. During extracorporeal circulation, the percent-increase in small platelets can be calculated by a mathematical formula:

$$(y = 77.1 \ e^{-\ 0.29 \ x}; \ r = 0.80).$$

When Protaminchloride was administered, a second platelet drop as well as a decrease of mean platelet volume occured. Deaggregating drugs like Acetylsalicyl acid or Bencyclan could not protect the platelets from the effect of Protamin chloride, but they did reduce the damage of platelets during extracorporeal circulation. Neither platelet aggregates nor microembolism were detected by histomorphological investigations in the sacrificed animals.

176

4.4. A membrane pump hooked up to an artificial circulation system
has proven to be extremely useful in our study on blood damage
caused by the blood's contact with blood foreign surfaces and
by particular stresses on blood during circulation. The technical parameters (narrowness of the stenosis, number of pulsations
of blood) were in correlation with coagulation parameters indicating platelet damage (platelet factor 3 and platelet factor 4
release). The mean platelet volume decreased in correlation with
the increasing concentration of hemoglobin in the plasma. When
blood filters were used, about 50 % of the platelets passed
through. Antithrombin III is activated, when plasma passed
through the filter system.

References

Bachmann, F., R. McKenna, E.R. Cole, H. Najafi, The hemostatic mechanism after open-heart surgery. I. The Journ. of Thorac. and Cardiovasc. Surgery 70, 76, 1975.

Bowie, E.J., J.H. Thompson, P. Didisheim, C.A. Owen, Mayo Clinic Laboratory Manual of Hemostasis, Philadelphia, 1971, W.B. Saunders Comp.

Brown, C.H., L.B. Leverett, C.W. Lewis, C.P. Alfrey Jr., J.D. Hellums, Morphological, biochemical and functional changes in human platelets subjected to shear stress. J. Lab. Clin. Med. 86, 462, 1975.

Büttner, W., S. Popov-Cenič, N. Müller, R. Kladetzky, Neutralization of Heparin after Extracorporeal Circulation. Anaesth. 24, 299, 1975.

Deutsch, E., Blutgerinnung und Operation. Urban & Schwarzenberg, München-Berlin-Wien, 1973.

Eckstein, P., Dissertationsschrift, 1979, Homburg/Saar.

Eika, C., On the Mechanism of Platelet Aggregation Induced by Heparin, Protamine and Polybrene. Scand. J. Haemat. 9, 248, 1972.

Encke, A., W. Hissen, M. Fichter, Der Einfluß des extrakorporalen Kreislaufs auf die Thrombozytenfunktion beim Menschen. Med. Welt 23, 28, 1972.

Ferbers, E.W., J.W. Kirklin, Studies of Hemolysis with a Plastic-Sheet Bubble Oxygenator. J. Thoracic Surg. 36, 23, 1958.

Friedman, L.I., H. Liem, E.F. Grabowski, E.F. Leonard, C.W. McCord, Inconsequentiality of Surface Properties for initial platelet Adhesion. Trans. Amer. Soc. Artif. Int. Organs XVI, 63, 1970.

Friedman, L.I., P.D. Richardson, P.M. Galletti, Observations of Acute Thrombogenesis in Membrane Oxygenators. Trans Amer. Soc. Artif. Int. Organs 17, 369, 1971.

Gans, H., A.R. Castaneda, Problems in Hemostasis during Open Heart Surgery: Changes in Fibrinogen Concentration during and after Cardiopulmonary Bypass with Particular Reference to the Effect of Heparin Neutralization on Fibrinogen. Annals of Surg. 165, 551, 1967.

Kramer, C., Künstliche Herzklappen und mechanische Hämolyse. Dissertationsschrift, 1973, TH Aachen.

Meyer-Bertenrath, J.G., Leitfaden der Labormedizin. Deutscher Ärzteverlag, Lövenich, 1975.

Salzman, E.W., Thrombosis in Artificial Organs. Transplantation Proceedings 3, 1491, 1971.

Vinazzer, H., Die postoperative Thrombosebereitschaft. F.K. Schat-
tauer Verlag, Stuttgart-New York, 1969.

Vinazzer, H., Gerinnungsstörungen in der Praxis. Fischer-Verlag,
Stuttgart, 1972.

Wenzel, E., E. Saavedra, I. Volkmer, H. Monadjemi, E. Pöhler, K. Sta-
penhorst, G. Harbauer, H. Isringhaus, Typical Changes of Platelet
Volume during and after Extracorporeal circulation. Thromb. Haemo-
stas. 38, 215, 1977.

Wenzel, E., M. Müller, Kh. Nienhaus, R. Hackhausen, Kinetics of Col-
lagen-induced platelet aggregation measured by volume distribution
in a Coulter Counter System. In: Collagen- Platelet Interaction.
Editor: H. Gastpar, F.K. Schattauer-Verlag, Stuttgart-New York, 1978.

Moderator: Wenzel

Born:    Have you checked your volumetric measurements
         with a coultercounter by one of the existing tech-
         niques to measure volume directly?

Wenzel:    We did, in fact, also study the volume distribu-
           tion of platelets with other methods. We have
           compared the results with those obtained by the
           group of Dr. Eckert in Hannover, working with the
           Laser-system. We are getting exactly the same
           volume distribution, however, one must also ana-
           lyse the same number of counts. It is not enough,
           if one only examines 20.000 or 30.000 platelets
           but rather about 120.000 as a minimum. If one has
           an abnormal platelet population one has to have
           much more counts since the method is also based
           on the rules of statistics.

Born:    With great respect, I would like to make a com-
         ment on the volume measurements on which so much
         turn; Dr. Wenzel and I have discussed this in
         the past. His conclusions depend on the so-called
         volume-measurements. I would like to ask you
         again, as I did some time ago, whether the coulter-
         counter measurement has been tested against a
         more direct technique determining volumes (see
         for example G.V.R. BORN et al., Journal of Phy-
         siology 209, 487-511 (1970)). We showed many years
         ago that it has been amply confirmed that changes
         indicated by the coultercounter do not in fact
         necessarily indicate changes in volume. The
         coulter-measurements are effected by changes in
         shape as well as in volume. It is quite easy to
         understand this, because when a platelet is shaped
         normally like a flat disk, it passes through the
         hole in the coultercounter oriented parallel to
         the streamline. And when it has changed shape it
         goes through as a spherical particle. This makes
         a measurable difference to the impedance effect

of the passing particle. On the basis of your
electronmicroscope pictures, one could interpret the Coulter results as due to shape rather
than volume changes. Therefore, caution would
suggest, that your conclusions be supported by
another technique. Thrombocrits have been developed for this very purpose, where one measures
total volume and the extracellular volume with
various markers and takes the difference. Until
this has been correlated with your measurements
I would have some doubts about their meaning. As
you put so much interpretation on these measurements their control  by another method would seem
to be essential.

Wenzel:     I think this is a very important question and I
can answer it. At first I would like to talk about
volume. If one is talking about a mean volume of
platelets, one summarizes many platelets of distinctly different sizes. This second method is
an electronical and statistical one. I think the
shape and the volume are influencing the measurements you have said but it is a question of the
number of particles one studies. If one has low
particle numbers one has a high error. We have
done more morphometric studies together with
Dr. Morgenstern, who is controlling our results
with measurements in the electronmicroscope pictures with morphometric techniques. These studies
indicate a limited accordance and we then say
that the shape of the platelets is influencing
the results more than the volume. Lastly one can
take of course Latex particles or any other material and can measure then by other methods and
control the Coulter results. This, of course, is
done every day because it is a clinical test and
we have to guarantee the quality of it daily. If
one measures that, one also gets a good correlation between the weight or the volume of the

particles and the volume measured in the Coulter. It is interesting to look at the differences of these particles, the distribution of their volumes mostly has a Gaussian shape, which is not seen with the thrombocytes.Their volume distribution is represented by a special curve which cannot be characterized by a simple mathematical function. Let me summarize: the signal is a volume and represents an electronically measured volume.

Born: With great respect, I still don't accept that. I would like to refer you to the paper of G.V.R. BORN, DEARNLEY, R., FOULKES, J.G. and SHARP, D.E., 1978, J. of Physiol., 280, 193-212, which describes the use of a very sophisticated apparatus to control aparent morphological changes. I believe that an analogous approach is necessary for electrical changes interpreted as changes in volumes.

Birnbaum: I would like to mention two points:
1. You do not measure electrical impedance, you measure the conductivity,
2. the volume of the particle replaces exactly a correspondent amount of electrolyte fluid. So the replaced electrolyte fluid is proportional to the volume of the particle.

Williams: Surely, you are wrong, it is not the volume, it is the cross-sectional area of the particle in the flow - not the volume which is measured. The pulse height proportional to the area of the particle and not the volume. What you are measuring is a change in the current which occurs when a non-conducting or a fully-conducting material goes through the pore of a Coulter counter That is the impulse height is going to be proportional to the decrease in the conducting area. The cell volume is going to be the integral of the pulse height and the pulse width. However, the machine only measures impulse height and not impulse width. And so you will not get cell volume measured directly. If you have a flat disk going through the orifice "face-on" it will give you a very high peak and a short pulse width. If you get the same cell going through the orifice "end-on" then it will give you a low peak which is wide. Since the machine does not measure the width of the peak, the size of the particle seems to be smaller, which is Dr. Born's point.

Birnbaum:    We don't analyse the crenation of particles by this. We know the so-called form factor in the calculation of the volume. For erythrocytes this form factor is somewhere between 1,01 and 1,02.

Williams:    I agree, but when you have a population of platelets some of which are discoidal and some of which are spherical (i.e. which may have undergone the release-reaction) there is no one single form factor that you can put in. How can you know how many you have got of any one particular type?

Birnbaum:    About the thrombocytes I would have to give the word to Dr. Wenzel. I only feel familiar with the erythrocyte counting in this system.

# 9. Electro-optical Investigations of the Fibrinogen-Fibrin Conversion in Artificial Membranes

P. Baurschmidt and M. Schaldach

Zentralinstitut für Biomedizinische Technik der Universität Erlangen-Nürnberg
(Geschäftsführender Direktor: Prof. Dr. M. Schaldach)

Since the introduction of extracorporeal blood circulation one of the most critical problems has been recognized in the foreign-surface induced interactions which frequently limit the functional life time of the device. The in-vivo or ex-vivo application of biomaterials induces an inevitable disturbance in the relation between the vessel wall and the coagulation system. The contact of blood with an artificial solid surface imposes a situation where adsorption, adhesion, activation or inhibition of cellular components and plasma proteins depend on some physico-chemical properties of the material used and on the special hydrodynamic situation given by the construction. The generally accepted process is that of a competitive adsorption of proteins leading to the deposition of a conditioning layer which controls the attachment and activation of platelets and, thus, the overall thrombogenic reaction (1-8).

There has been a strong evidence that the thrombogenicity of a material is coupled to the electronical structure of the surface. A key to the solution of the problem has been given by electrochemical studies, first carried out by Boddy, Brattain and Sawyer (9). On the basis of a purely electrostatic model it was shown that negatively charged surfaces exhibit an antithrombogenic behaviour. In the following years several investigations of individual clotting proteins have been performed, showing that thrombosis is related to positive potentials, that fibrinogen is converted to a fibrin-like product and that an electron transfer takes place at the interface which depends on the energy of the charge carriers present at the surface (10-16).

## The Interface: Solid-Surface - Fibrinogen

In order to study electrochemical reactions of proteins
an electrolyte cell is employed in which the proteins are
subjected to various potentials ( see Fig. 1). Changes of
the protein adsorption and identification of the type of
reaction (oxidation, reduction) are deduced from the measurement of the current passing the cell and the impedance
of the interface. These data lead to a quantitative eval-

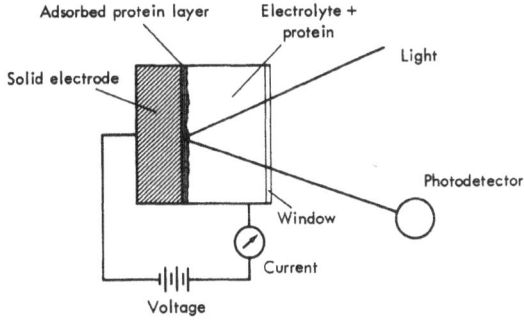

Fig. 1  Schematic experimental set-up

uation of the concentration of the exchanged charge carriers.

Additional information are achieved from the optical behaviour of the adsorbed and/or activated protein film by
measuring the optical density and the light scattering
properties. This is an in-situ method and applies very
specifically to structural changes of macromolecules.
Changes in the reflectivity of the test electrode as a
function of the applied potential allow a determination of
the energy of the charge carriers. Both methods combined
give a simultaneous measure of the electronical structure
of the solid and of the polymerisation processes in the
protein layer close to the surface (17).

The optical properties of a fibrinogen solution during
the clotting process with thrombin is shown in Fig. 2 as a
function of time. The adsorption of untreated fibrinogen
is given by the thick line, whereas the thin ones  show an
increase of the light scattering with the increasing size

of the polymeric molecule at time intervals of 1 min. Deviations from the theoretical line (dashed curve) occure
with increasing coagulation time and decreasing wavelenght
due to a transition from linear to cross-linked molecules
(18).

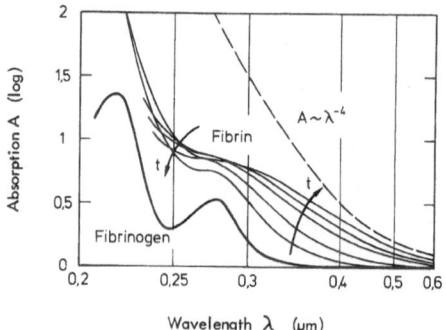

Fig. 2  Absorption and scattering intensity of fibrinogen
        during coagulation with thrombin

The generally observed behaviour of the fibrinogen system in contact with a semiconducting Germanium electrode
is given in Fig.3. The potential is swept from cathodic to
anodic values and the change of the scattering intensity
is recorded which is indicated in the figure  as a qualitative change in the degree of polymerisation. The re-
cording shows that the polymerisation process proceedes
only in the anodic range of potential and that no changes
in the structural state of the fibrinogen molecule are to
be seen in the negative range. This is confirmed by prolonged cyclic polarisation leading to a stepwise build-up
of successive fibrin layers.

The concentration of polymerized molecules and the position of the 'onset'-potential depend on the material and
the charge carrier concentration. The compatibility of a
material depends on the difference of the 'onset'-potential
and the rest-potential which is established when the material comes in contact with blood. For materials such as
titanium or pyrolytic carbon differences in potential
have been found which range from +100 mV to +200 mV. With
that, the rest-potential lies on the cathodic side and an

electro-activation of fibrinogen will not occur. This is
in good agreement with clinical findings from prosthetic
heart valves where these materials are in use.

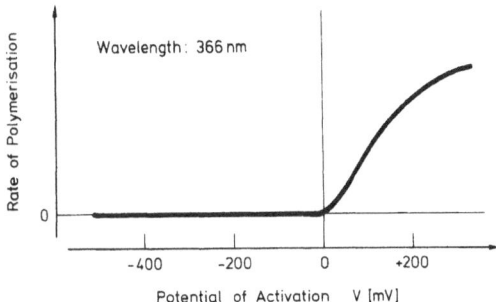

Fig. 3   Electro-polymerisation of fibrinogen

## The Electronical Model

The mechanism of coagulation-specific reactions will only
be understood in complete when the electronical structure
of the solid body is taken into account. Thus, it is a
necessity for interpretation that a single set of parameters is to be found which permits the description of
both the biological and the solid phase. An appropriate
model is that of the electronical band structure for redox systems, from which the reciprocal exchange of charge
carriers between the solid surface and the electrolyte
can be extended to the protein system.

   The charge carriers of the solid which take part in reactions with the proteins are grouped together in bands of
well defined energy. Between the lower and the upper band
there is a zone in which no charge carriers are to be
found: an energy gap. According to the width of the energy
gap, which ranges from zero for metals to up to 3 eV for
insulators, we find different carrier concentrations and
with that different electrical conductivities.

   The electronical structure of proteins are described by
a concept which goes back to Szent-Györgyi (19) , who in the
early forties  assumed a similar band model. This model

has been extended by Eley (20) and others. They measured
the value of the energy and the carrier concentration and
confirmed the existance of an intramolecular conductivity
mechanism.as a result of the periodicity of the helical
protein structure. The value of the band gap for fibrinogen
is in the order of 1 to 2 eV.  Fig. 4 shows both band
structures of the adjacent solid and protein. The effect
of an externally applied potential to the interface results in a vertical shift of the bands relative to each
other. The situation shown here is that for an anodic potential. The lower bands of the solid and the protein over-
lap energetically which results in an exchange of charge
carriers. In the case of cathodic potentials the bands of
the protein are shifted upwards. Since the lower protein
band has no corresponding energy level in the range of the
energy gap of the solid an exchange of carriers is pro-
hibited. From this model, the cathodic behaviour of
fibrinogen can be understood, where no activa-

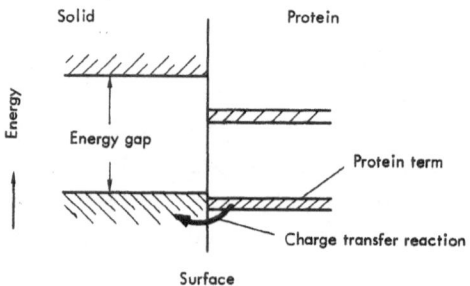

Fig. 4   Schematic energy term distribution and transfer
         of charge carriers

tion of the fibrinogen molecule is found and in which there
will probably be only adsorption without conformational
changes.

To summarize these effects, it can be said that the fibrinogen conversion shows a correlation with the characteristic parameters of the electronic surface structure.
It was shown that electro-polymerisation of fibrinogen is
comparable to the proteolytic action of thrombin(21). As a
consequence, the ability of a material to initiate poly-

merisation depends on the interfacial potential which is a characteristic of the individual material.

Taking the electroactivating effects of prothrombin and others into account (13,14), it can be stated that the first steps to thrombosis which are induced by the introduction of an artificial surface are not necessarily depending on the activation of one of the primary factors of the cascade, like Hageman, but might be a consequence of electronic processes, activating one of the late factors like prothrombin or fibrinogen. The cause is a shift in the equilibrium state of these clotting proteins which results i) from the missing regulatory action of the vessel wall and ii) from interferences with the electronical properties of the artificial surface.

## Material Development

The model described can be applied to the development of blood-compatible materials on the premises that an improvement of the material is correlated with an inactivation of the last stages of the clotting mechanism. Materials with rigid or polymeric properties are of special interest for cardiovascular applications.

As there would be a widespread use of ceramics for implantable and extracorporeal devices, a procedure has been found to overcome the rather thrombogenic behaviour of alumina when in contact with blood. These materials have been coated with semiconducting oxides which fullfill the requirements of an inhibition of protein activation by means of their electronical band structure. Fig.5 shows the principle of selecting a suitable material. The energy bands are given for various materials as well as the important protein band which is indicated by a dot. From the possibility of inhibiting an exchange of charge carriers it is obviously that metals like silver are not advantageously whereas semiconducting materials get the more suitable the more the lower band lies energetically beneath the the protein term. On this basis, a stannic and titanium coated alumina has been developed which has been tested mechanically and in dog experiments. Blood

compatibility is evaluated by implanting rings into the
femoral veins of dogs. The results show an appreciable
improvement in comparison to non-coated rings.

An improvement of flexible polymers is possible by es-
tablishing organic semiconducting properties on the sur-

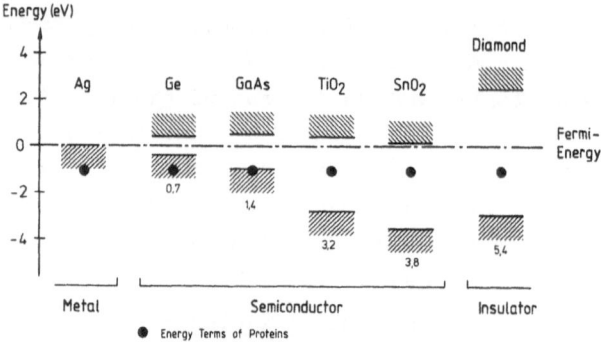

Fig. 5   Band gaps of various materials

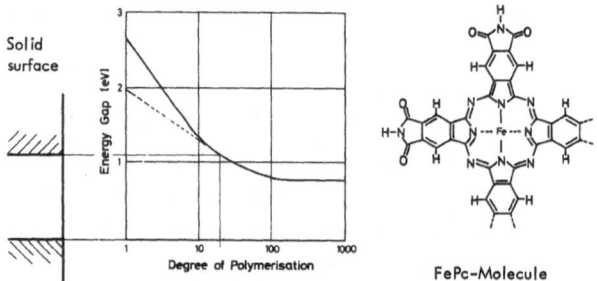

Fig. 6   Band gap of iron-phthalocyanine

face. As an appropriate material oligomeric iron-phthalocyanine has been found which can be grafted onto a poly-
urethan matrix and other polymers (22). Iron-phthalocyanine
has the great advantage that the energy bands can be pre-
determined according to the manufactoring parameters. Fig.
6 shows the energy gap as a function of the degree of
polymerisation. The chemical structure of the molecule is
shown on the right and is closely related to the hem of
the hemoglobin. The application of this polymer coating
process results in an inhibition of a charge transfer between the plasma clotting proteins and the artificial surface.

## Summary

Thrombogenic reactions at the surface of implantable materials are related to the electronical structure and are potential dependent. The initiation of thrombosis may as well occure without the need of a prior surface-induced activation of Hageman or other factors. The degree of compatibility of a prosthesis is determined by the conditioning layer of proteins which depends on physico-chemical parameters of the material. Criteria for the development of blood compatible materials have been deduced and have led to the realisation of rigid and flexible compound systems for the use in cardiovascular implants and extra-corporeal devices.

## References

1. Vroman,L.,A.L.Adams, J.Biomed.Mater.Res. 3,43(1969)
2. Lyman,D.J., et al., Trans.Amer.Soc.Artif.Int.Organs 14,250(1968)
3. Kim,S.W., et al., Trans.Amer.Soc.Artif.Int.Organs 20,449(1974)
4. Baier,R.E.,R.C.Dutton, J.Biomed.Mater.Res.3,191(1969)
5. Morrissey,B.W.,R.R.Stromberg, J.Colloid Interface Sci. 46,152(1974)
6. Roohk,H.V., et al., Trans.Amer.Soc.Artif.Int.Organs 22,1(1976)
7. Chiu,T-H., et al., Trans.Amer.Artif.Int.Organs 24,389 (1978)
8. Schmid-Schönbein,H. et al.,in: Blood Vessels p. 57, Springer Verlag, Berlin-Heidelberg-New York (1976)
9. Boddy,P.J.,W.H.Brattain,P.N.Sawyer,in: Biophsical Mechanism in Vascular Homeostasis and Intravascular Thrombosis p.30, Appleton-Century-Crofts(1965)
10. Stoner,G.,L.Walker, J.Biomed.Mater.Res. 3,645(1969)
11. Gileadi,E., et al., J.Biomed.Mater.Res. 6,489(1972)
12. Ramasamy,N., et al., J.Electrochem.Soc. 120,354(1973)
13. Duic,L., et al., J.Electrochem.Soc. 120,348(1973)
14. Ramasamy,N., et al., Electrochem. Acta 19,137(1974)
15. Schaldach,M., et al., Ber.Bunsenges. phys.Chem. 77, 795(1973)
16. Baurschmidt,P. et al., in: Blood Vessels p. 177, Springer-Verlag, Berlin-Heidelberg-New York (1976)
17. Baurschmidt,P.,M.Schaldach, J.Bioeng. 1,261(1977)
18. Ferry,J.D.,P.R.Morrison, J.Amer.Chem.Soc.69,388(1947)
19. Szent-Györgyi,A. Nature 148,157(1941)
20. Eley,D.D.,D.Spivey, Faraday Soc. 56,1432(1960)
21. Baurschmidt,P.,M.Schaldach, Biomed. Technik 23,169(1978)
22. Brauner,H.,M.Schaldach, 1.Europ.Conf.Evaluation of Biomaterials, Strasbourg 25.-28.9.1977

Müller-Mohnssen:       Because the majority of the members of this
symposium do not work every day in electroche-
mistry, I try to interpret some basic ideas of
this paper. At first, one should differentiate
between membrane potential, which is better
known by biologists, and membrane surface potential. The cell *membrane potential (M.P.)* depends on a concentration difference of cations
between the intra- and extracellular space and
- according to the common interpretation - originates from diffusion in the direction of the concentration gradient. The polarity of the extracellular phase is (in case of resting potential)
*positive* with respect to the intracellular phase.
In understanding the approach of surface protection done by Prof. Schaldach and his group,
M.P. can be neglected (forming of a surface of
living cells on the arterial prosthesis - re-
endotheliazation - is neglected in this model).
The *membrane surface potential (S.P.)* which is
usually measured as electrokinetic potential
(and which must be considered in discussions
about hydrophilic properties) depends on the
density of fixed surface charges. Normally there
is an excess of. fixed anions; the polarity of
surface potential is, therefore, *negative* with
respect to the extracellular fluid. The stronger
the negativity of the S.P. the better the endothelium is protected against thrombogenesis,
firstly, because most of the membrane material
is hydrated (large thickness of the layer of
hydrating water dipoles), and the membrane surface is secondly protected against heteropolar
bonding (electroadsorbtion) of negatively charged
proteins as fibrinogen. Counterions as $Ca^{++}$ or
$H^+$ tend to adsorb at the membrane surface there-

by decreasing the surface potential. If the isoelectric state is attained, hydrophility and protection against protein adsorption is lost.

At the surface of a normal endothelium active processes care for "cleaning" the surface from counter-cations which had adsorbed in excess, so that a stable negative S.P. is attained. In trying to copy this mechanism also for artificial vessels, Prof. Schaldach and his group search for an inorganic semiconductor in which the energy niveau of the electron in the valency band and the conductivity band are adapted to the respective energy bands of the fibrinogen, such way that the free negative surface charges which are screened by adsorption of fibrinogen can be substituted by carrying electons to the surface. This way the S.P. is kept constant and adsorbtion is limited. The energy sources for this electrical current, normal to the surface plane, necessary for this electron transfer are thought to be identical with some enzymatic redox systems present in living tissues. In the basic experiment shown by the first slide of Dr. Bauerschmid's presentation the path of electrical current necessary for stabilization of the negative S.P. was normal to the surface plane. The electric energy source for this current was an external generator. To maintain a stationary current also at the inner surface of an implanted artificial vessel a closed electrical loop is needed consisting of 1. an electrical battery with a polarity opposite to that of the surface area considered, and 2. the passive electrical conduct connecting battery and surface to a closed electrical circuit. Can you draw an equivalent circuit diagram of your model to answer the following questions: Firstly, where is the battery located in your model and secondly, where are the current paths by which the electrical circuit elements are connected to a closed electrical loop?

Bauerschmid: At first, I would like to comment that you are totally correct in the point that the membrane potential is negative and the FERMI-niveau is shifted thereby in a direction inhibiting the protein reactions. Secondly, my paper deals with two points. First I have demonstrated the method we used to test the reactions in order to evaluate the parameters of the material which influence the reactions. We have done this by applying an external potential. This is not what we intend to do after    implantation of the material. Secondly, after finding a fundamental model, I tried to explain how we applied criteria for the development of a material which in contact with blood exhibits a negative potential. It is of our prime interest not to apply any potential but to handle a material which in contact with the blood proteins and the electrolytes shows a negative potential thereby inhibiting adsorption and conformational changes.

Schmid-Schönbein: Dr. Bauerschmid, I think we have to come back to Fig. 3    of your talk. I took the liberty of selecting it again. You have on your ordinate "rate of polymerization". What is actually being measured? I think you have to prove to us that in fact a "fibrin polymerization" (chain formation and crosslinking of fibrin-monomers into fibrin-networks) occurs in the sense that fibrin monomers form crosslinks and that you have a fibrin network. As an alternate explanation, I would suggest that you may have

194

an electrophoretic motion of the proteins towards the wall and something like an adsorption. In other words, I would like to see better evidence for "fibrin formation".

Hemker:
I, too, do think so, and if I may add to this, when we try to think of all the types of effects you could get on a charged surface in your set-up, such as pH-effects, temperature effects, effects of ionic strength , also the effects you create by having a combination of positively and negatively charged proteins and so on, I think you would need rather a lot of control experiments to allow interpretation of your data - I haven't seen any. You claim to have seen fibrin polymerization but I see no reasons to exclude trivial protein precipitation.

Bauerschmid:
To the first question. We have measured the optical density at a wavelength of 360 nm, this is just the light energy where no UV-absorption is caused by untreated fibrinogen. If you add thrombin for example, you will have as a cause of the cross-linking of fibrin-monomers to polymers a time-dependent increase in light-scattering which reduces the intensity of the transmitted light. The same phenomena are observed in the case of an external potential applied to a solution of fibrinogen.

Hemker:
How do you ever know where the increase in absorption comes from?

Bauerschmid:
The process is the following:
By the influence of electropotential there is some splitting off of fibrinopeptides, as we have shown. I have some slides which demonstrate their existence. So, if we accept this as correct, you get fibrin monomers. These

monomers are able to aggregate and built a chain of linear polymers.

Hemker: But I am asking, where does the increase of absorption comes from?

Bauerschmid: It comes from the scattering of the light by large polymers. This is just a matter of the techniques applied.

Hemker: Now any denaturated protein will precipitate, aggregate and scatter light. How do you differentiate between fibrinogen that aggregates because of some type of denaturation at the surface on the one hand and polymerization of fibrin monomers on the other?

Bauerschmid: I have to refer to an experiment done by BODDY, BRATTAIN and SAWYER or by STONER and WALKER (BODDY,P.J., W.H. BRATTAIN, P.N. SAWYER, in: Biophysical Mech. in Vasc. Homeostasis and Intravascular Thrombosis; STONER,G., L. WALKER, J. Biomed. Mater. Res. 3,645 (1969)).
They have applied a potential and have looked at the interface by electronmicroscopy and have shown that the generated product is of a fibrin-like type. The crosslinking and the structure is similar to the morphology of thrombin-clotted fibrin.

Hemker: As a matter of fact there is some doubt in my mind as to the specificity of these methods. The only way to show that you get fibrin monomers is when you demonstrate that fibrinopeptides do appear. Did you determine fibrinopeptides?

Bauerschmid: We did. We investigated our fibrin solution at a positive potential where we observed an increase of the optical density. We kept the solution at this potential for some time, say for about 5 minutes, and then transfered the solution after centrifuging and addition of

196

ninhydrin at alkaline pH-values into a spectro-
fluorimeter and measured the amount of arginine
produced in this solution. This certainly is
a rough measure and gives only the sum or the
concentration of the fibrinopeptide A and B
but is in any case an identification for their
existence.

Hemker:        That depends upon what you define as a fibrinopeptide. If you mean that any peptide coming
from your solution would be a fibrinopeptide
than I agree, but then it is no longer a measure for polymerisation. Fibrinopeptides are
specific peptides cleaved off by thrombin and
some snake venoms. If you agree to that then
you will have to show that they appear in your
experiments and I don't know any other method
to do that, except the immune techniques as
developed a.o. by Blomback.

Bauerschmid:   The peptides are obviously splitted off at
the arginine-glycine bond since the fluoro-
metrical signal which we get is significant
for arginine and     therefore a measure of
release of the fibrinopeptides. This is an
evidence for the occurence of the same peptides     you get when you add thrombin .

Müller-Mohnssen:   Of which magnitude are the currents necessary
to keep the surface potential at 200 mV (this
potential you obviously need for protecting
the surface)? Which units are used to indicate the current $(A/cm^2)$?

Bauerschmid:   The current is determined by the electrode
potential and the current which is flowing
depends more or less on the material used.
The difference in current with or without
fibrinogen solution is very very small; it is
beneath  10 to 29 milliamperes. It is very
hard to detect, so I haven't shown you any
pictures.

197

Müller-Mohnssen:    This small current difference is on top of
the negative electrode. Here, the current den-
sity is in the range of milliampères and it
usually shows some instabilities.

At surfaces carrying negative fixed charges
an adsorption of cations of strong electrolytes regularly takes place. For the deple-
tion of adsorbed cations according to your
system an electrical current is necessary
to flow. Where is the redox electrode located with respect to the surface in vivo? Where
are the current paths connecting the redox
electrode and the surface layer?

Bauerschmid:    Since the condition for inhibiting a charge
transfer from the protein to the solid is that
of a low concentration of electron acceptor
states, it will be sufficient to have an excess
of negative charges at the surface. This can
be achieved by an external current with external electrodes, but in a much more appropriate way by the equilibrium state of the
interface where no net current flows and which
is a result of anodic and cathodic partial
current densities. These are determined by the
redox systems of the blood and the properties
of the material such as solubility or special
features like catalytic activity and specific
adsorption.
This would be correct, if we implant copper
material which is thrombogenetic just like
LUCAS et al. have shown.

In this case you have to apply a negative
current and now all the things we just discussed about inhibition of protein activation
come into action. But what we are looking for

is a material which in contact with the blood
exhibits a spontaneous negative potential. So
you don't have to apply any current to the
implant.

Müller-Mohnssen:    I thought, you already got such a material.

Bauerschmid:    Yes, by coating rigid and flexible materials
with semiconducting materials, we get a material exhibiting a negative potential when
in contact with blood.

Schmid-Schönbein:    We have to start really from Dr. Sawyer's experiments. They were done at a time and age
which is over, when the "clotting scheme"
you showed was quite uncontested. In the mean-
time, the role of platelet in the initiation
of thrombo-embolic events is so clear that any
theory which excludes him is no longer useful.
I think on a meeting which took place about
three years ago (BLOOD VESSELS, Problems Arising at the Borders of Natural and Artificial
Blood Vessels, 8th Scientific Conference of the
Gesellschaft Deutscher Naturforscher und
Ärzte, Edited by S. Effert and J.D. Meyer-
Erkelenz, Springer Verlag, 1976), in which
Dr. Schaldach and Dr. Sawyer were present,
it was well agreed that one has to re-think
the Sawyer-experiments. It is perfectly
possible, that negative charge produces a
repulsion of platelets rather than an inhibition of actual coagulation. Then if one cuts
off the current in the copper rings the platelets will adhere better; and then, a very
long series of biochemical events begins en-
ding in the formation of fibrin. I tend to believe that there is, among many other materials,
an amorphous material, platelet residues and
some fibrin. However, I think it by no means
proven that the fibrin formed there first and

then the platelets settled. There is much
evidence now indicating that neither in artificial nor in normal vessels thrombotic
events are possible without the action of
platelets (this holds at least for arterial
thrombosis). This is the point where our
interpretation should start rather than at
a late step that you call polymerization, an
interpretation which was challenged by
Dr. Hemker.

Bauerschmid:       Certainly, this is correct for the arterial
system. But the amount of adsorbed platelets
and a subsequent activation depends very
strongly on the composition and the conformational variability of the deposited protein
film. My paper had been de-
dicated to the conversion of the fibrinogen-
fibrin system from an electrochemical point
of view. The plasma protein fibrinogen is
preferentially adsorbed and thus establishes
the conditioning layer for platelet adhesion
and activation. The evaluation of the layer
properties depends on the material, and to
some extent on the electrical properties.
You see, what I wanted to show is that apart
from adhesion of platelets and the introduction of thrombosis via aggregation of
platelets there is a second possibility not
yet discussed by direct action of the interfacial potential and energy of the material upon the plasma clotting proteins.

Schmid-Schönbein:    There is no doubt that proteins adsorb to
surfaces - the problem arises whether or not
the adsorption of proteins (including fibrinogen) promotes a platelet deposition or protects
against it. Certainly, I can visualize the
layering of a monolayer onto any of these

surfaces and electrical effects on such
layering which does not require a cleavage
of parts of the molecule. If you talk about
polymerization, you have to prove that this
is actually occurring.

Hemker:                 Are you able to solve the material you de-
                        posited in urea or in acetic acid?

Bauerschmid:            Well, to some extent. Not all. So there is
                        evidence of some type of denaturation. We
                        were able to solve some of them.

Hemker:                 And the material that remains, when you
                        look at it through a microscope would you
                        call it a polymerisate or not?

Bauerschmid:            Yes, I would call it this way. It is very
                        similar to the protein film found by
                        STONER. The morphology is very similar to
                        crosslinked fibrin.

Hemker:                 O.K., when you have a polymerisate of fi-
                        brinogen which cannot be dissolved in urea
                        or in acetic acid you must have had active
                        factor XIII around somehow. And you cannot
                        activate factor XIII unless you have throm-
                        bin around. So, you must have had thrombin
                        in your experiment, which then can be held
                        responsible for the fibrin generation as
                        well.

Bauerschmid:            Well, actually I can't comment on this be-
                        cause there has never been an investigation
                        up to now showing the influence or the
                        effects which are created by a potential
                        upon proteins. The enzymatic way of looking
                        at the activation is something different
                        and not applicable. You mentioned the necessi-
                        ty of factor XIII. In the enzymatic system
                        it is certainly necessary but the situation
                        at the interface with an applied potential

is quite different.

Hemker:    This actually is not completely true, because many proteins among which many pro-
enzymes can be subjected to strong electrical fields without any damage, e.g. in pre-
parative electrophoresis. Now, I am buying
that you form fibrin by some electric action. I am just assuming that you could get
fibrin monomers. I don't believe it for
other reasons but that is something else.
Now when I asked you if your fibrin monomers
crosslink and you say they presumingly do
so, then I won't buy that your electrons in
the first place wil imitate a serine pro-
tease and then in a second set of reactions
they will simulate the crosslinking action
of factor XIII a, as well. That is a bit
too much of a good thing for me.

Bauerschmid:    Well, I wanted to demonstrate what happens
if for some reason you find a charge trans-
fer reaction of proteins with the implanted
material. This possibility is not seldom,
in fact, we believe that it always plays
a crucial role at artificial surfaces.
Whether it is fibrinogen in the usual way
of looking at it from the enzymatic description or not should be left to further
discussions. In any case you find some deposit. And you find, and that has been
confirmed by clinical investigation, a
rather thick film of fibrin on the surface
of the implant.

Schmid-Schönbein:    I think that serious re-orientation is necessary in the analysis of thrombus formation
in devices with artificial polymers in contact with flowing blood. Most engineers working in this field have been brainwashed

202

to take as factually very brilliant, very useful but very biased coagulation hypotheses which are very useful for analysis of coagulation deficiencies but not for excessive coagulation. We do one of two things, either one should go ahead pragmatically ("anything goes" in this respect) and just try to think and try out some polymer which works. But then, of course, there is the other goal, the attempt to find out what is actually meant by "thrombogeneicity" or "non-thrombogeneicity" of polymer surfaces. And here, I think, we have to start from scratch.

Feijen:

I think the interaction of materials with blood is a very complex problem. But the rheological aspects are very complex too. And I think if we are looking for improvement of oxygenation or dialysis we have to deal with both aspects. You can put it one way, say we look only at the influence of the flow conditions; then I would say probably something goes wrong because I think the materials certainly influence the occurrence of blood trauma in artificial organs. On the other hand if I say we have to look at the biomaterials only, something goes wrong because we cannot test biomaterials without defining the flow conditions (this will be detailed in my paper).

Müller-Mohnssen:

The disagreement may be due to the following difficulties. From the interdisciplinarity of this symposium one can conclude that the problems involved in extracorporeal circulation (as for instance thrombogenesis) shall be discussed under different aspects (pluralism of aspects). This implicates tolerance to serious approaches which are different with respect to the methods (pluralism of methods). The organizing committee of this symposium obviously (see program) has considered that the problem of thrombogenesis involves not only the *blood* with its cellular and molecular components of clotting system but also the *vessels* (properties of the wall) and the physics of *flow*.

This pluralistic view may prevent us from narrowing our mental horizon to doctrins as for instance from reducing firstly, the whole clinical problem of thrombo-genesis to tests of some factors of the enzymatic clotting system and secondly, the problem of biocompatibility of ma-terials to the results of only tests mentioned in 1. (as done in the bioma-terial program of the German ministry of Research and Technology).
In Germany the group of Dr. Schaldach is one of the very few groups working here on the electrochemical effects involved in haemostasis. Since the work of Sawyers we permanently have learned new facts about electrochemical inter-action of blood components with the vessel wall from many authors. It follows from this material that the approach is still a serious one.

# 10. FLUID DYNAMIC ASPECTS OF MECHANICAL HAEMOLYSIS [*)]

### by Alexander Naumann

Prof. emerit. for Fluid mechanics, Institute of Aerodynamics,
Rhein. Westf. Techn. Hochschule Aachen

Dr. Schmid-Schönbein asked me to give a short report on the work
we are doing at Aachen in the problems of the biomedical technique,
and to tell you somewhat about the history and the way, how this work
has been developed.

## 1. General remarks

The initial ignition was awaked by a question of doctors at Essen and
Düsseldorf in 1966. They told me that after the implantation of artificial heart valves a relatively high mortality rate occurred after longer
delay, perhaps some months after the implantation date. This effect
was accompanied by a high haemolysis rate, that means by an unphysio-
logical high rate of destruction of the red blood cells. Influenced by
the idea of US scientists they asked whether a turbulent flow might be
the reason. I proposed to make a model test at first in order to know
the flow pattern, namely to use a bigger ball model of the heart valve
in a water flow. I believe this was the birth-hour of our interest in the
biotechnical engagement. But also this was the step to become acquainted
with the different terminology in the physical-engineering and the medical languages; and, much more than this, with the different professional
comprehension, the difference in the working methods in view towards
the aims of the research; all this affected by a difference in the professional ethos.

In 1967 a Medical Faculty was founded at the Technical University at
Aachen. This became a very fortunate step for our collaboration, because those professors were ready to come to such a purely technically

---

*) Dinner Speech, Nov. 21 - 23, 1978

orientated institution, who had recognized the utility of such a combination for the medical progress in diagnosis and therapy. So an excellent prerequisite for success was given. Some time before the Medical Faculty started its research, a working group of institutes in Aachen and clinics of the University of Düsseldorf begun with a program related to the development of a blood pump, not designed for implantation. It was soon found to produce a small haemolysis rate; therefore it will not be able to replace the roller pump in the heart-lungs-engine.

The first results obtained the Institute for Fluid Dynamics on the artificial heart valves and the basic phenomena of flow-induced haemolysis were presented in Paris in 1968 and at the Academy of Sciences at Düsseldorf[1] in 1969. I think these efforts and successes contributed taking the decision to establish a new Institute for Biomedical Technique and attach it to the Technical University. This institute was sponsored by the Volkswagenstiftung, which gave several million D-Mar as a starting help. The institute bears the name "Helmholtz-Institut für Biomedizinische Technik". Now we have an extended group of different working teams, which are sharing a common interest for biomedical tecl niques. These include from the engineering side the following institutes of the Technical University:

> Fluid Mechanics, Pneumatic and Hydraulic Control, Chemical Engineering, Plastics, Electrotechnique, Electronics;

from the medical side the departments of the Medical Faculty of the Technical University Aachen:

> Internal Medicine I and II, Pathology, Physiology, Cardio-Surgery, Urology;

---

1) A. Naumann, Arb.-Gem. Forschg. Nordrhein-Westf. 203 (1969).

from the Medical Faculty Düsseldorf the departments:

Internal Medicine, Physiology, Experimental Surgery;

and

the Helmholtz-Institute for Biomedical Technique.

In the first phase we obtained financial help from the government of our state Nordrhein-Westfalen and of the Deutsche Forschungsgemeinschaft (German Research Society). Then we were able to constitute – not without strong efforts – a "Sonderforschungsbereich" (freely translated a particular research program): "Artificial Organs – Models and Organ substitutes". The research programs of such "Sonderforschungsbereiche" are supervised and confirmed by the German Council of Science, and then organized by the DFG. They are of great help, since they provide for several years a budget.

This is perhaps the moment to briefly give an overlook of the work we are doing in Aachen **).

A. Fluid dynamics in vessels:
        pulsatile flow at ramification, stenosis, arterio-venous anastomosis; flow pattern, arterial sound; microcirculation, biorheology.

B. Cardiac assistance systems:
        intra aortic balloon pulsation, pacemakers.

C. Artificial heart valves:
        fluid dynamics, blood damage, cardiologic problems, new types.

D. Artificial blood pumps:
        design and development, control, fluid dynamics, plastics.

E. Artificial kidneys:
        improvement in the quality of the dialysates and ultra-filtrates and supply of the method of ultrafiltration.

---

**) In this dinner speech only a few references are given; most of the results are presented in papers at the Annual meetings of the Dt. Ges. f. Biomed. Tech.

F. Damage of blood cells by blood flow itself:

>    damage by shear stresses, mocrorheology of haemolysis
>    and thrombosis.

G. Biotechnique of the respiration.

H. Urodynamics:

>    artificial ureter and substitution of the peristaltic transport
>    phenomena.

J. Measuring techniques.

K. Education:

>    methods of educating young people, courses for students;
>    also the cooperative education of medical and engineering
>    people.

All these questions need the cooperation of medical and engineering
people. Success can be expected only by a reciprocal action of both
parts; an interdisciplinary communication is necessary. Whereas the
doctor tries to find the correct diagnosis and the best way to therapy
mainly from his profound knowledge of phenomena at work within the
human body, the engineer tries to compare the analogous elements in
different phenomena, to find out common features and on this basis
to apply in practical medicine the methods of physical sciences. It is
not necessary to expess that this approach has serious limits, which
result from the very different boundary conditions in the animated and
unanimate nature. Because it is nearly impossible to copy the natural
systems, in other words, because we are unable to duplicate all the
initial and boundary conditions and all the secondary actions, which
are occurring in nature, it is mandatory to study the principal features
which are securing the physiological effects. In order to illuminate the
principle of engineering aspects in our branch, I would like to choose
one example only; and I hope you will agree, when I tell you somewhat
about one part of our special work in the fluid dynamics aspects.

One of the important questions is: what happens with the erythrocytes
in the streaming blood? The blood cells are elastically deformable
208

structures of a very small size; because their density is not much different from that of the carrier-fluid, the plasma, they comply easily to the local movement of the plasma. Here however the considered fluid elements must be of the order of magnitude of the erythrocyte-size. For the deformation of such elastic particles the stresses, the particles are exposed to, are chiefly responsible. Since Newton they are described by the relation

$$\tau = \eta \, \frac{du}{dy} \, ,$$

for laminar flow, that means they are bounded to the velocity gradient normal to the local main flow, or (naturally) by a corresponding law of a rheological fluid. So it is necessary to know the flow pattern, to recognize where are the regions of a high speed, stagnation regions, vortex formations and so on.

The differential equations of the fluid dynamics are so complicated, that no exact solution can be given. When we write the variables in a dimensionfree form, we are able to derive characteristic dimension-free numbers, which are determining the physical behaviour. If we gain the dimensionfree laws, for instance by experiments, than we will be able to transfer these results to our special case. This method is called the similarity method; and this is the base of the model test method, but its application needs a longer practical experience. The best known parameter is the Reynolds number, representing the ratio of the inertial force acting on a volume element of the fluid.

## 2. Artificial heart valves

In the following I should like to show some results concerning flow behaviour in artificial heart valves; and here I must restrict myself to the ball prosthesis. I believe that from all organ substitutes the artificial heart valve is the best investigated one; on the other hand it presents the danger of haemolysis under critical circumstances.

Using the similarity method we are able to observe the flow pattern in
a _water_-stream with __bigger__ poppets than in the reality, and we can
measure the pressure losses in an air stream[2)3)]. Fig. 1 is to show

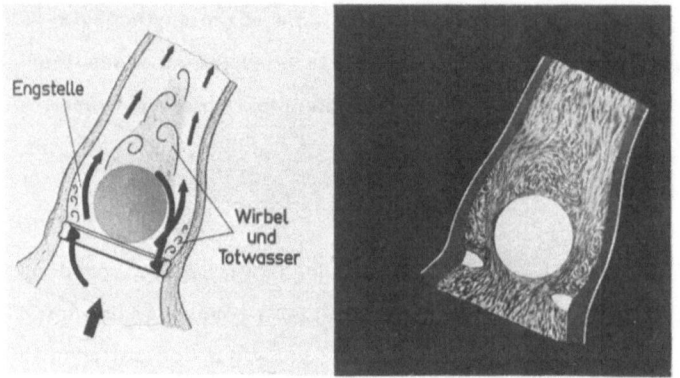

Fig. 1

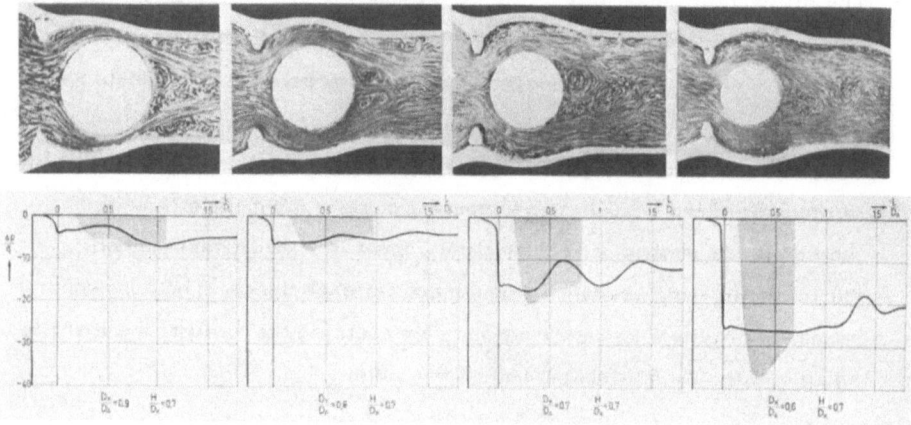

Fig. 2 : Smeloff-Cutter valve. The influence of the ball size on the
flow pattern and the pressure loss.

2) C. Kramer, A. Naumann, W. Bleifeld, S. Effert, Thoraxchir.,
   Vasc. Chir. 16 (1968) p. 269.

3) A. Naumann, Klin. Wochenschr. 53 (1975) p. 1007.

the principle. The vortices behind the sphere, the separation downstream on the aortic wall, and – this is important – the wakes behind
the valve ring can be seen; this is an important site for thrombogenesis. The critical places for the sedimentation of the erythrocytes
are not the wakes themselves, as often said, but the places of stagnation, i.e. where small velocities are occurring in the neighbour-
hood of stagnation points. Fig. 2 shows – again as an example – the
Smeloff-Cutter valve, and the influence of the ball size. We realize
the great effect of the size made visible by the wake sizes, the amount
of local speed and the secondary effects at the aortic wall as well as
the separation behind the ring. This wake formation can be prevented
by a simple collar giving a guidance to the streamlines. In the lower
part of the figure the measured pressure courses along the aortic wall
are plotted; the pressure drop at the right end is the effective pressure
loss (in the medical literature "pressure gradient"). These losses are
summarized in Fig. 3; the abscissa is the poppet diameter $D_K$ related

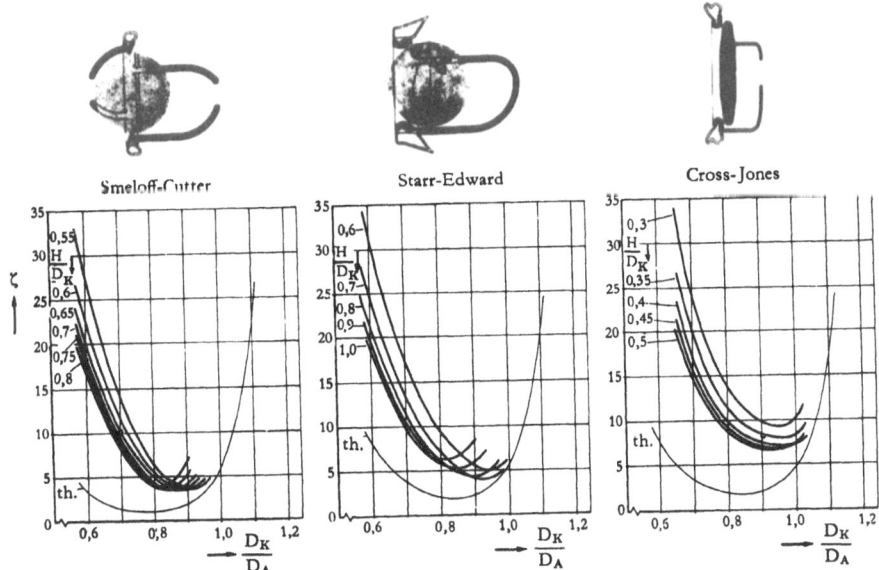

Fig. 3: The pressure loss of heart valves

211

to the aortic diameter $D_A$, the ordinate is the total pressure loss related to the cinetic energy of the flow in the aorta. Parameter is the stroke H of the ball, related to the ball size. We recognize the great influence of the size on the losses and thereby on the mechanical performance of the heart.

It may be of interest to take a look at the mitral valve as an example of the influence of the boundary downstream. Whereas the aortic valve is located in the inlet of a tube, the mitral valve opens into an enlarged and enlarging space, the ventricle. Besides this the wall is expanding during the inflow, producing a velocity component normal to the wall. This must be simulated in the model test. We did not do this by moving the wall, but by perforating the wall of the ventricle model and by suction from outside. Two significantly different flow patterns are occurring (Fig. 4). At a small gap between the ball and the ring the flow

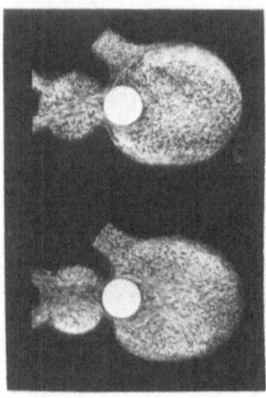

Fig. 4

Starr-Edwards valves as mitral valves.
$D_K/D_o = 0.75$

above $H/D_K = 0.5$

below $H/D_K = 0.4$

is adjacent to the ball wall a long way downstream; at a wider gap the flow separates from the ball and is adjacent to the wall of the collar or the ventricle. The transition occurs unsteadily and suddenly, depending on the ratio of the gap width to the curvature radius of boundaries. These phenomena can be explained by means of the Coanda effect, which is well known in technical problems. In our case this effect becomes of interest for the washing of the ventricle wall, which means avoiding the danger of erythrocyte sedimentation.

212

A few words now on the dynamics of the poppets movement. We have measured the time dependent movement, the acceleration and deceleration, the oscillations of the balls and their end position during the systole[4]. It is not possible to go into details here; sufficient to say the following: The acceleration of an aortic valve ball during the systole reaches values as high as sixty g's, and the striking speed into the cage can be in the order of 1 m/sec. And nearly in all cases the ball does not reach its designed end position. This particularly occurs in the pendulum valves such as the Björk-Shiley or the Lillehey-Kaster valves; this effect is caused by the flow forces on the poppet. It is hoped to overcome this difficulty by a changed flap form, designed according to the aerodynamic laws for the airfoils.

### 3. Influence of fluid dynamics on haemolysis

The first question, we have been confronted with, was to study whether or not the flow itself is able to destroy red blood cells. To this end we used various special equipments. The blood was periodically pumped through disks with a central hole of different diameters (orifices) or through perforated disks; the rate of haemolysis was measured as free haemoglobin concentration in the blood plasma (mg haemoglobin/100 $cm^2$ plasma). The results disclosed a strong effect, i.e. a high release of haemoglobin from the cells into the plasma. Details on the methods and results may be found in the literature[5].

One of the characteristic results is summarized in Fig. 5. The increase of plasma haemoglobin $\Delta PHb$ is plotted against the dimension-free pressure drop $\zeta$ over the stenosis [ $\Delta p$/stagnation pressure of the flow] for 5000 working cycles, corresponding to a heart action of nearly 3 hours. The dimensionless pressure drop is chosen in order to characterize the fluid dynamics behaviour. Without going into details it is shown that the haemoglobin increase in the plasma is considerable at increasing pressure loss coefficients. At small disturbances $\zeta$ no

---

4) J. Köhler, doct. thesis Aachen 1978
5) C. Kramer, W. Bleifeld, H. Pelzer, Acta Medicotechn. 18 (1970) p. 10
   C. Kramer, Habil. thesis Aachen 1973. See also ref. 1) und 3).

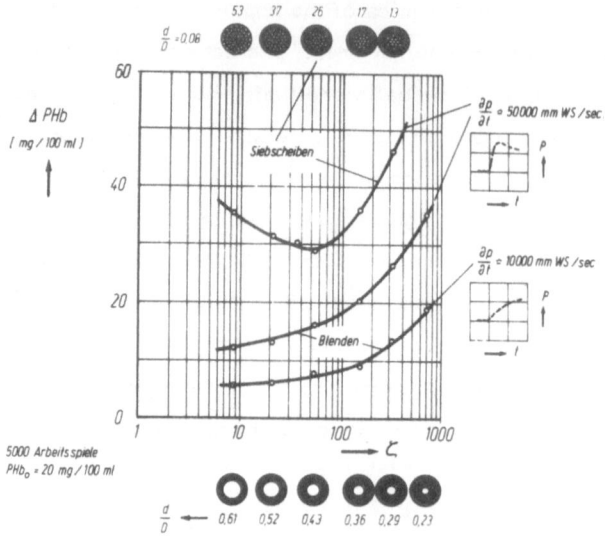

Fig. 5: Haemoglobin increase at orifices (Blenden) and perforated discs (Siebscheiben) vers. dimensionfree pressure loss for 5000 cycles.

danger of haemolysis arises; this corresponds to the fact that the flow cannot induce haemolysis in physiological conditions. The diagram indicates two essential and interesting features. A comparison between the orifice and the perforated disk confirms that the drag itself is not responsible for the haemolysis rate but rather the mechanism of the drag. Additionaly the results show a very great and unexpected increase of the released haemoglobin at increasing steepness of the oncoming wave $(\frac{\partial p}{\partial t})$. The first influence can be easily explained by the mixing process downstream of the obstacles. The second influence was tested in long series, using different forms of pulse waves. As one example this increase is plotted in Fig. 6; parameter is the pressure loss.

It is considered that destruction of erythrocytes occurs, when the shear stress, the erythrocytes are exposed to, exceeds a certain critical amount. The existence of such a critical value is physically plausible and significant, because the dilation and the disruption of the membrane

214

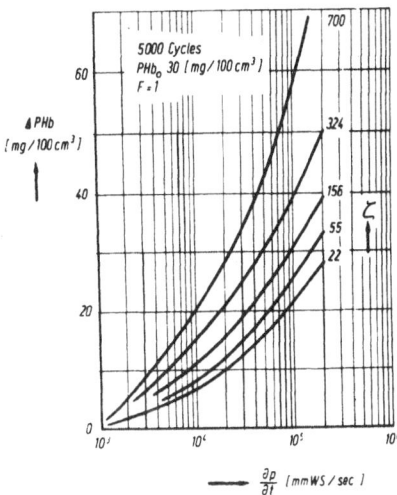

Fig. 6

The haemolysis increase caused by the steepness of the pulse wave.

requires a certain amount of external force. But till now we do not know exactly the relationship between shear stress and tearing tension. The critical value is mostly assumed to be $\tau = 1500$ to $2000$ dynes/cm$^2$; it has been measured by several authors using rotational viscosimeters. According to this test methods however, this value can be valid for laminar flow only, because the Couette-flow corresponds to a solution of the laminar differential equation only.

We do not know either whether the shear stresses in turbulent flow – or better the tangential forces caused by turbulent fluctuations – produce an analogous effect as the Newtonian shearstress. It must be expected that if at all the damage must depend on the structure of the turbulence. Homogeneous turbulence in the classical sense cannot be expected in the blood circuit because the turbulence needs a certain length for its development which does not exist in the arteries. In the tube inlet, at arterial branchings as well as behind an obtacle (stenosis) or prostheses etc. the separated discontinuity surface rolls up into vortices. There are two systems of vortex formation. Beyond a moderate Reynolds number dependent on the shape of the edge periodic small vortices are formed; they are drawn into the big vortex which surrounds the wake, the so-called dead water. One must start from the assumption

215

that the rolling up into small vortices takes place from laminar stream-lines within the discontinuity layer so that these vortices have bended streamlines of a laminar character. The red blood corpuscles are swimming within laminar stream; they are exposed to laminar stresses. With regard to the tiny dimensions of the erythrocytes it must be stated that vortices are not equivalent to turbulence. On the other hand these small vortices can exhibit a considerably high, locally limited circu-lation at a small diameter; therefore they could have an essential signi-ficance for the damage of the blood cells.

Summarizing these views: in the big arteries and veins, bifurcations as well as in artificial organs, vessel prostheses or stenoses neither a fully developed laminar flow nor a homogeneous turbulence occurs, there exists rather a disturbed flow with embedded vortices.

But there is another very important problem – in my opinion more im-portant than the question turbulent or laminar; namely the extent of the shear stress, which becomes critical for haemolysis, which also de-pends on the ecposure time of erythrocytes to shear stress. In most experiments this duration was in the order of minutes. But in our body the erythrocytes are mostly exposed to higher shear stresses, how-ever for very short periods only. It can be estimated that this ex-posure time lies within one thousandst and perhaps one hundredst of a second; regarding this question relatively little work has been done (e. g. Williams; E. Richardson; Coakley; Roshke, Leverett). It is known that the critical shear stress increases considerably for such small durations.

So we used a new method, which has been described in the doctoral thesis of my former coworker Lambert[6]. We could reach exposure times in the range of $10^{-5}$ to $10^{-2}$ secs. at laminar shear stresses near the wall as high as 80 000 dynes/cm$^2$. The erythrocytes (here fresh human blood given by the test person during the test) are suspended in a solution of Dextran in saline, which flows through a micro-channel

---

6) J. Lambert, doct. thesis Aachen 1976.
  J. Lambert, A. Naumann, 3rd Ann. Meeting ESAO London 1976.

(300 μm × 1000 μm × 100 μm) with a parabolic velocity profile. The channel was mounted on the stage of a microscope. The erythrocytes are
stretched to a spindle-like shape when an adequate high shear stress
is reached, as it has been shown by Schmid-Schönbein for small shear
stresses. From the contour of the deformed cells, taken from pictures
the cell content   could be approximately determined. The cell volume I
exhibits a linear dependence on the product of shear stress $\tau$ and the
square root of the exposure time $t_B$:

$$I \sim \tau \sqrt{t_B} \; .$$

It may be related to the paper given by Dr. Lambert at this symposium.
This parameter seems to be the essential haemolysis parameter, at
least for a short duration, even though we do not know till now its
dimensionfree description.

There arises another problem; but this is not a fluid dynamics problem.
We know that the physiological haemoglobin release from RBC is in the
order of 6400 mg per day; but we also know that the human body is able
to digest a higher amount of free haemoglobin, if released. But almost
nothing is exactly known on the total amount of free haemoglobin
which can be tolerated by our body. From animal experiments Bernstein and Blackshear made a somewhat risky extrapolation to the human body, namely that the free haemoglobin in the plasma can reach the
maximum amount of 0, 1 mg Hb per min and per kp body weight. E. G. a
man of 60 kp would be able to tolerate up to 8600 mg each day. Therefore the additional nonphysiological rate of haemoglobin would be of
2000 to 2500 mg. This amount of haemoglobin is not reached by the
flow through artificial heart valves, if they are well operating (estimated 200 till 500 mg Hg per day). However if a leakage of the valve
(regurgitation) occurs caused perhaps by a thrombus at the valve ring,
the critical value can be exceeded and become very dangerous. The
rolling blood pump, particularly in a not occluding function or used for
the ultrafiltration which requires a high pressure ratio represents a
very critical element in an extracorporal circulation. A substitute of

217

arterial ramifications can become critical because of the secondary flow
in the branching region. A acting as a stenosis, particularly if it is
sharp-edged, produces easily shear stresses as high as 4000 or 5000
dyn/cm$^2$ and thereby a considerable haemolytic rate.

In the following a list of unsolved problems connected with the sketched
blood flow aspects may be given:

The haemolysis rate and in correlation with it the amount of the critical shear stress are dependent on:

> the loading time, because the critical shear stress is
> depending on the loading time,
> the hardness of the pulse walve,
> the form of the stenosis producing the discontinuity
> surface,
> the age of the erythrocytes,
> the number of passages through the stenosis; can the
> repeated passage through critical zones produce a
> presensibilization of the erythrocytes?
> the state of the coagulation of the cells,
> the atmospheric pressure.
> The connection between the critical shear stress and
> the rupture tension of the membrane is poorly known.
> The influence of haemolysis on the thrombogenesis is
> detected, but not all known; here the formation of
> microthrombi is of a particular interest.
> The flow inside the cells must be important for the cell
> deformation.

## 4. Final remarks

Finally I should like to make a basic remark about the philosophy of
engineering, physical or chemical work in biomedicine. Contrary to
the basic scientific research, which we call the really profound
sciences, the bioengineering, biophysical, biochemical research is
218

not a research in itself. In the actual state of medicine, our work must be directed towards medical application. More than in other disciplines our work is standing in the focal point of public interest. And the public demands for practical success. On the other side the doctors are living more and more in a certain anxiety, not to find the pace to remain in contact and get acquainted with the technical progress, particularly with the invasion, the penetration of physical apparatus or methods; they are perceptive of their significance; but their application brings them sometimes into discord with their medical responsibility. Here perhaps some limits may be seen; and herefrom derives also our duty to provide for an alternate bilateral education. But above all, we must bear in mind that the human relationship doctor – to – patient remains the most important and indispensable feature of medicine.

# 11. Cellular Blood Damage Caused By Foreign Materials: An Engineer's View Of The Problem

J. Olijslager[+], J. Feijen[+], J.C.F. de Jong[*] and
Ch.R.H. Wildevuur[*].


+   Department of Chemical Technology, Twente University
    of Technology, P.O. Box 217, 7500 AE  Enschede, The
    Netherlands.

*   Department of Experimental Surgery, State University
    of Groningen, The Netherlands.

## INTRODUCTION

It is well known that extracorporeal circulation causes damage of the circulating blood. At this moment there is a lack of information about the mechanisms which are involved. In general three factors contribute to the phenomena which are observed. These are the surface properties of the blood contacting materials, the flow conditions in the extracorporeal circuit (ECC) and the blood chemistry.

The interaction between blood and foreign materials has been described before in terms of protein adsorption, activation of the intrinsic coagulation and adhesion, aggregation and release reactions of blood cells (11). Depending on the flow conditions, a convective transport of blood elements and metabolites to and from the surface can be established. In this way activated clotting factors, release products from blood cells and activated cells can rapidly be distributed in the blood. Butruille et al. (7), Turitto et al. (37), Feuerstein et al. (10) and Nyilas et al. (28) studied the adhesion rate of thrombocytes on different surfaces under varying flow conditions. It was concluded that the experimental data can be described by taking into account the enhanced diffusion (compared to Brownian diffusion) as well as the adhesion reaction at the surface.

Shear forces in flowing blood can directly activate or damage blood elements. This has been investigated in well defined _in vitro_ systems by for instance Schmid-Schönbein et al. (32), Blackshear et al. (2), Goldsmith (13) and Williams (40). Few _in vivo_ experiments were carried out to investigate the influence of the material surface properties on the blood damage caused by ECC under identical flow conditions (3, 15, 19).

In this paper we will describe the results of some _in vivo_ experiments with different commercial membrane oxygenators (MO) using dogs. The influence of flow and materials on thrombocyte numbers during ECC has been studied. Also some experiments were carried out with a model of an experimental Couette type MO, developed by Oomens et al. (29). In this MO different materials and different shear stresses can be applied. Finally the bloodcompatibility of both clinically used and experimental MO's is discussed with respect to shear stresses and membrane materials.

MATERIALS AND METHODS

Three different MO's were compared in an _in vivo_ experimental set up (ECC, fig. 1): the Travenol Microporous Teflo Membrane Oxygenator (Teflo MO), the Modulung Membrane

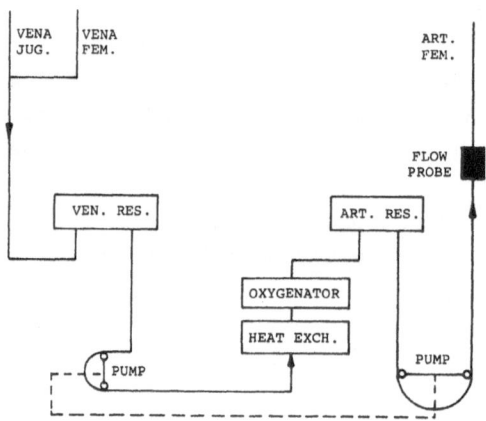

Fig. 1. Schematic presentation of the experimental set-up consisting of PVC tubing, roller pumps, heat exchanger and oxygenator.

Oxygenator (Modulung; Travenol) and a Spiral Coil Membrane
Oxygenator (Kolobow MO; Sci. Med.). Table 1 shows some
characteristics of the different MO's.

Table 1. Characteristics of membrane oxygenators.

| Type | Membrane Material | Surface area $m^2$ | Max. shear rate $sec^{-1}$ |
|------|-------------------|----------------|--------------|
| Teflo MO | porous teflon | 2.25 | 2000 |
| Modulung | silicone rubber | 2.25 | 2000 |
| Kolobow MO | silica free sil. rubber | 2.50 | 5000 |

Mongrel dogs weighing about 30 kg were premedicated with
0.5 mg atropine sulphate and 50 mg pethidine HCl. Anesthesia was effected with sodium pentothiobarbital (30 mg $kg^{-1}$
BW i.v.) and continued with fluothane (Halothane ® ) 0.5%
in a gas mixture of nitrous oxide 4 l $min^{-1}$ and oxygen 2 l
$min^{-1}$ after tracheal intubation. The right femoral artery
and vein and the external jugular vein were cannulated and
connected to an extracorporeal circuit (ECC) in a V-A shunt.
The experimental set-up of the ECC (Fig. 1) was composed
of a PVC tubing system with 2 buffer reservoirs (Travenol
Lab. Int., Deerfield, Ill., USA), two coupled non-occlusive
roller pumps (Dreissen, type Modul pump, Hellevoetsluis,
The Netherlands), a heat exchanger (Travenol Lab. Int.)
and an oxygenator. An extravascular flow probe (E.M.F. Trans-
flow 600, Skalar, Delft, The Netherlands) was included to
maintain a blood flow of 3000 ml.$min^{-1}$ for a period of 2
hours.

The ECC was primed with equal volumes of heparinized
donor blood and gelatin plasma expander (Haemaccel®
The priming volume for the ECC was 2.5-3 l; during perfusion a gas flow of 5-6 l $min^{-1}$ ($O_2$ : $CO_2$ = 95 : 5) was
needed to ensure physiological blood gas levels in the
animal. During the experiments systematic heparinization
was employed (200 IU $kg^{-1}$ BW initially and 100 IU $kg^{-1}$
every hour) and neutralized by protamine chloride ( 2 mg.

kg$^{-1}$ BW) after disconnection of the ECC. Each type of M.O. was tested by perfusing six animals.

Blood samples were taken from an indwelling catheter in the left femoral artery: before cannulation, after 5, 15, 30, 60 and 120 min. during ECC, after 60 and 120 mins. post ECC. By means of vena puncture blood samples were taken daily in the recovery period during the first week, on day 14 and on day 21. Only hematologically normal dogs were used for the experiments. Thrombocytes, leucocytes and erythrocytes were counted with an automatic cell counter (Coulter Counter, Dunstable, England) calibrated for canine blood cells. ADP-induced thrombocytes aggregation was performed by means of an adapted Born technique (5). Bleeding times were determined in the upper hindleg according to a modified method of Borchgrevinck (4). Standard laboratory techniques were used to measure hemoglobin, hematocrit, SRE (39), fibrinogen (22), PT (31), APTT (30), thrombin time (38) and reptilase time (34). Plasma hemoglobin levels were determined by means of the method of Lee Kum Tatt (23). Cellular counts, thrombocyte aggregations, hematocrits and hemoglobin levels are expressed as percentages of the preoperative values. To eliminate the effect of hemodilution caused by the priming of the ECC, cell counts, fibrinogen and plasma hemoglobin levels were corrected for changes in hematocrit on the day of the experiment. For thrombocyte counts under 80.000 $mm^{-3}$ the ADP-induced aggregation was corrected according to a normogram as previously described (18).

Statistical analysis of the results included the Student t-test for 2 means and the paired Student t-test. We will only discuss here platelet count and hemolysis (plasma hemoglobin). The other data will be presented elsewhere (17).

In a second experiment an experimental model of a new type of MO was tested. This model was previously described by Oomens et al. (29) and can be used to impose well defined shear stresses on the passing blood. The Couette type model contains a rotating cylinder in a housing made of stainless steel

The cylinder and the inside housing were coated with RTV silicone rubber (Dow Corning type A, no. 891). Silicone rubber membranes (120 µm; Edwards Lab.) were attached to the housing. Blood is transported between the cylinder and the membranes either by viscous drag building up two thin and stable blood layers (high shear; fig. 2), or by gravity action when the cylinder is not rotated (low shear). Table 2 shows the characteristics for the Couette MO.

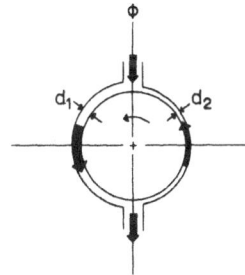

Fig. 2. Cross section of Couette type MO at high shear conditions. $\emptyset$ = blood flow, $d_1$ and $d_2$ are thicknesses of blood films

Table 2. Characteristics of Couette MO

| Shear | Membrane materials | surface area $m^2$ | shear rate $sec^{-1}$ |
|-------|--------------------|--------------------|----------------------|
| low   | silicone rubber    | 0.1                | 0 - 1000             |
| high  | silicone rubber    | 0.1                | 4000 - 5000          |

Mongrel dogs weighing between 20 and 30 kg were given Halothane® anesthesia. After an initial dose of heparine of 300 IU $kg^{-1}$ BW a vena jugularis and a vena femoralis were cannulated (Portex, 5 mm Atrial Cannula, Hythe-Kent, England) and connected to the ECC in a V-V shunt. The ECC (fig. 3) composed of silicone rubber tubing (5 x 8 mm, Talas B.V., Ommen, The Netherlands), flow probe (Trans flow 660, Skalar, Delft, The Netherlands), MO, blood reservoir (silicone rubber), and a roller pump (Dreissen, Hellevoet- sluis, The Netherlands) was flushed with carbon dioxide and primed with saline. During 120 mins of perfusion a blood flow of 400 ml.min$^{-1}$ was established.

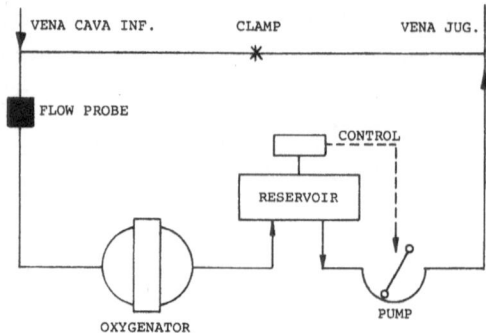

Fig. 3. Schematic presentation of the experimental set-up,
consisting of silicone rubber tubing, Couette type
MO and roller pump.

The MO was internally heated to maintain the blood temperature on 38°C. During the experiment the silicone membranes were exposed to air. After termination of the perfusion an appropriate amount of protamin chloride (Hofman -
La Roche) was administered. The same hematological parameters were followed as in the first experiment. We will
only discuss here platelet count and hemolysis (plasma
hemoglobin). In this series 3 animals were perfused under
high shear and 3 under low shear conditions.

   RESULTS

Although many hematological parameters were measured we
are focussing on thrombocyte behaviour. For all experiments
differences in thrombocyte numbers correspond with differences in thrombocyte function as measured by ADP aggregation (16). Therefore we only present the thrombocyte numbers.
   The results for the three MO's tested are given in fig:s
4 and 5. During perfusion all three MO's show the same performance. When the Teflo MO is compared with the Modulung,

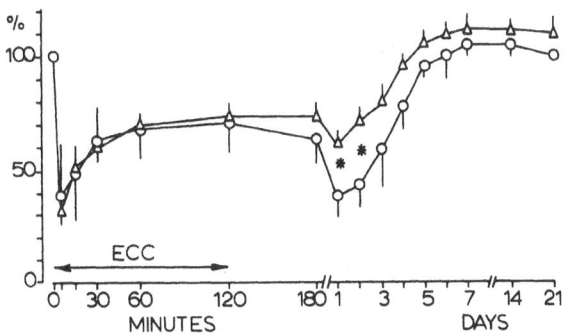

Fig. 4. Mean values and standard errors of the number of
circulating thrombocytes as related to the preoperative values, during and after ECC with a
Teflo MO (Δ) and a Modulung (o).
Statistically significant differences (p< 0.05)
between the groups are indicated with an asterisk.

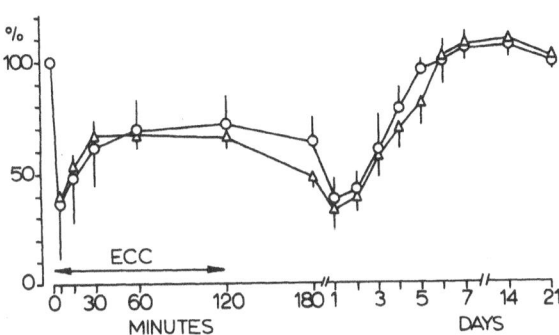

Fig. 5. Mean values and standard errors of the number of
circulating thrombocytes as related to the preoperative values, during and after ECC with a
Modulung (o) and a Kolobow MO (Δ)

significant differences are observed on the first and second post-operative days, the Teflo MO showing higher throm-

bocyte numbers than the Modulung. This difference is also
observed on the following days but is not statistically
significant. When the Modulung is compared with the Kolobow
MO no differences are observed. In all cases plasma hemoglobin levels were not exceeding 20 μ mol.1$^{-1}$.

Fig. 6 shows the thrombocyte numbers for the Couette
type MO. In this case we see differences between low and
high shear conditions during and after termination of perfusion up to the fifth post-operative day. The differences

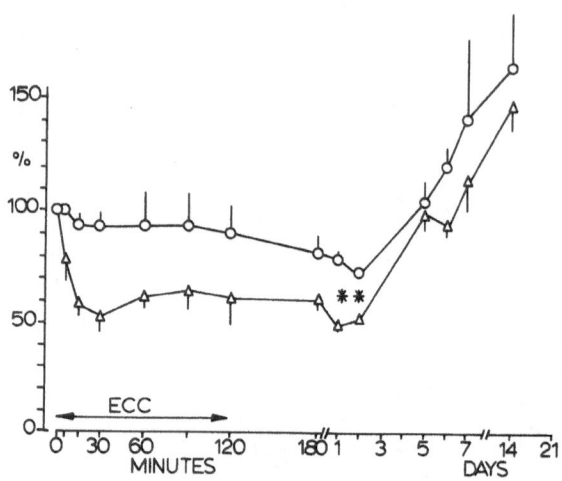

Fig. 6. Mean values and standard errors of the number of
circulating thrombocytes as related to the preoperative values, during and after ECC with a
Couette type MO at high (Δ) and low (o) shear conditions. Statistically significant differences
(p< 0.05) between the groups are marked with an
asterisk.

on the first and second post-operative days are again significant. During perfusion the plasma hemoglobin level at
high shear attained a level of about 100 μ mol.1$^{-1}$.
From the first post-operative day normal levels of about

$2 \mu$ mol.$l^{-1}$ were measured.

## DISCUSSION

Fig. 4 shows that on the first and second post-operative days the use of a Teflo MO leads to better maintained thrombocyte numbers than the Modulung. Those two days can be considered as an indication of the hemocompatibility of an ECC with respect to the thrombocytes. Because the Teflo MO and the Modulung have the same design and were tested in an identical set-up, it can be concluded that the differences in thrombocyte numbers are only due to the application of different membrane materials: Microporous teflon versus silicone rubber. Bloom et al. (3) found that platelet counts during the V-V perfusion of lambs with spiral coil MO's containing ethylcellulose perfluorobutyrate membranes remained higher than during perfusion with spiral coil MO's containing silicone rubber membranes. No significant differences were observed after termination of the perfusion (24 h).

Despite the absence of screens in the blood path and the use of silica free silicone rubber membranes in the Kolobow MO design it can be seen from fig. 5 that the Kolobow MO shows the same performance as the Modulung.

When the Couette type MO at high shear conditions (fig. 6) is compared with the MO's mentioned before (fig.'s 4 and 5) the platelet counts are similar. Despite the small membrane surface area the Couette type MO is almost as traumatic as the much larger clinically used MO's.

Leverett et al. (24) have presented a literature survey on hemolysis as a function of applied shear stress and exposure time in in vitro experiments. It was shown that there is an absolute threshold in the shear stress of about $15 \text{ N m}^{-2}$ for the onset of hemolysis. We have collected literature data on the serotonin release of human thrombocytes as a function of shear stress and exposure time in similar in vitro systems. The results are plotted in fig. 7.

In the area below the line, damage of thrombocytes by fluid dynamical factors is not expected. From fig. 7 it can be seen that for blood exposure times of about 10 seconds, which are common in clinically used MO's, thrombocytes will be activated by shear stresses higher than 20 N m$^{-2}$. For blood this amounts to shear rates of about 7000 sec$^{-1}$.

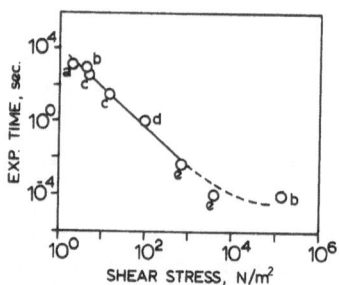

Fig. 7. Serotonin release from human platelets in platelet rich plasma as a function of shear stress and exposure time: a. capillaries (14), b. hemoresistometer, jet (1), c. couette (6), d. capillaries (12) and e. capillaries (9).

In the Kolobow MO and the Couette type MO the maximum shear rates are very close to 7000 sec$^{-1}$. Therefore it is possible that the lower platelet counts observed with the use of these two MO's are due to the occurence of high shear stresses. The Couette type MO shows a relatively high rate of hemolysis. Because direct hemolysis by the shear stresses in the blood is not likely - the shear stress is about 10 times lower than the treshold value of 150 N m$^{-2}$ mentioned by Leverett et al. (24) - we expect that the hemolysis is caused by the seals at both sides of the rotating cylinder. The necessity of seals in MO's which contain rotating systems makes them less attractive with respect to hemocompatibility. Stormorken et al. (35) reported that the occurence of hemolysis influences the

230

behaviour of thrombocytes, which complicates the interpretation of the data.

In view of the data presented in fig. 7 it is quite
surprising that new MO designs with even higher shear
stresses were proposed. In these so called secondary flow
designs, gas transport is improved by breaking up the thin,
highly saturated blood layer adjacent to the membranes.
Table 3 shows a comparison between some experimental
designs of MO's and some clinically used MO's with respect
to the maximum shear rate which can be expected.

Table 3. Shear rates in Membrane Oxygenators

Clinically used

| system | type | max. shear rate, $sec^{-1}$ |
|---|---|---|
| sandwich | Lande, Edwards (21) | $10^3$ |
| enveloppe | Travenol (36) | $2.10^3$ |
| spiral coil | Kolobow (19) | $5.10^3$ |

Experimental

| system | type | max. shear rate, $sec^{-1}$ |
|---|---|---|
| toroidal (Taylor mixing) | Drinker (26) | $10^4$ |
| oxford (pulsatile flow) | Bellhouse (27) | $2.10^3$ |
| double capillary (pulsatile flow) | Clevert (8) | $2.10^3$ |
| annular (Taylor mixing) | Gaylor (33) | $10^5$ |
| annular (shear mixing) | Oomens (29) | $2.10^4$ |

It can be seen that except for the Bellhouse and the
Clevert MO's, the experimental designs apply shear rates
beyond the already mentioned critical level, of 7000 $sec^{-1}$.
This implies that these designs are less attractive with

respect to hemocompatibility.

When shear stresses are well below the critical level of direct mechanical damage of the blood elements, the membrane materials will dominate in the cause of blood trauma. As mentioned in the introduction, flow conditions are then most important with respect to the transport phenomena (11, 7, 37, 10, 28). In this case it is worthwile to improve the hemocompatibility of membrane materials which are used in MO's. The following possibilities are under investigation:

A thin layer of a new blood compatible material on a microporous support e.g. Bloom et al. (3) used ethylcellulose perfluorobutyrate on Celgard ®.

A non-thrombogenic coating on non-porous materials, which have a high oxygen and carbon dioxide permeability e.g. Lagergren et al. (20) and Hagler (15) have coated silicone rubber with heparin complexes.

Controlled release of blood protecting agents from the material surfaces. This possibility looks promising especially for short term applications. The function of blood cells can be locally inhibited at the wall where the concentration of the protecting agent will be highest. Some prostaglandines are very promising and might find an application in clinically used MO's (25).

ACKNOWLEDGMENT.


We want to thank the members of the group of Experimental Surgery of the University of Groningen for their assistance in carrying out the experiments, **Mrs. Bergsma** for typing the manuscript and Mr. Arends for drawing the pictures.

1. Bernstein, E.F., U. Marzec, M.D. Clayman, S. Swanson, G. Gilbert Johnston, Platelet function following surface injury and shear stress: adhesion, aggregation release. and factor 3 activity, in: Annals of the New York Academy of Sciences vol. 283, ed: L. Vroman, E.F. Leonard, New York Academy of Sciences, New York (1977).
2. Blackshear, jr. P.L., R.J. Forstrom, F.D. Dorman, G.O. Voss, Effect of flow on cells near walls, Federation Proceedings 30 (5), 1600 (1971).
3. Bloom, S.R., M.T. Snider, R. Peterson, T.R. Wonders, W.M. Zapol. Platelet lifespan and gas exchange during perfusion with spiral coil membrane lungs coated with ethylcellulose perfluorobutyrate, Trans. Amer. Soc. Artif. Int. Organs, 22, 119 (1976).
4. Borchgrevinck, C.F. and B.A. Waaler, The secondary bleeding time - A method for the differentation of hemorrhagic diseases, Clin. Chim. Acta, 6, 538 (1961).
5. Born, G.V.R., Aggregation of blood platelets by adenosine diphosphate and its reversal, Nature 194, 927 (1962).
6. Brown, C.H., R.F. Lemuth, J.D. Hellums, L.B. Leverett, C.P. Alfrey, Response of human platelets to shear stress, Trans. Amer. Soc. Artif. Int. Organs 21, 25 (1975).
7. Butruille, Y.A., E.F. Leonard and R.S. Litwak, Platelet interactions and non-adhesive encounters on biomaterials, Trans. Amer. Soc. Artif. Int. Organs, 21, 609 (1975).
8. Clevert, H.D., R. Mohnhaupt, K. Affeld, F. Wallner, E.S. Bucherl, The double capillary oxygenator, Trans. Amer. Soc. Artif. Int. Organs 18, 391 (1972).
9. Colantuoni, G., J.D. Hellums, J.L. Moake, C.P. Alfrey, The response of human platelets to shear stress at short exposure times, Trans. Amer. Soc. Artif. Int. Organs 23, 626 (1977).
10. Feuerstein, I.A., J.M. Brophy, J.L. Brash, Platelet-transport and adhesion to reconstituted collagen and artificial surfaces, Trans. Amer. Soc. Artif. Int. Organs 21, 427 (1975).

11. Feijen, J., Thrombogenesis caused by blood-foreign sur-
    face interaction, in Artificial Organs, Proceedings
    of a siminar on the clinical applications of membrane
    oxygenators and sorbent-based systems, R.N. Kenedi,
    J.M. Courtney, J.P.S. Gaylor and T. Gilchrist editors
    MacMillan Press Ltd, London 1977, Chapter 26, p. 235.
12. Forst, R., Published in this book.
13. Goldsmith, H.L., The effect of flow and fluid mechanical
    stress on red cells and platelets, Trans. Amer. Soc.
    Artif. Int. Organs 20, 21 (1974).
14. Goldsmith, H.L., J.C. Marlow, S.K. Yu, The effect of
    oscillatory flow on the release reaction and aggre-
    gation of human platelets, Microvascular Res. 11, 335
    (1976).
15. Hagler, H., Study of the blood's interactions with
    heparin bound plastic surfaces, Ph.D. Thesis: Southern
    Methodist University (1975).
16. Jong, J.C.F. de, J.M. Nelems, C.Th. Smit Sibinga,
    Ch.R.H. Wildevuur. The influences of tranexamic acid
    on thrombocytopenia caused by artificial surfaces,
    Trans. Amer. Soc. Artif. Int. Organs 20, 596 (1974).
17. Jong, J.C.F. de, To be published, J. Thor. Cardiovasc.
    Surg.
18. Jong, J.C.F. de, C.Th. Smit Sibinga, Ch.R.H. Wildevuur,
    Platelet behaviour in extra corporeal circulation
    (ECC). in: Artificial Organs, ed. R.M. Kenedi,
    J.M. Courtney, J.D.S. Gaylor, T. Gilchrist, The
    MacMillan Press Ltd., London (1977) p. 27.
19. Kolobow, T., T. Tomlinson, J. Pierce, L. Gattinoni,
    Platelet response to long-term spiral coiled membrane
    lung bypass without heparin using a carbon silicone
    rubber membrane, Trans. Amer. Sic. Artif. Int. Organs
    22, 110 (1976).
20. Lagergren, H., P. Ollson, J. Swedenborg, Inhibited
    platelet adhesion: A non-thrombogenic characteristic
    of a heparin-coated surface, Surgery 75, 643 (1974).
21. Landé, A.J., R.G. Carlsson, R.H. Patterson jr.,
    J. Baxter, C.W. Lillebei, Cardiac surgery with dis-
    posable membrane lungs, Trans. Amer. Soc. Artif. Int.
    Organs 18, 532 (1972).
22. Leclerc, M. and A. Khodabandeh, Micromēthode de dosage
    de fibrinogène plasmatique, Ann. Biol. Chim. (Paris)
    2, 596 (1953).
23. Lee Kum-Tatt and Ai-Mee Ling, Determination of micro
    quantities of haemoglobin in serum, Mikrochim. Akta
    (Wien) 5, 995 (1969).
24. Leverett, L.B. J.D. Hellums, C.P. Alfrey, E.C. Lynch,
    Red blood cell damage by shear stress, Biophysical
    J. 12, 257 (1972).
25. Mc Rea J.C., S.W. Kim, Characterization of controlled
    release of prostaglandin from polymer matrices for
    thrombus prevention, Trans. Amer. Soc. Artif. Int.
    Organs, 24, 746 (1978).

26. Murphy, D.A., K. Norris, M. Martin, The in vitro characteristics of a toroidal flow membrane oxygenator Trans. Amer. Soc. Artif. Int. Organs 17, 337 (1971).

27. Nelems, J.N., B.J. Bellhouse, C.M. Curl, T.I. MacMillan, S.B. MacMurray, Prolonged pulmonary support of new-born lambs with the Oxford membrane oxygenator, Trans. Amer. Soc. Artif. Int. Organs 20, 293 (1974).

28. Nyilas, E., W.A. Morton, D.M. Lederman, T.H. Chin, R.D. Cumming, Interdependence of hemodynamic and surface parameters in thrombosis, Trans. Amer. Soc. Artif. Int. Organs 21, 55 (1975).

29. Oomens, J.M.M., J.E.A. Spaan, A.P.P. Donders, Annular membrane oxygenator with tangential flow, in: Physio-logical and clinical aspects of oxygenator design, ed: S.G. Dawids, H.C. Engell, Elzevier North Holland Biomedical Press (1976).

30. Proctor, R.R. and S.I. Rapaport, The partial thrombo plastin time with kaolin, Am. J. Clin. Path. 36, 212 (1961).

31. Quick, A.J., Hemorrhagic diseases and thrombosis, ed. 2, Philadelphia, 1966, Lea and Febiger, p. 39.

32. Schmid-Schönbein, H., J. v. Gosen, L. Heinich, H.J. Klose, E. Volger, A counter-rotating "rheoscope chamber" for the study of the microrheology of blood-cells aggregation by microscopic observation and microphotometry, Microvascular Res. 6, 366 (1973).

33. Smeby, L.C., The Taylor-vortex membrane oxygenator, in: Artificial Organs, ed. R.M. Kenedi, J.M. Courtney, J.D.S. Gaylor, T. Gilchrist, The MacMillan Press Ltd. London (1977).

34. Soria, J., G. Soria, J. Yver and M. Samana, Temps de reptilase, ètude de la polymerisation de la fibrine en prèsence de reptilase; Coagulation 2, 173 (1969).

35. Stormorken, H., Platelets, thrombosis and hemolysis, Fed. Proc. 30, 1551 (1971).

36. Trudell, L.A. L.I. Friedman, M. Kahvan, P.M. Galetti, P.D. Richardson, Evaluation of a disposable membrane oxygenator, Trans. Amer. Soc. Artif. Int. Organs 18, 538 (1972).

37. Turitto, V.T., H.R. Baumgartner, Platelet deposition on subendothelium exposed to flowing blood: Mathemetical analysis of physical parameters, Trans. Amer. Soc. Artif. Int. Organs 21, 593 (1975).

38. Vermijlen, C., and M. Verstraete, Antithrombin V: Critical evaluation of its assessment and properties, Thromb. Diath. Haemorrh. 5, 267 (1961).

39. Westergren, A., Ergebn. inn Med. Kinderheilk., 26, 577 (1924).

40. Williams, A.R., Shear-induced fragmentation of human erythrocytes, Biorheology 10, 303 (1973).

DISCUSSION          Moderator: Engell

Engell:          You call your paper "Cellular blood damage in-
                 flicted by foreign biopolymer ", but you have
                 worked with oxygenators of different construction
                 as well as of different material. Therefore, you
                 have not only to evaluate the properties of
                 different materials, but you must also take the
                 influence of different shear rates into considera-
                 tion. Your really have tried to disentangle what
                 is due to foreign material and what is due to
                 difference in shear rate. I was beforehand, as
                 you know, a bit skeptical as to whether this was
                 possible. But I think you did very nicely and I
                 invite comments from the audience.

Williams:        I am afraid I must disagree very strongly with
                 regard to that slide you showed on the effect on
                 platelets of hydrodynamic shear stress and time
                 of exposure (see Fig. 7 , page 230, paper presen-
                 ted by Dr. Feijen). My point is that a lot of
                 other data do not fit at all on a relationship
                 like that. Most of my own work, particularly the
                 work I presented earlier, that is, my
                 in vivo production of thrombi using an oscillating
                 wire system, which gave us an exposure time of the
                 order of milli seconds, and the shear stresses
                 were only of the order of 300 dyn/cm$^2$, which is
                 completely off a curve like that. That relation-
                 ship holds both in vitro and in vivo.

Feijen:          We have only taken the data we have seen in the
                 literature and this is all for its worth. If you
                 have other data then we have to change this curve.
                 So I really cannot make any other comment on that.

Olijslager:      I want to say that these data are from the lite-
                 rature, I can also add some that fit this curve.
                 It will change a little bit. I think that yours
                 would also fit. It will be somewhat below but

236

not so much as you state.

Tillmann:   I would like to underline the comment of
Dr. Williams. The data Dr. Feijen presented in
Fig. 7   may be not that important as the measured data of Dr. Williams, because if you look
at the exposure times, they are out of the range
you are interested in. If you look at your plot
you have there exposure times of $10^4$ sec and on
the other hand very short exposure times ($10^{-5}$ sec).
But if you look at the time which is necessary for
a platelet to pass an artificial organ you might
be in the order of 1-10 milliseconds. And I think
this is the exposure time of interest. Therefore,
the measurement data of Dr. Williams are very
important because they give the real critical
threshold.

Engell:   I think what you want to say is, that you have
just indicated the ranges we are working in or
those we will be interested in. Is that true?

Schmid-Schönbein:   I would also like to underline Dr. William's
statement. In the past, for reasons of clarity,
we have looked separately for red cells and for
platelets. Now, we have to put them back together
again. Many data in the literature, I am especially thinking of the work of BAUMGARTNER's
group (BAUMGARTNER et al., Thromb. Diath.
Haemorrh. 18, (1967)) clearly demonstate that
the presence of red cells greatly changes the
platelet behaviour. Firstly, the platelets are
more reactive and secondly, they are more sensitive to increases in shear stress ; this may be
due to either physical or chemical reasons or to
a combination of both.

Motthagy:   A question regarding the oxygenators of
S. GAYLOR and J. OMEN. How do you define the
shear rates in this instrument? How do you compare them with non-rotating oxygenators?

237

| Feijen: | We have of course shear rates which tend to be constant over the whole gap if you have no influence from the laminar flow. So it depends on the influence from the laminar flow on the correct flow which is induced in the device. |
|---|---|
| Motthagy: | You were speaking about the improvement of oxygenators. You were suggesting, for instance, an omission of secondary flow. I would say this might be beneficial for reducing blood trauma but at the expense of gas-exchange capacity. Thus we have to separate the two different aspects of the problem and then aim at an optimum. |
| Feijen: | We have to discuss the requirements for improved gas transfer during the workshop in Groningen. |
| Schmid-Schönbein: | I was very much impressed by your presentation, Dr. Feijen. For intellectual clarification it is necessary to differentiate flow conditions and surface properties. But in real life, obviously these two interact. I believe that if we have a material which is so well designed that it avoids the deposition of just one platelet, it is better than the one which allows this to happen. As we have seen especially from the work of RICHARDSON and MÜLLER-MOHNSSEN and his group this first platelet acts as a landing place for other platelets. This is quite understandable, because however small the deposited platelet, it does affect the flow around it. For example, condensation of flow lines occurs as Dr. Müller-Mohnssen has shown, a flow condition which has great effect on the platelet-platelet interaction. My argument is probably naive, but if we would have a material which has the ideal surface chemistry in molecular terms it could still be insufficient if, for any activated platelet, it provides a potential landing point. That first deposited platelet triggers both the aggregate growth and |

238

possibly an activation of coagulation processes. Dr. Feijen's paper showed very nicely that in our *research* the distinction between surface materials and flow condition is absolutely necessary to understand the processes underlying thrombotic events in artificial organs. The users and/or the biochemists and physiologists interested in blood-trauma will have to tell the design-engineers to construct oxygenators and pumps in such a fashion that both criteria are met: Flow and surfaces should be made as natural "as possible". We are talking about events, which, at least in my opinion, always start near the wall, where we have high shear stresses and where activated materials exhibit important biophysical and biochemical functions. Therefore, in our struggle for the design of non-thrombogenetic internal artificial organs we have to put all these factors together again which, for research purposes, were separated to get clear inside details.

Wildevuur:           I fully agree with Dr. Schmid-Schönbein. I would like to add some more evidence. COOPER demonstrated that even when you use silica-free silicon rubber material which is supposed to have a very smooth surface, it still will contain microbubbles on the surface after it is primed. Only when he performed so-called vacuum priming, which is laborious to do, the microbubbles could be released from the surface. He showed that under these conditions only very little platelet loss was observed as compared to the non-vacuum prime. So, indeed, even microbubbles appeared to be "landing places" for platelets. Also LYMAN believes that it is practically impossible to obtain an absolute smooth surface like endothelium on artificial surfaces. I personally feel that utilization of prostaglandin could contribute more to decrease the platelet aggregation on "landing

239

places" in ECC. When platelet aggregation is inhibited, they are unable to "land" and to aggregate. In this way they will not lose unnecessari-
ly their function in the repeated surface contacts
in ECC.

Feijen:              I fully agree with that, but I think it does not
                     only depend on the landing of platelets. In the
                     earlier presentation we have seen that besides the
                     landing of platelets on the surface there is also
                     the cohesion factor (which was called $K_{pw}$). So
                     there the properties of the materials are coming
                     in again; it might be possible that you have pla-
                     telets landing on the surface but that the sur-
                     face has such a property that the platelets are
                     washed away again with a tangential shear stress.
                     So it depends on the cohesion parameters. But we
                     would like to know what is the cohesion parameter
                     for different surfaces and what influences the
                     cohesion parameters.

Agostoni:            I need more information on hemolysis. We have
                     some experience with long-term extracorporeal
                     oxygenation using a Kolobow membrane and during
                     the priming according to the Kolobow indications;
                     in these conditions hemolysis is practically
                     irrelevant. Can you give me some information about
                     the technique you use in your circuit?

Feijen:              The details can better be given by Olijslager, but
                     I want to say that when you use only the circuit
                     then you don't rotate the cylinder. In this case,
                     the hemolysis is very low. The same experimental
                     setup is used in the higher shears and in the low
                     shear conditions. So in our opinion there are only
                     two possibilities: One is that the shear stress
                     used in the treatment of the blood is inducing
                     hemolysis, the other is that the seals which are
                     placed against the cylinder are actually causing
                     the damage. At this moment, we cannot separate

between the two of them.

Dawids:    I would like to turn myself a little away from
           what we said on design aspects and ask a perhaps
           silly question. We have heard that protein settles
           down on the surfaces and covers them totally.Now,
           my question is, if you have such a covered mem-
           brane what will the difference of the different
           materials be, when you attempt to have, let us
           say, the same physical surface properties in it
           as e.g. Silastic$^R$ and Teflon$^R$?

Feijen:    If I understood your question, you ask me what is
           the influence of the material on the composition
           of the protein layer  on the material. Is that
           your question?

Dawids:    No, my question was: Will you not achieve a si-
           milar surface using different materials when you
           have a protein layer covering it?

Feijen:    No, I don't think so. I think this can also be
           asked to Dr. Hemker. This morning we already have
           indicated that if you adsorb for instance fibri-
           nogen on a hydrophilic surface and compare this
           with the adsorption on a hydrophobic surface then
           the fibrinogen conformation is different in the
           two cases. We have one other major problem. What
           is the relevance of protein adsorption studies
           using one single protein or a mixture of two for
           predicting how the surface will actually be
           looking after contact with plasma. I think, we
           have to carry out more protein adsorption studies
           and in this respect we try  to label proteins in
           our department. When you know the behaviour of
           the labelled proteins you can mix them with plas-
           ma and see how they behave in this mixture. You
           are, of course, familiar with the work of
           VROMAN, who has used immunological studies to
           trace down these effects. I believe  that the
           protein composition on different surfaces is

241

different and also the conformation of these proteins as well as the reversibility of the adsorption. It is well known that if you have hydrophilic materials, in general proteins are exchanged more easily as compared to proteins at hydrophobic surfaces. We have also seen in our laboratory and this work was carried out by the group of Dr. Smolders that even on hydrophobic surfaces when you adsorb albumin you can have a more or less reversible adsorption because lipids can take off albumin from the surface. At the moment we need information about the initial formation of the protein layer also in plasma and we need information about how this layer is changed as a function of time. In general, it can be said that from very complicated mixtures of proteins such as plasma surfaces with different properties will adsorp a different selection of individual proteins. Any one of these proteins, once it has been adsorbed can display different properties depending upon the properties of the surfaces. But in this context, I would like to ask a question. I saw that you are still working with heparin - coated surfaces or polymers on which heparin was adsorbed. Now, if I want to purify activated coagulation factors or antithrombin in my lab what I use are columns in which heparin has been immobilized because clotting factors selectively adsorb on it. So on theoretical basis one could think that what heparin actually does is to collect activated prothrombotic factors at the surface rather than prevent coagulation.

I think, the question is if you pick up the activated factors. First of all, it is known that heparinized surfaces pick up antithrombin III, the heparin analogues do the same. And then you can pick up for instance thrombin. So, if for instance

thrombin is formed at some place, the surface
acts in this way that it picks up thrombin and
possibly other clotting factors and in this way
prevents the formation of clots at the surface.
So, I believe, that we probably have to use a
combination of drugs like prostacyclins  and
maybe heparin.

# 12. MICROMECHANICS OF THE RED CELL IN VISCOMETRIC FLOW

T.M. Fischer, M. Stöhr-Liesen and H. Schmid-Schönbein

## 1. INTRODUCTION

It is known that red cell damage is an undesired phenomenon
in the use of artificial organs. There have been different
experimental approaches to study this phenomenon in vivo
and in vitro. However, there is very little information to
date on the actual events leading to red cell damage. The
method of rheoscopy lends itself for their study since it
allows the observation of cells subjected to quantifiable
shear stresses. Using high spatial and temporal resolution this method has previously supplied basic information
about the mechanical properties of the mammalian red blood
cells. The present report summarizes these studies which
may lead to a better understanding of mechanical haemolysis
as a phenomenon akin to droplet burst.

## 2. THE RHEOSCOPE

Fig. 1 shows a schematic drawing of our instrument - the rheoscope. It consists of a cone-plate-chamber in which a maximum shear rate of about 1200/sec can be achieved. Cone and plate are in counterrotation creating a stationary fluid layer half way between them. If we focus the microscope on red cells in this stationary layer we can observe individual cells for a relative long time. This cone-plate-chamber is adapted to an inverted microscope (diavert, objective 100x, interference contrast, Leitz, FRG). For registration we use stroboscopic illumination (Strobex, Chadwick-Helmuth, Monrovia, Calif., USA) and a high speed movie camera (Locam, up to 500 frames/sec., intermittent transport, Redlake, Santa Clara, Calif., USA).

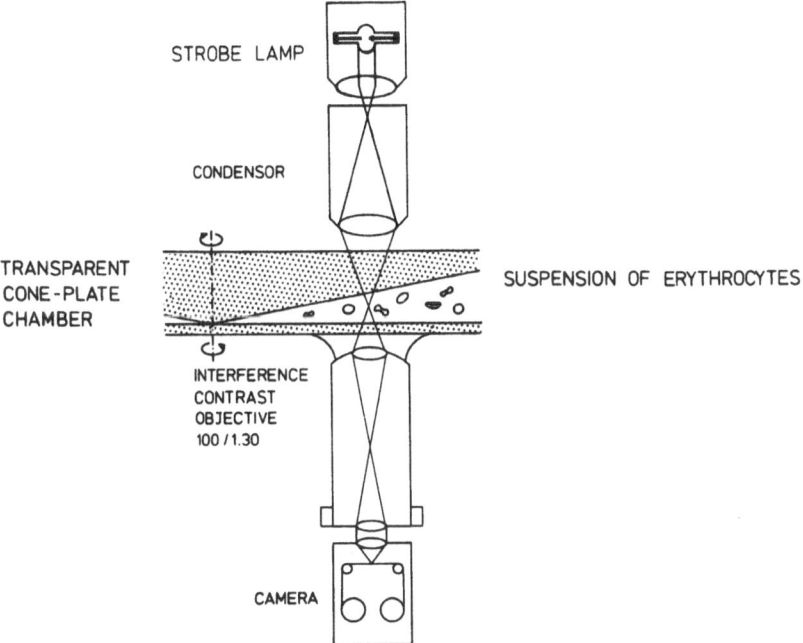

STROBE LAMP

CONDENSOR

TRANSPARENT
CONE-PLATE
CHAMBER

SUSPENSION OF ERYTHROCYTES

INTERFERENCE
CONTRAST
OBJECTIVE
100 / 1.30

CAMERA

Fig. 1: Schematic drawing of the rheoscope (for details see text).

245

## 3. MECHANICAL BEHAVIOR OF RBC  IN SHEAR FLOW

### 3.1. QUALITATIVE RESULTS

Fig. 2 shows whole blood at a shear rate of 940/sec in
the rheoscope. Two effects can be observed:

1. An elongation of the red cells into flat ellipsoidal
   shapes
2. An orientation of these cells with their flat sides
   parallel to cone and plate and their long axis parallel
   to the flow direction.

These effects become more prominent with rising shear rate
and/or rising haematocrit. Because of the predominance of
cell-cell-interactions in the flow of whole blood, the
fluid dynamic boundary conditions for an individual cell
are very complex. In order to simplify  these conditions
we suspended the cells at a low haematocrit in dextran
solutions with about 10 times the plasma viscosity.

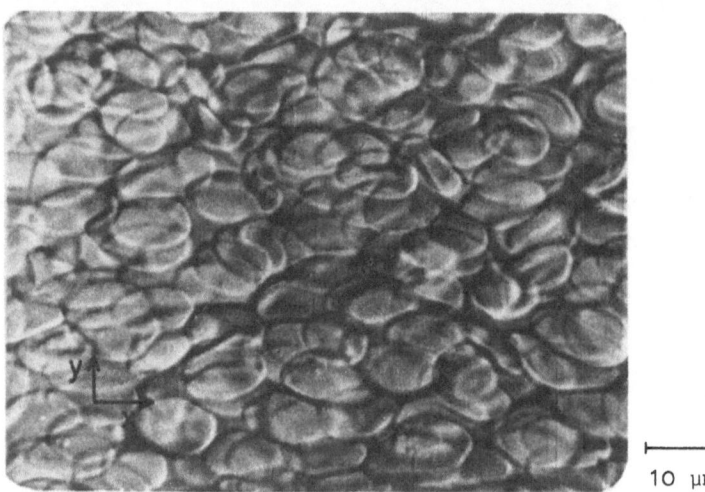

10 µm

Fig. 2:  Whole blood (Hct. 45%) subjected to viscometric
flow ($\dot{\gamma}$ = 940/s). Elongation and orientation of
red cells.

Care was taken to make the dextran solutions as physiologic as possible. The dextran (DX60, Knoll, Ludwigshafen, FRG) was first dialized and freeze-dried in order to eliminate the stomatocytic agents found in the material as supplied by the manufacturer. The dextran was then dissolved in hypotonic phosphate-buffered saline; this is necessary in order to end up with isotonicity of the concentrated dextran solutions. Osmotic pressures of the dextran solutions were adjusted within a 10%-error by measuring the vapour pressure (Dampfdruckosmometer, Knauer, Oberursel, FRG). To prevent crenation of the RBC human albumin (0.1 to 0.3 g per 100 ml) was added to the dextran solutions.

Fig. 3 shows a RBC suspension in a dextran solution of 20 cP subjected to a shear rate of 50/sec in the rheoscope. A steady state orientation and elongation of the cells is seen. The system thus mimicks the two effects observed in whole blood, but in a much more regular way. The dynamic nature of these phenomenona, however, remains hidden because of the uniformity of the membrane and the cytoplasm but it can be made visible by marker particles.

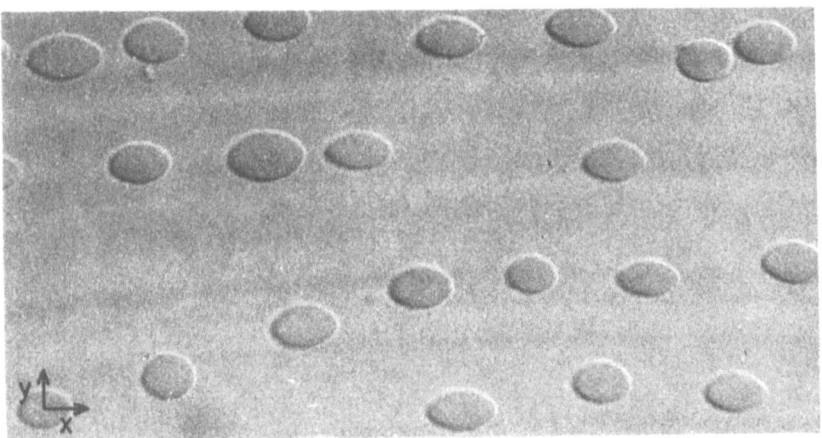

⊢——⊣  10 μm

Fig. 3: RBC (Hct. 1%) in dextran solution (20 cP) subjected to viscometric flow ($\dot{\gamma}$ = 50/s).

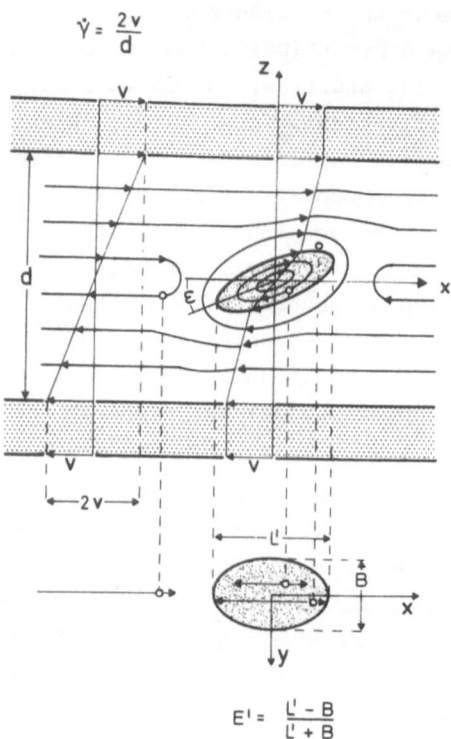

$$\dot{\gamma} = \frac{2v}{d}$$

$$E' = \frac{L' - B}{L' + B}$$

<u>Fig. 4:</u> Schematic drawing in two sections of an elongated
and oriented RBC (mottled) in the shear field of a
viscous solution showing intracellular and extracellular flow lines, a membrane-bound, a cytoplasmic and a freely suspended marker particle (o),
velocity profile of the unperturbed and perturbed
shear field, definition of the apparent shear rate
$\dot{\gamma}$ and of the elongation index E'.

For gaining a three-dimensional interpretation of the
motion of such marker particles which are observed in the
rheoscope in two dimensions only, Fig. 4 schematically
shows the situation in two sections. The plane shear flow
between two parallel plates moving in opposite directions
is perturbed by the presence of a RBC and shear flow is
generated within its cytoplasm. The membrane is driven into

248

a periodic motion around the cell content - the so-called tanktread motion. This can be demonstrated by the motion of Heinz bodies (haemoglobin precipitates produced by incubation of RBC (haematocrit 2.5%) in acetylphenylhydrazine (2 mg/ml) in phosphate-buffered saline at 30°C for 4 hours) adhering to the cytoplasmic side of the membrane. In the rheoscope, not the cross section (x,z) but rather its projection upon the plate (x,y) is seen. The circular motion of a Heinz body on its path around the cell appears in the rheoscope as a back and forth linear motion. Fig. 5 shows this back and forth motion in a photomontage from a motion picture.

The direct visual demonstration of membrane tanktreading of red blood cells in *whole blood* is technically very difficult because of the crowding of cells. We succeeded, however, in filming some sequences. Fig. 6 is a photomontage which shows half a period of the tanktread motion of a cell membrane in whole blood.

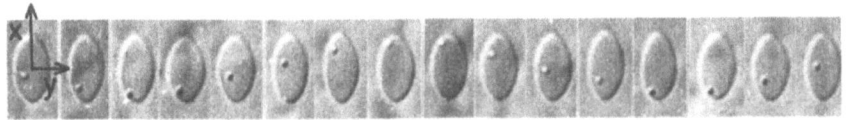

├───────┤  10 μm

Fig. 5: RBC in the shear field ($\dot{\gamma}$ = 46/s) of a dextran
        solution (35 cP). Tanktrading of a membrane-
        bound Heinz body. Photomontage from a motion
        picture (time interval 40 ms).

If, in addition to the membrane-bound Heinz bodies, there are also such ones freely suspended in the cytoplasm, one is able to visualize also the cytoplasmic shear flow. It is evident from Fig. 4 that cytoplasmic Heinz bodies should reverse the direction of their motion before they reach the edge of the cell and that they should have a lower frequency of motion than the membrane-bound ones. This is demonstrated in Fig. 7.

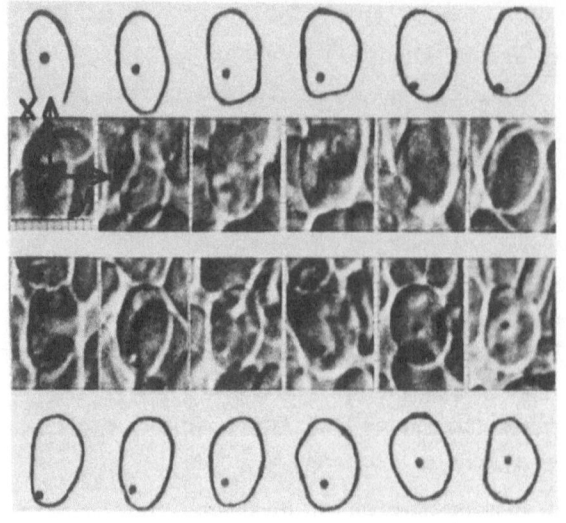

10 µm

Fig. 6: Whole blood (Hct. 45%) subjected to viscometric
flow ($\dot{\gamma}$ = 700/s). Tanktreading of a membrane-bound
Heinz body. Photomontage from a motion picture
(time interval 15ms). Schematic drawings of the
outlines of the cell and positions of the Heinz
body.

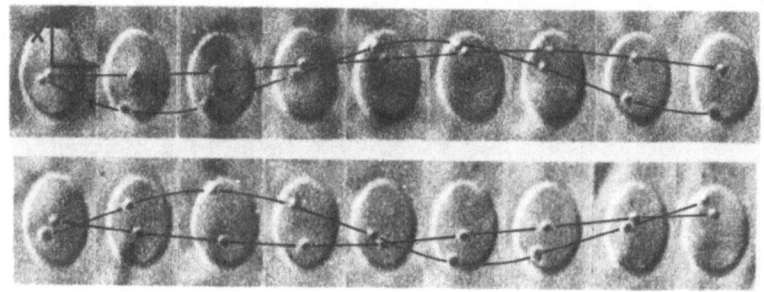

10 µm

Fig. 7: RBC in the shear field ($\dot{\gamma}$ = 22/s) of a dextran
solution (35 cP). Motion of a membrane-bound and
of a cytoplasmic Heinz body. Photomontage from a
motion picture (time interval 120 ms). Heinz
bodies of successive frames are connected by
lines.

250

The Heinz body on the left is a membrane-bound one. It moves with about twice the frequency of the cytoplasmic Heinz body. The membrane-bound Heinz body reverses its motion at the edge of the cell whereas the free one in the cytoplasm does it before reaching this edge.

We studied also the local flow field outside the RBC. We found freely moving Latex spheres which approached the RBC and then turned and moved backwards. The interpretation of this behavior is again given in Fig. 4. There are three different regions of streamlines outside the RBC:

1. closed streamlines around the RBC,
2. open streamlines above and below the RBC,
3. half open streamlines at the leading and the trailing edge of the RBC.

These three streamline regions are bounded by limiting streamlines which end in a stagnation point at the leading and trailing end of the RBC. Fig. 8 shows the motion of a small latex sphere on such a half open streamline. Of course, this observation cannot simply be extrapolated to whole blood, because there, the cells are so crowded. Convective motion of platelets by this mechanism in whole blood might add to platelet motion by diffusion alone such as it occurs in platelet rich plasma.

## 3.2. QUANTITATIVE RESULTS

### 3.2.1. *Elongation Index*

To quantify the elongation of RBC observable in the rheoscope we use the elongation index E' which is defined in Fig. 4. E' varies between $o$ for a circular outline and 1 for a straight line.

Fig. 9 shows the dependence of E' on the shear rate $\dot{\gamma}$ and the dextran viscosity $\eta_o$. The data portrayed result from the analysis of one blood sample. For a constant $\eta_o$, E' increases with $\dot{\gamma}$. When $\dot{\gamma}$ is held constant E' increases with $\eta_o$. To describe this twofold dependency on the

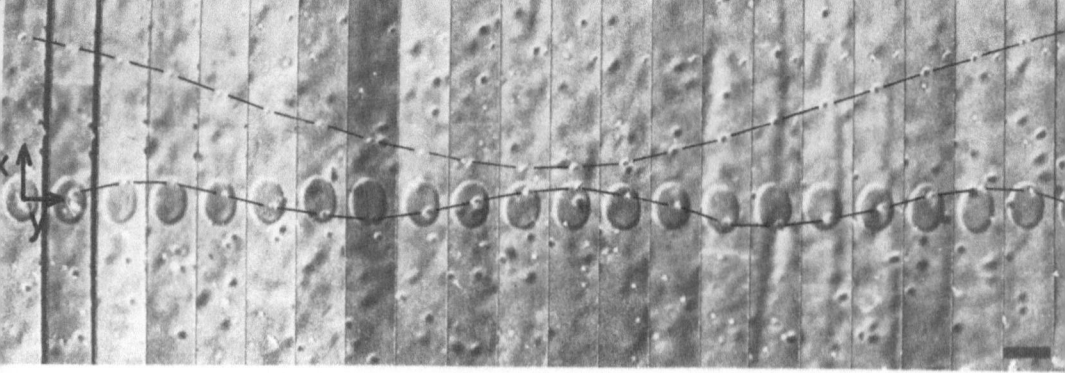

⊢—⊣ 10 μm

Fig. 8: RBC in the shear field ($\dot{\gamma}$ = 22/s) of a dextran
solution (21 cP). Motion of a membrane-bound and
of a freely suspended latex sphere (diameter
0.8 μm). Photomontage from a motion picture
(time interval 160 ms). Latex spheres in succesive
frames are connected by lines.

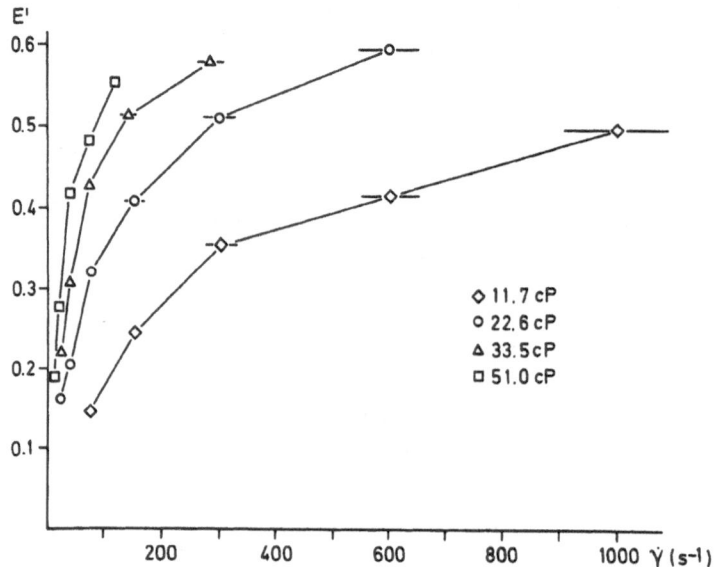

Fig. 9: Elongation index E' (definition see Fig. 4) of RBC
suspended in dextran solutions of different viscosities vs. shear rate $\dot{\gamma}$. Experimental result of one
blood sample. Values are means (n=40) ± SEM.

variable $\eta_o$ and also $\gamma$ as a function of a single variable we tested a combined variable of the form $\eta_o^s \dot{\gamma}$. By fitting the data of 12 blood samples we found within our range of viscosities (10 to 50 cP) and shear rates (3 to 1000/sec) an exponent equal to 1.5 with a standard deviation of 0.2. This means that the viscosity of the suspending medium has a greater influence on the elongation index than the shear rate.

In Fig. 10 the elongation index of all 12 blood samples is plotted versus $\eta_o^{1.5} \dot{\gamma}$. The curve shows for small values of the product a linear increase and levels off for high values. Morris and Williams (1) proposed that the levelling off is due to the build up of isotropic stresses in the membrane. To obtain more evidence for this proposition we made a two parameter curve fitting. Formally, it is the same as the fitting of saturation kinetics according to Michaelis-Menten. The insert in Fig. 11 shows the resulting equation. $E'_{max}$ is the maximum elongation index and K is the value of $\eta_o^{1.5} \dot{\gamma}$ where we have $E'_{max}/2$. The graph in Fig. 11 shows the method for parameter fitting for one blood sample. It is the so-called Hofstee plot. The circles are the experimental points and the dots are representing the corresponding computed regression line. The intercept of the regression line with the ordinate gives $E'_{max}$, K is given by the slope of the regression line and the intercept with the abcissa is proportional to the initial slope of the elongation curve versus the product $\eta_o^{1.5} \dot{\gamma}$ (Fig. 10).

Fig. 12 shows the regression lines of 12 blood samples. There is a wide spread in the intercept at the abscissa whereas the spread of the ordinate intercept is much smaller. This supports the notion that the levelling off of the elongation curve is dominated by the high isotropic modulus of the membrane. For this we have to assume that the ratio of surface area to volume of the RBC does not vary strongly between the different blood samples. The wide range of the abscissa intercepts indicates, however,

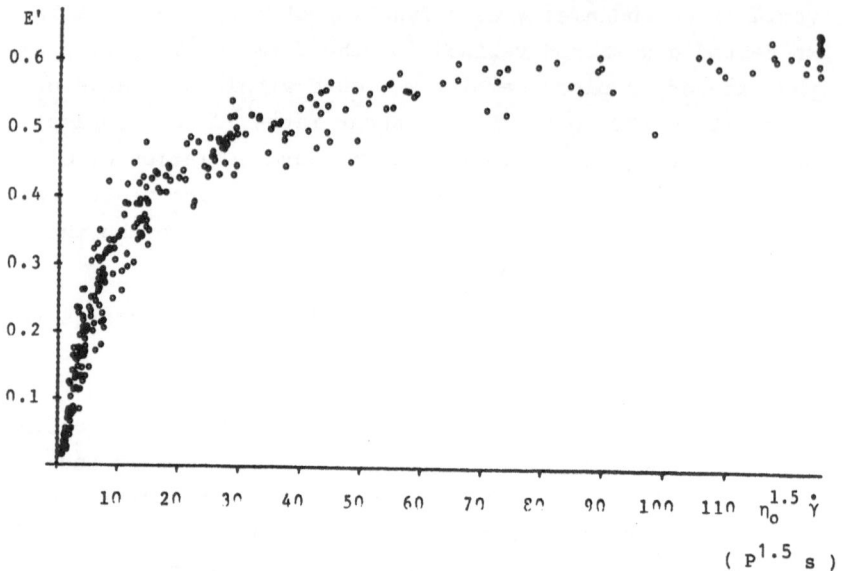

Fig. 10: Elongation index E' versus $\eta_o^{1.5}\dot{\gamma}$ of RBC in
dextran solutions in the viscosity range 10 to
50 cP. Experimental result of 12 blood samples.
Values are means (n = 20 to 40).

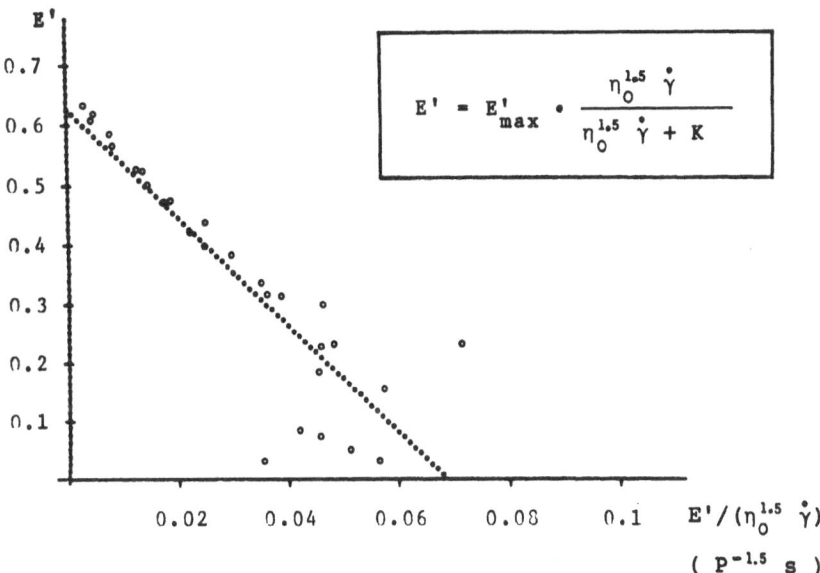

Fig. 11: Determination of $E'_{max}$ and K with the Hofstee-plot. Experimental result (circles) of one blood sample and regression line (dots). The insert shows the two parameter equation to which the data are fitted.

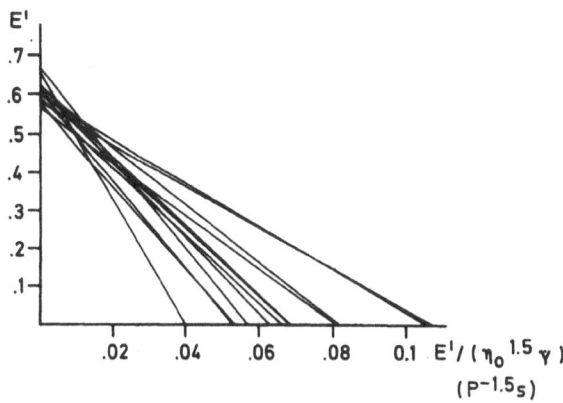

Fig. 12: Regression lines from a Hofstee-plot for 12 different blood samples.

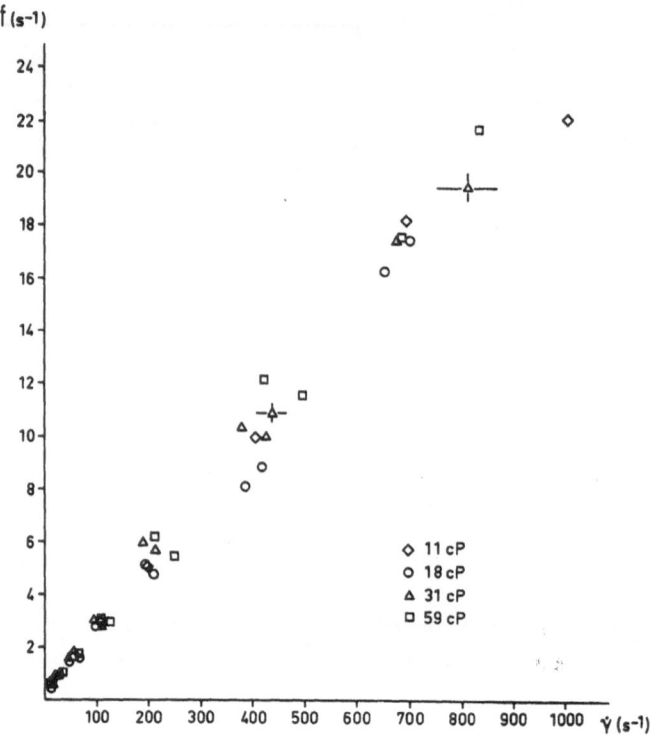

Fig. 13: Tanktread frequency f of RBC suspended in dextran
solutions of different viscosities vs. shear rate
$\dot{\gamma}$. Experimental result of 3 blood samples. Values
are means (n = 5 to 20) ± some representative
SEM.

that there is a big scatter in the membrane shear modulus
for the 12 analyzed blood samples.

### 3.2.2. *Tanktread Frequency*

To quantify the dynamic behavior of RBC in the shear field
we measure the frequency of the tanktred motion (f). Fig.13
shows the data obtained from three blood samples. Within
the measured range of $\eta_o$ and $\dot{\gamma}$ f increases linearly with
the shear rate. The slope of this increase is independent
of the dextran viscosity between 10 and 50 cP.

# 4. DESTRUCTION OF RBC BY SHEAR FORCES

## 4.1. THEORETICAL CONSIDERATIONS

There are two main mechanisms through which RBC can be destroyed mechanically in the shear field:
The first one is yielding of the membrane under isotropic stresses. By this mechanism membrane pores could be opened for potassium, ATP or even haemoglobin without actual fragmentation of the cells. This has been shown by Chien and coworkers under quasi-static conditions, namely for the passage of red cells through small pores. As we heard from Dr. Schmid-Schönbein yesterday there is no experimental evidence for such a process for a cell in an extended shear field.

The second possible mechanism is fatigue of the membrane under alternating bending or shear deformations. Due to tanktreading each membrane element undergoes an alternating load with two load cycles for one cycle of tanktread motion. For fragmentation of red cells, with resulting spheres still containing a high haemoglobin concentration, fatigue and consequent creep of the membrane represent a probable mechanism.

Morris and Williams proposed that the continous bending (1) of the membrane around the tip of the deformed cell is the major fatigue mechanism. Another possibility is fatigue of those membrane structures bearing the two dimensional shear resistance of the membrane. To obtain evidence for this possibility we estimated for a tanktreading cell the energy dissipation in the membrane due to two dimensional membrane shear $\dot{\gamma}_{mem}$ and related it to the energy dissipation in the cytoplasm due to ordinary shear $\dot{\gamma}_{cyt}$. For this calculation we used the intrinsic material constants as found in the literature and the geometric and dynamic parameters as measured in the rheoscope.

The energy dissipation ED in the membrane and cytoplasm per RBC is given by:

$$ED_{cyt} = V \, \eta_{cyt} \dot{\gamma}^2_{cyt}$$

$$ED_{mem} = F \, \eta_{mem} \dot{\gamma}^2_{mem}$$

where F is the surface area and V the volume of a single RBC. From the literature we have:

$$\eta_{cyt} = 9 \text{ cP} \qquad\qquad (2)$$

$$\eta_{mem} = 0.05 \text{ cP cm} \qquad\qquad (3)$$

The cytoplasmic shear rate is approximated by

$$\dot{\gamma}_{cyt} = v/H$$

where $v$ is the linear velocity of the membrane during tanktreading (obtained from analysis of motion pictures) and H is the thickness of the cell in the $z$ direction (estimated indirectly from the surface area and volume of the RBC in question).

The determination of the membrane shear rate $\dot{\gamma}_{mem}$ is detailed in Fig. 14 in the form of an example. The top row shows schematically the silhouette of an elongated RBC in two subsequent states of the tranktread motion (A) and (B), which are a quarter cycle apart. The position of a certain part of the membrane in state (A) and (B) is indicated by a mottled band. The circumference along this band increases from 8 µm in state (A) to 12 µm in state (B). Since the surface area of the membrane remains constant this band becomes narrower when going from state (A) to state (B). Therefore, a samll piece of the membrane which is a square in state (A) becomes a rhomb in state (B). The shear angle $\gamma_{mem}$ between state (A) and (B) can be obtained as indicated in Fig. 14. From this we get as a rough approximation for the membrane shear rate:

$$\dot{\gamma}_{mem} = \gamma_{mem} \cdot 4 \cdot f$$

where f is the tanktread frequency of this cell.

The actual values which may occur in the rheoscope are illustrated in Fig. 15. The first row shows microphotographs of a cell at rest. The second row shows the same cell subjected to different shear rates in the shear field

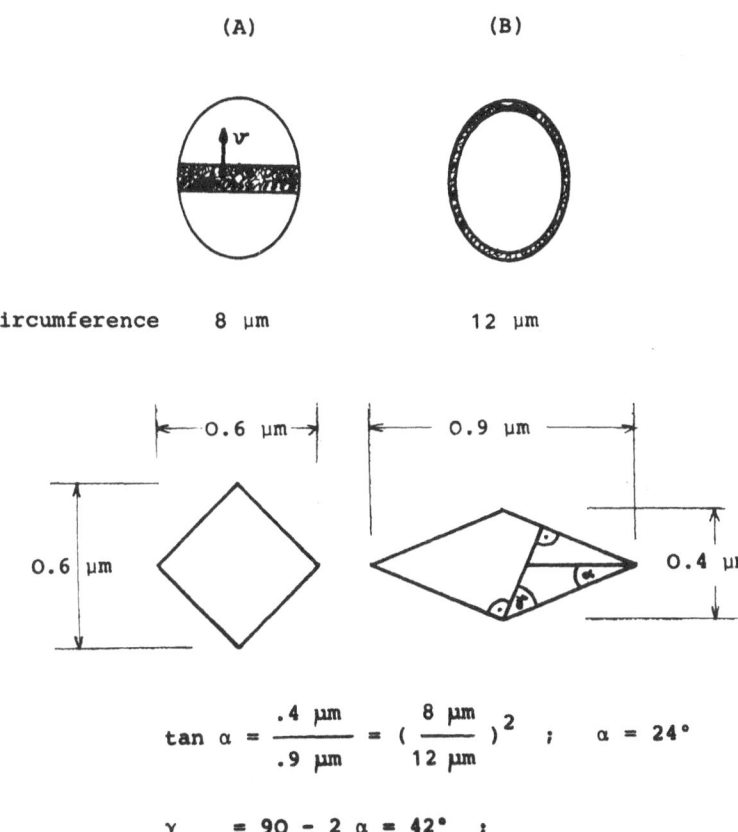

$$\tan \alpha = \frac{.4 \ \mu m}{.9 \ \mu m} = (\frac{8 \ \mu m}{12 \ \mu m})^2 \ ; \quad \alpha = 24°$$

$$\gamma_{mem} = 90 - 2 \alpha = 42° \ ;$$

Fig. 14: Determination of the two dimensional membrane shear angle $\dot{\gamma}_{mem}$ during tanktreading (for details see text).

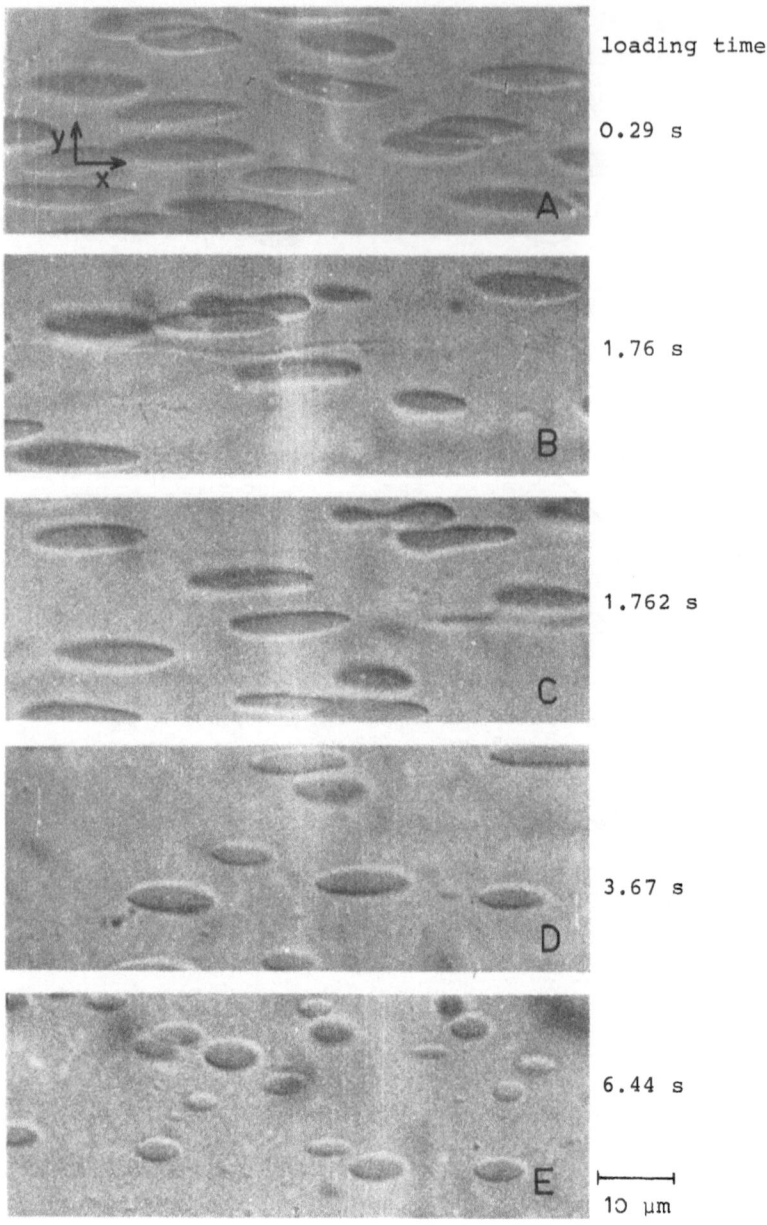

loading time

0.29 s

1.76 s

1.762 s

3.67 s

6.44 s

10 μm

Fig. 16: Red cells in the shear field ($\dot{\gamma}$ = 12090/s) of ⌐
dextran solution (60 cP). Increasing number of
fragments with increasing loading times.

260

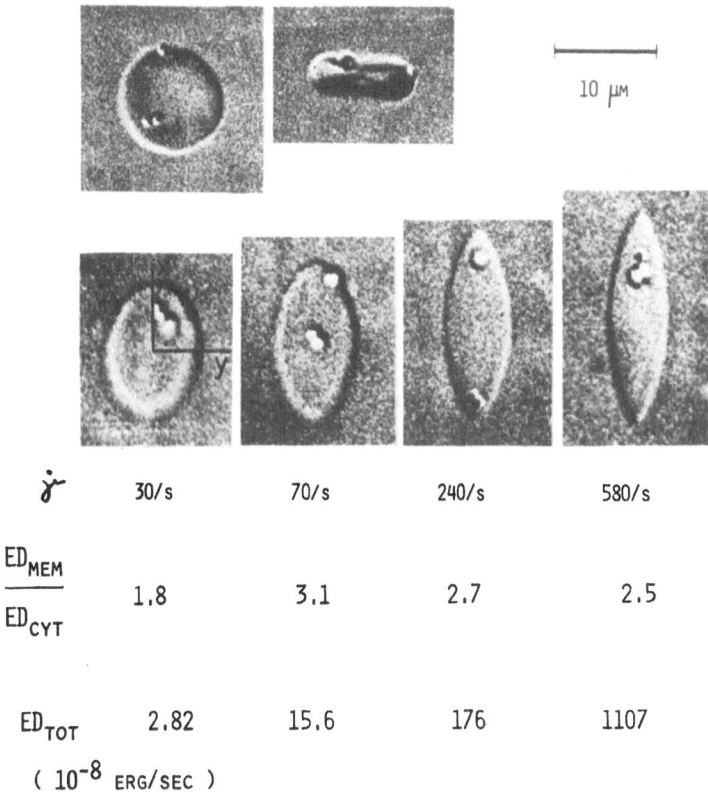

| $\dot{\gamma}$ | 30/s | 70/s | 240/s | 580/s |
|---|---|---|---|---|
| $\dfrac{ED_{MEM}}{ED_{CYT}}$ | 1.8 | 3.1 | 2.7 | 2.5 |
| $ED_{TOT}$ | 2.82 | 15.6 | 176 | 1107 |

( $10^{-8}$ ERG/SEC )

Fig. 15: Microscopic pictures of a single RBC in the rheoscope suspended in a dextran solution (23 cP) at rest (top row) and at different shear rates $\dot{\gamma}$ (second row). Values of the calculated ratio of membrane and cytoplasmic energy dissipation and of the total energy dissipation per cell (for details see text).

of a dextran solution of 23 cP. The shape of the cell
changes from an ellipsoid to a spindle when the shear rate
increases from 30 to 580/sec. We determined the experimental values of F, V, $v$, H and f from the motion pictures
and calculated the energy dissipation in the membrane
$ED_{mem}$ and in the cytoplasm $ED_{cyt}$. The sum of both is the
total energy dissipation $ED_{tot}$ of this RBC (Fig. 15). It
strongly increases with shear rate. The ratio

$$\frac{ED_{mem}}{ED_{cyt}}$$

is essentially independant of $\dot{\gamma}$ with a value of about 2.

This is quite a surprising result because this ratio is
calculated per cell. If the same ratio is calculated per
volume of the respective cell components we end up with
an energy dissipation due to membrane shear which is two
orders of magnitude higher than that due to shear in the
cytoplasm. This indicates that fatigue of the membrane
structures bearing the shear elasticity should not be
excluded from consideration.

## 4.2. EXPERIMENTAL RESULTS

To induce fragmentation of red cells we suspended the RBC
in 60 cP dextran solution. Fig. 16 shows what happened,
when we sheared this suspension with 12000/s. At the beginning the cells showed a very high elongation (Fig. 16A).
Their integrity, however, seemed to be unchanged at least
at the beginning. In the next seconds we saw a progessive
increase of the number of fragments (Fig. 16D,E), Fig. 16
B,C shows how such a fragmentation could occur. It shows
a cell with a central tapering in two subsequent frames,
which are 2 msec apart in time. It is interesting to note
that the cell does not immediately fragment after the
necking down. If the measured linear increase of tanktread frequency with shear rate in Fig. 13 is extrapolated to this shear rate the cell should make approximately
half a cycle of tanktread motion between these two frames.

The fact that the cell does not change its shape during this time interval shows that fragmentation is a slow process compared to tanktreading. This in turn indicates that fragmentation is due to a fatigue mechanism. During shearing the membrane of the cells or fragments respectively still looks very smooth, Fig. 16. However, when we observe the cells during the stop of shear flow the membrane looks different (Fig. 17).

*At first* probably due to the release of the isotropic tension the membrane of these cells or fragments relaxes and shows a crumpled appearance (Fig. 17, second line) indicating that irreversible changes in membrane structure have occured during shear.

*Afterwards* most of the fragments turn into some spheres of varying size (fig. 17, third and fourth line) thus bringing the membrane again under isotropic stress and pulling it smooth.

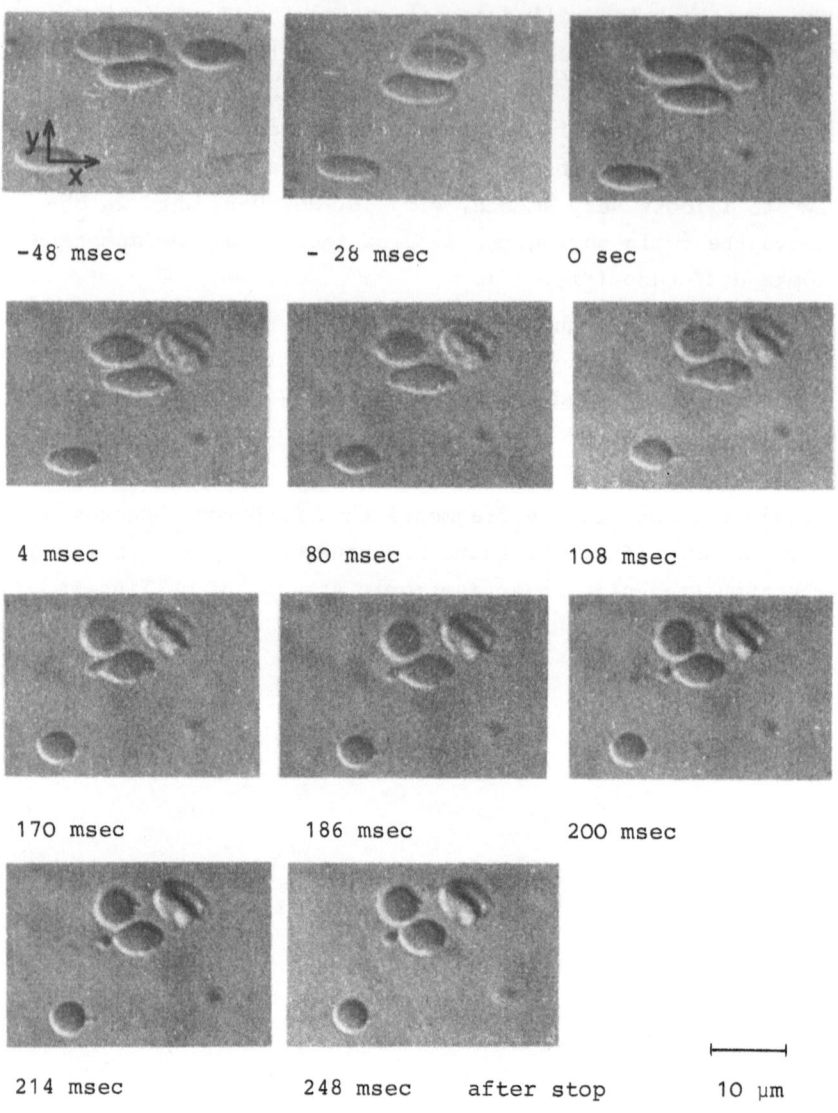

-48 msec       - 28 msec      0 sec

4 msec      80 msec      108 msec

170 msec      186 msec      200 msec

214 msec      248 msec    after stop      10 μm

Fig. 17: Red cells in a dextran solution (60 cP). Stop of
shear flow ($\dot{\gamma}$ = 10260/s) at t = 0 sec after a
loading time of 6 sec. Relaxation of RBC shape
and formation of microspheres.

264

*Acknowledgements:* It is a pleasure to acknowledge
valuable discussions with Dr. P.L. Blackshear, Jr. of the
University of Minnesota, (concerning the problem of membrane versus cytoplasmic energy dissipation) and with
Dr. P.D. Richardson and Dr. S.K.F. Karlsson of the Brown
University (concerning the problem of the external flow
field of the RBC.).

REFERENCES

(1)    Morris, D.R. and Williams, A.R. (1978): Membrane
         Fatigue as a Parameter in Shear induces Lysis of
         Erythrocytes, Biorheology, AICHE Symposion Series
         182, Vol. 74, pp. 27-30.

(2)    Chien, S., (1975): The Red Blood Cell, Vol. II in:
         Surgenor, D. Mac N. (ed.), New York, pp. 1066.

(3)    Hochmuth, R.M., Worthy, P.R., Smith, S. and
         Evans, E.A., (1978): Surface Viscosity of Red Cell
         Membrane, Biorheology, AICHE Symposion Series 182,
         Vol. 74, pp. 1-3.

Moderator: Williams

Deggeler:              I was wondering if collision between cells is
                       causing the fragmentation of the cells. I got
                       this impression and in that case it will be
                       dependent on the concentration of cells, so
                       the moment of fragmentation depends on this
                       concentration.

Fischer:               We have a real low concentration anyway. We
                       don't think that collision does play a role
                       with these cells in the high viscosity dex-
                       tran for the following reason. I showed you
                       a schematic drawing of the flow field around
                       the cell. There are closed streamlines which
                       are going around the cell. This flow pattern
                       separates the cells in the shear field and
                       dampens collisions. I don't think that the
                       membranes of two red cells can touch one another
                       under our conditions because they are separa-
                       ted by layers of the suspending fluid.

Dawids:                Have you measured the release of hemoglobin
                       and been able to correlate this to the frag-
                       mentation?

Fischer:               No, we are not able to do that because the
                       volume, which we fill into the rheoscope, is
                       too small. But I think Dr. Williams can ans-
                       wer this. He and Dr. Morris have studied that.

Williams:              We have been correlating fragmentation with
                       hemolysis and we find that there is reasonable
                       correspondence. If the cells stretch in a
                       shear field and break up, we do get hemoglobin
                       coming out provided that they do not form
                       microspheres. This is why I have some little
                       problems with the interpretation of
                       Dr. Fischer's film. It seemed to give the im-
                       pression that the cells were breaking up to

form these microspheres while still within the shear field. This is not what we find in our work. We use lower shear stresses, lower shear rates and lower viscosity media. We find that cells elongate in the shear field, their membrane tank treads and the cells slowly stretch. As long as you keep absolutely laminar flow conditions, the membrane fatigues and then breaks, releasing the hemoglobin contents of the cell. But the cells do not break up to form microspheres. However, when you remove the shear field, then the cell relaxes and breaks up to form microspheres exactly as you have shown so excellently in that film. However, in your film we apparently saw cells breaking up to form microspheres. I also noticed that the cells did not appear to be in laminar flow. There seemed to be many instabilities present, possibly bubbles, which could result in a transient perturbation of the field. This caused any given cell to oscillate around in the plane of the field. In this case you may have had transient interruptions to the flow field which could have been enough to allow the relaxation phenomenon to occur and permit the red cells to break up to form microspheres.

Fischer:     There are no gas bubbles in our cone-plate chamber at least at that place where we make the observations, because we would see them. Furthermore, we have a laminar flow. What you see as oscillations is probably imposed from the outside by mechanical imperfections of the rheoscope itself (the ball bearings, the cone and so on).

Williams:    It does not matter what the cause is. If you have any small perturbation of the shear field it could be enough to permit this relaxation so that the cells appear to break up while still within the same shear field. When we view cells under shear by means of optical diffraction patterns, we see the cells aligning in a certain direction. The cells maintain that same shape and orientation until the membrane breaks and all of the hemoglobin is released. We can see from the diffraction patterns that we do not get microspheres formed until we remove the shear stress (or transiently interrupt it) when this relaxation phenomenon occurs and enables the cells to fragment.

Fischer: What suspending medium was used - was it plasma?

Williams: No, it was a saline/dextran medium but at a lower viscosity (only 30 cP) than that used in the film.

Schmid-Schönbein: If we accept the red cell as a fluid droplet we should be prepared that there could be two types of droplet burst, one with the formation of microspheres and one without. I am referring to the work done by Mason's group and I think this question is open. As Dr. Fischer has mentioned, we have an upper limit of shear rates in the present rheoscope. Dr. Fischer has constructed a special rheoscope for much higher shear stresses and will go to much higher rates to answer that question.

Fischer: We also tried with lower shear stresses and there we did not get fragmentation. Therefore, I think that if you increase the shear rate in your instrument, or if you increase the viscosity, you should also get fragmentation during shear. My guess is that the break up

268

|  |  |
|---|---|
|  | into spheres in your system and ours is due to the same mechanism. In analyzing your diffraction patterns you must keep in mind that many of these spheres are still connected to each other. We see that, when we observe the fragments microscopically under a low shear flow. |
| Williams: | I agree, we have also seen these chains of microspheres in scanning electron micrographs of cells after they have been taken from the shear field, i.e. looking like a series of beads held together with membrane remnants. |
| Birnbaum: | Do you have any idea whether during the shearing the hematocrit alters? |
| Fischer: | No, I don't. |
| Williams: | Our measurements suggest that it does not alter. We have a technique whereby we pass a laser beam through the entire cell population as it is being sheared. From the resulting diffraction pattern you can work out the dimensions of the cell. Even under shear there is no measurable change in the cell volume, it cannot be seen to increase or decrease, so therefore, we say that the hematocrit remains the same under shear. |
| Birnbaum: | How do you know,whether the liberation of hemoglobin corresponds to the occurrence of microspheres? |
| Williams: | It does not. Because you can get a population of erythrocytes to break up to form microspheres without the concomitant release of much hemoglobin. But, the conditions that you have to subject the cell to must be enough to first "disarrange" its membrane  so that it can form microspheres by this relaxation |

269

process. The mechanical variability within the population is such that the conditions necessary to "disarrange" the membrane of the average cell will have disrupted the most fragile cells which incidentally are the youngest cells within the population and not, as one would expect, the oldest cells. Therefore, you usually get hemolysis of some cells under the conditions where others are only just "altered" so that they could fragment if the shear field is removed or perturbed. But fragmentation itself, at least in our hands, seems to occur with the loss of relatively little hemoglobin.

Schmid-Schönbein: This is not at all surprising; it is known from the biochemist's work by FUHRMANN (G.F. Fuhrmann, Blut 16, 321 (1968)) that one can form microspheres from red cells by suspending them in a 1-3 molar urea solution and the amount of hemoglobin released is surpringly low. In other words the membrane is so constructed that out of one discoid erythrocyte two spheres can be formed and the membrane fuses before too much of the liquid cytoplasma escapes.

Hakim: What do you mean by "fatigue". As a biochemist I would like to know if it is a decrease in erythrocyte ATP and/or a specific membrane damage?

Fischer: I use fatigue in its mechanical sense. Under a constant load which is above the elastic region the cell membrane creeps and shows plastic flow. It does not yield immediately to break but it flows plasticly. Under a cyclic load above a certain limit we also can have irreversible changes of the mechanical properties of the membrane. This in technical language is called fatigue.

Hakim: Could you tell me what are the objective criteria of "fatigue"?

Fischer: We observe in the rheoscope an altered mechanical behaviour of these cells which we
refer to as fatigue since we impose a cyclic
load by tanktreading. I don't know the biochemical reason for this alteration. My guess is,
that the cytoplasmic layer of proteins - the
spectrin - is involved, but I don't know, how.

Williams: I would also agree with that. We seem to be
trying to ascertain what the actual mechanism
of the fatigue process is; my thoughts were
that it is strain at the tip of the stressed
ellipsoid; but, as we have heard from
Dr. Fischer, there are alternative explanations. In any case it would appear to be
that we are putting a strain or a dislocation
upon those factors within the membrane responsible for its architecture. This is presumably the spectrin meshwork. By repeated tension,
flexion or whatever mechanism, the energy of
the shear field is coupled into this so that
you are either breaking cross-links or
causing rearrangement of this structural architecture. This is clearly seen when you
first remove the cells from the shear stress
field, you get "crumpled" cells.
The fact that they are crumpled means that you
have now got portions of that membrane which
have different mechanical properties to other
parts around it. If one assumes that the normal biconcave disc shape of the cell is because
every part of that membrane is exactly the
same, and each part wishes to be as flat as
it can, then we have the nice symmetrical
shape of a biconcave disc. If you induce

271

asymmetry into that membrane, then you will no longer get a nice smooth biconcave shape, you will have a crumpled cell. In this case those portions of the membrane having the least "resistance to bending" will be forced into a high radius of curvature and would form the peaks of the ridges or protrusions from the surface.

We have no mechanism for obtaining detailed information as to what is actually happening within the membrane. We know there must be some structural entity there since the physical properties of the cell (i.e. its ability to resist high shear stresses) cannot be due entirely to a lipid film which would not have great mechanical integrity when subjected to these forces. There must be some physical entity which restrains and constrains the cell and gives rise to its elastic and viscous parameters. These properties cannot be ascribed to the lipid portion of the cell and so must be ascribed to the protein. We do not as yet have enough biochemical information as to what the structural entity within the membrane proteins are, and so it must therefore remain a hypothesis since we do not know how the structure is perturbed by the shear field. Once the biochemists tell us what the structure is, then we will suggest how this structure could be perturbed by the shear forces.

Deggeler:      Did you analyse the lipid bilayer of the membrane and correlate its composition with the behaviour of the cells?

Fischer:       We didn't do any correlation between changes in the lipid bilayer and the mechanical behaviour of red cells. We modified, however,

272

the membrane by SH-reagents thus modifying the proteins and here we get a strongly reduced elongation index of the cells. This reflects - as we interpret it - changes in the shear resistance of the cell membrane which is due to the proteins at the cytoplasmic side of the membrane (spectrin and maybe some others). (T.M. Fischer et al., Biochim. Biophys. Acta 510, 270 (1978)).

Williams:

I would like to go on record as saying that I disagree with that interpretation by Dr. Fischer. I do not disagree with the experimental observations - just the interpretation. In our experience these differences in cell lengths at the same applied stress are more likely to be due to a distribution of internal viscosities within the cell population. Because there is a vast difference in internal viscosity between young red cells and old red cells from the same individual. The cellular distortions seen in the first part of your movie film (in a medium of eleven centipoise at the low velocity gradient of eighty reciprocal seconds) show some cells being quite ellipsoidal whereas others are almost circular in profile. At 11 cP you would expect that some cells would not be distorted because their internal viscosity is higher than that of the suspending medium. Other cells in the same population have internal viscosities of less than 11 cP and so would be distorted. Thus, I propose that we could see the internal viscosity distribution of the population displayed for us in your movie film.

Fischer:

Even if you know that the internal viscosity is increased, you don't know whether this is

the reason for a decreased deformability if
you don't measure the membrane parameters in-
depently. In experiments not reported here,
we compared the theoretical behaviour of liquid droplets with the experimental behaviour
of red blood cells in shear flow. In this
study we came to the conclusion that the viscosity of the cell interior is of minor importance for the mechanical behaviour of the
red cell and that it is mostly the membrane
of the red cell which dominates its behaviour.
This conclusion rests mainly on the opposite
behaviour of liquid droplets and red blood
cells in elongation index as well as in tanktread frequency after a change of the internal
viscosity (T.M. Fischer et al., Biorheology,
AI CH E Symposion Series 182, vol. 74 (1978),
p . 38). The big scatter in the elongation
of cells in the film sequence you are referring to could as well be explained by
different membrane properties.

Schmid-Schönbein:    Before we have an independent control  of the
surface area to volume ratio or non-sphericity
and of the internal viscosity from elongation
alone we are unable to differentiate the reason for abnormal mechanical behaviour of old
and young cells. Would you agree or not?

Williams:    I think we are beginning to degenerate into
an argument getting deeper and deeper into
points which will not be either black or
white but will be somewhat grey and so I have
some points of agreement and some points of
disagreement with you.

Olijslager:    I want to know whether the system that you
are using is comparable to the situation of
whole blood flow. That means that you can
derive a shear stress at which red cells release their content and I am asking you

274

whether you are using whole
blood flow this type of things will happen?

Fischer:
I don't think a quantitative number can be
derived from these experiments, because similar to elongation also in fragmentation
an increase of the viscosity of the suspending medium is more effective than an increase
of the shear rate. Firstly, the dextran solution we used in the fragmentation study had
a viscosity of more than 10 times that of whole
blood. Secondly in whole blood due to the
high hematocrit we have a prevalence of
cell-cell interactions, which are nearly excluded in our system.

Williams:
I agree with that. The shear stress required
to rupture cells in a very low viscosity medium like blood plasma or saline is so large
that you are now coming into a turbulent
regime. All the work that I know of which has
been shearing blood in its own plasma or in
saline, where values have been obtained for
the shear stress needed to rupture the cells,
can be seriously criticised on the grounds
that the shear fields were either turbulent
or at least in a Taylor vortex region. Therefore, the estimates of shear stress and the
estimates of the residence time within that
stress must be somewhat suspect and so the
numbers obtained cannot be given great cre-
dence.

Olijslager:
In designing a new oxygenator, we don't have
to be so careful for the red cells that they
will lyse because of their high shear stress.

Schmid-Schönbein:
We are here investigating a basic mechanism
and we are pushing the shear forces to a point
of rupture. Before that, the cells suffer

275

from what has been called a subhemolytic
damage and we will come back to that after
Dr. Lamberts paper. I think, therefore, that
it is absolutely necessary in the future to
design artificial organs in such a fashion
that high shear stresses must be avoided.

Williams:

I am fully in agreement. In practice one
should attempt to design a pump system so as
to get the applied velocity gradient as low
as possible. Certainly, gradients of the order
of $10^4$ reciprocal seconds ought to be avoided
at all costs.

Kratzer:

Is there any relationship between the behaviour of whole blood, as observed in your
rheoscope, and the dissipation of energy in
the red cell?

Fischer:

For an individual tranktreading erythrocyte
in whole blood, we calculated from its shape
and its measured tanktread frequency a similar
ratio of energy dissipation in the membrane
and cytoplasm as for a single cell in dextran.
It is interesing, however, to go further. We
made a model of the whole suspension ("blood")
and compared it to its measured viscosities.
The result of these very rough estimations is
a theoretical viscosity of 2/3 of the experimental viscosity, which is an adequate coin-
cidence. But more important, it turned out
that there is ten times more energy dissipation in the blood plasma than in the red cells
at a shear rate of 700/s (unpublished).

Kratzer:

Does this explain that suspension viscosity
decreases with increasing shear rate?

Fischer:

The energy dissipation is proportional to the
apparent viscosity and to the shear rate
squared. Therefore, despite of the decreasing

276

viscosity, the overall energy dissipation
increases with increasing shear rate.

# 13. Effect of extracorporeal circulation with different oxygenators on the volume of red blood cells

D. Birnbaum, R. Thom, J. Billich, E. S. Bücherl


Titel zur Veröffentlichung des Vortrages von Stolberg 1978.
Autor: Dr. D. Birnbaum (Ass. Prof.)


Department of Surgery (Director: Prof. Dr. E. S. Bücherl) and
Laboratory of Experimental Haematology (Prof. Dr. R. Thom),
Klinikum Charlottenburg, Free University of Berlin

# 1. INTRODUCTION

Extracorporeal circulatory systems for oxygenation of blood are an important tool of modern heart surgery (1, 10, 17, 18). In addition, those devices became recently applicable for therapeutic assist in patients with pulmonary insufficiency (9, 25).

Many studies are done in concern of oxygenator and capacity function, however the illumination of side effects of those devices became of increasing interest; postperfusional morbidity was at least partly referred to the oxygenators.

The traditional parameter indicating deteriorating effects of those systems is haemolysis, as being determined by rising levels of free haemoglobin in plasma. With the improvements of heart-lung-machines, especially with the advent of membrane oxygenators, this parameter lost of its value to characterise the quality of an extra-corporeal perfusion (8). The clinical experience tought, that maintenance of extracorporeal perfusion with oxygenators is possible for weeks without hazard to patients and without threatening increase of plasma haemoglobin levels. This gave impulses to search for more sensitive parameters that would help to decide wether membrane oxygenation is justified even for short open heart operations.

Shear forces acting on red cells under in vitro conditions lead to alterations of the ion concentrations intra- and extracellularly on the basis of which consecutive volume alterations were hypothesised (15, 16). The direct effects of shear forces upon the volume of the red cell has been demonstrated by the authors: Human erythrocytes, which are exposed to shearing in a Cylinder-Viskosimeter in the range of $20 - 200 \times 10^{-5}$ $N/cm^2$ are subjected to an initial process

of shrinkage followed by a status of swelling (6). These processes
are strictly dependent on shear intensity and duration of exposure.
As long as a certain level of shearing has not been exceeded, these
effects are reversible (6). The increase of the volume of erythrocytes in pure plasma suspensions correlates with the liberation of
LDH, ADP and haemoglobin; of course also the haematocrit increases with the swelling of the cells (7). These findings are in
accordance with the results of others (13).

Assuming analogous shear forces being possibly present within
the blood paths of oxygenators and extracorporeal circulation systems a series of experiments with different oxygenators were performed in dogs by the authors. Gasdispersion oxygenation led to a
distinct volume alteration of the circulating red cells. This effect
was also seen in one out of four different types of membrane oxygenators (5).

On the basis of these experiments we were interested wether volume changes of the red cell population do occur during the open heart
surgery in man and wether there are differences if different oxygenator types are in use. Furthermore the question was raised,
wether cell volume distribution is a worthful parameter to search
for oxygenator side effects and wether possible volume alterations
are in any relation to the postoperative morbidity.


2.  METHODS


This study was undertaken on patients undergoing open heart surgery. The extracorporeal circulations (ECC) were performed by
random using either a gasdispersion oxygenator of the type 6-LF,
TRAVENOL (= group I) or a membrane oxygenator of the type TMO,
TRAVENOL (= group II). Evaluation of the red cells volume and
distribution was done in 30 patients, 15 in each group.

For reasons of the discussion during the seminar in Stolberg
(near Aachen, Germany) in November 1978 the method is described

extensively: The analysis of the mean cell volume of the erythrocyte and the volume distribution was performed by the Particle-Volume-Analyser M5 MP 1 (TELEFUNKEN). This device is a proceeded development of coulters principle. It is distinguished from the original arrangement by removing multiple sources of systemic errors and by an essentially more intense rate of dissolution (23). As shown in figure 1 the transducer allows a hydrodynamic focusing of the cell suspension, which means that all cells form a single file in the axis of the sensing aperture.

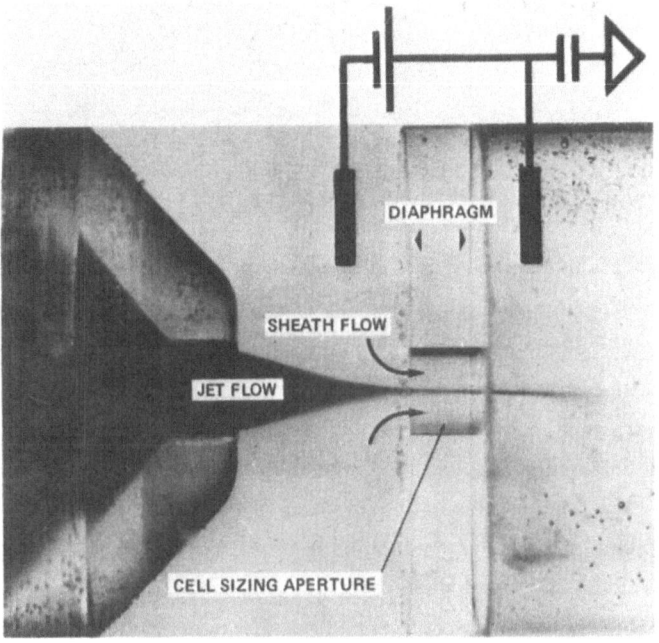

Fig. 1: Model of transducer. Negative pressure behind the sensing aperture effects a particle free sheat flow as well a centralized particle jet flow passing the aperture. Electrode 1 within the electrolytic tank behind, electrode 2 within the particle free electrolyte in front of the aperture.

For reasons of the laminar profile of velocity here the erythrocytes are oriented virtually unique and stretched out longitudinally (Fig. 2).

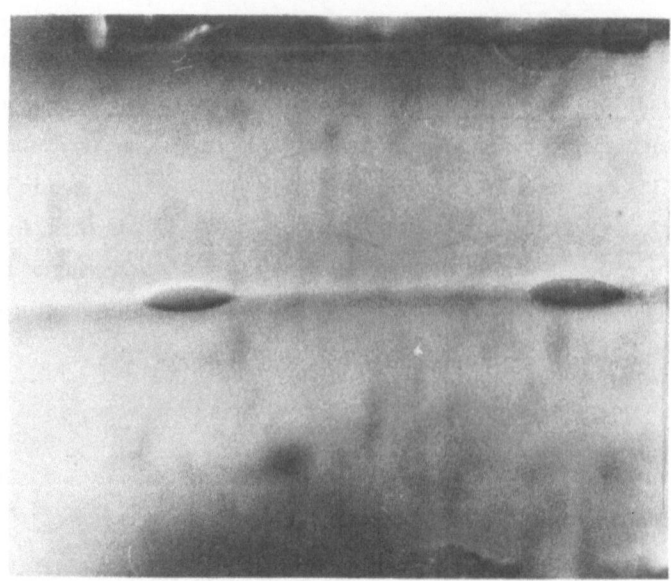

Fig. 2: Native blood cells during passage through the sensing
aperture.

A constant-current-generator prevents deviations of the current
between the electrodes which may occure by temperature dependent
changes of the conductivity of the electrolyte. The cells, while passing the area of the sensing aperture with electric equipotentials,
generate changes of the resistance proportional to their volume.
The uniform shape and length of the electric impulses according to
the function of the sheath-flow-detector allows, that the delivering
process of the measured impulse amplitude to the analyser for hight
of impulses is dependent from the shape of the impulses (21). By
this means exclusively those impulses are registered which were
generated by single erythrocytes and distorsions of the distribution
of the hight of impulses in consequence of statistical coincidences
and jamming are impeded. Because of electric isolation between the
cell suspension and the electrolyte, no alterations of the cells are
possible by a suspension media decomposed of electrolytes (24).

The data of 143 patients were collected to receive information
about the postoperative blood loss with the purpose to reveal possi-

ble correlations between volume alterations and enhanced sequestration of the red cells. Blood loss via drainage tubes placed into the operative area as well the amount of transfused blood were registered and blood haemoglobin analyses were performed daily, by the method according to the ICSH (12).

Statistical statements are based on the Wilcoxon test, which was choosen for reasons of expected alternatives. The level of significances is marked on the figures which are obtained directly from the digital plotter.

3.  RESULTS

The volume distribution of a population of red cells can be characterised mathematically by some parameters such as mean (MCV), variation coefficient and slope of the distribution curve. These data were obtained from the patients red cells before, during and two

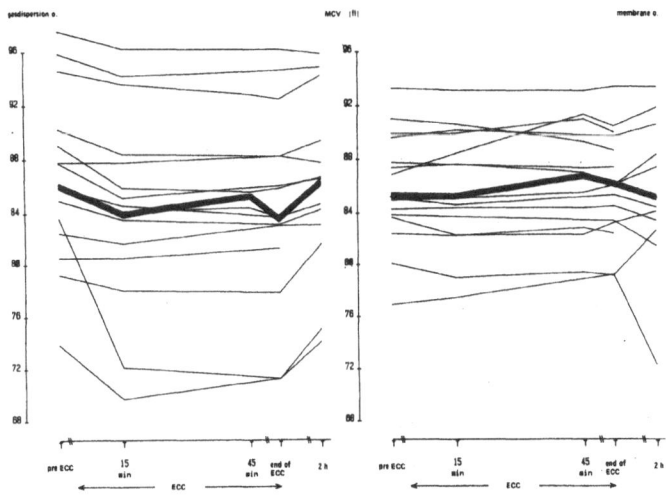

Fig. 3: Mean cell volume of erythrocytes of the patients of group I (gasdispersion oxygenator) opposing those of group II (membrane oxygenator).

hours after the end of the ECC and they were put together in figures 3 - 6, each opposing the different oxygenator groups. Figure 3 shows, that the mean volume of red cells is not different between the two groups of patients. Before ECC the means of the red cell volume are identical within the methodological error ($\tilde{x}$ = 86.44 fl in group I, $\tilde{x}$ = 85.83 fl in group II; Fig. 3).

The curves in figure 4 reflect the differences between the measurement before ECC and each measurement there after from all sin-

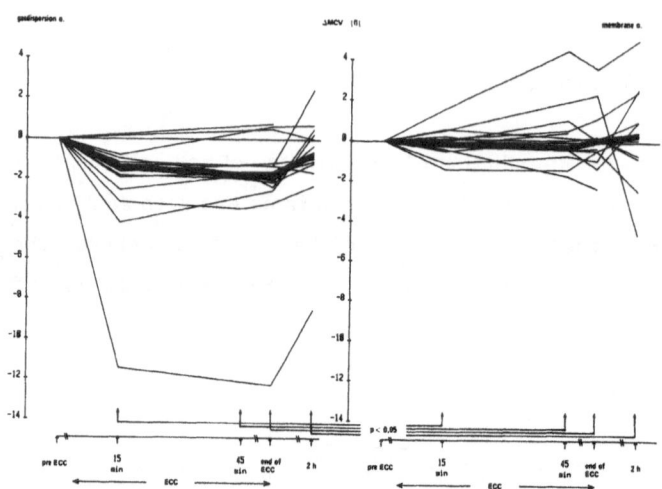

Fig. 4: Deviation of MCV from the values obtained before ECC.

gle patients with the superposed statistical mean. There is a definite decrease of the MCV in most patients with gasdispersion oxygenation, which is significantly different to the corresponding values under membrane oxygenation; after the ECC has been stopped, the red cell volume tends to normal.

The values of all other parameters are not different among the two groups, which means that a broadening or asymmetry of the population curves did not occur (Fig. 5, 6).

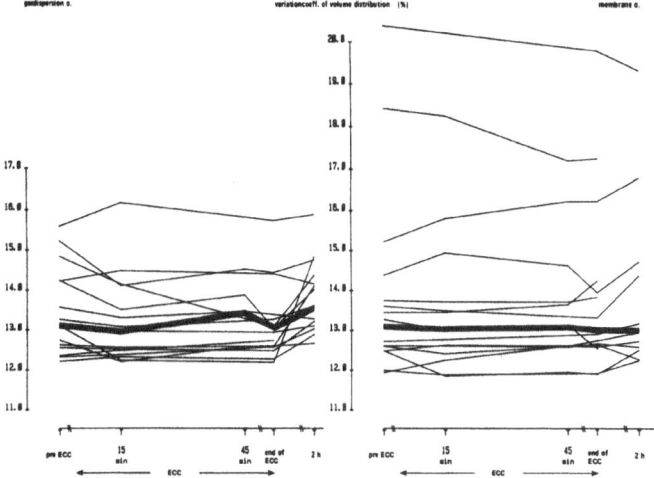

Fig. 5: Variation coefficients of the red cell volume distribution curves.

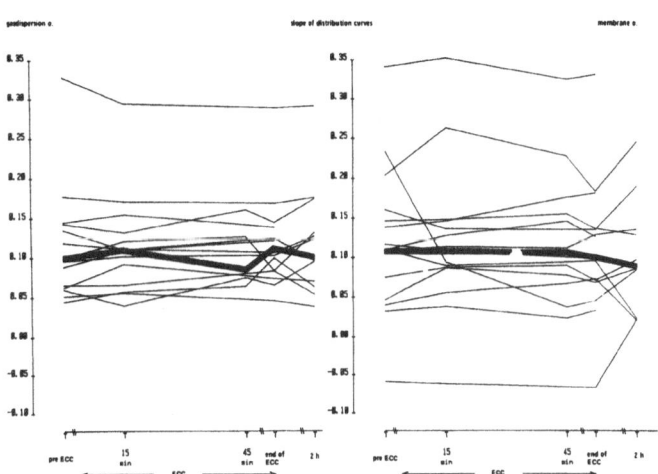

Fig. 6: Slope of the red cell volume distribution curves (dimension less).

In patients under heart surgery with a gasdispersion oxygenator (6-LF Travenol) the volume of all (the total population) red cells undergoes a shift to the left, which means a shrinkage of the cells.

The figure 7 and 8 summarise the data of 143 patients devided into the group membrane and gasdispersion oxygenator. Blood loss

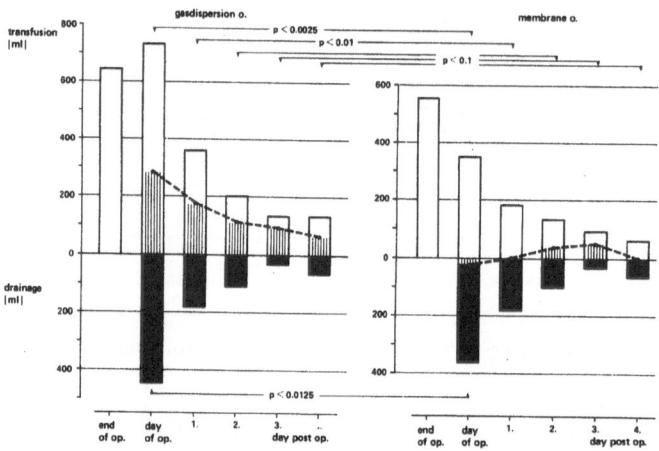

Fig. 7: Balance: blood drained to blood transfused in 76 patients under gasdispersion and 67 patients under membrane oxygenation.

via drainage tubes is high on the day of operation but higher in the cases of gasdispersion oxygenation. Later on there is no difference of the average amounts between the two groups. Supposing a uniform indication for blood transfusion of all patients (low CVP and/or Hb levels $< 9.0$ g%, in patients under 45 ys. $< 8.5$ g%), the amount of transfused blood could serve as an indirect measure for blood loss out of the vascular bed. Patients with gasdispersion oxygenators received more blood postoperatively. The balance between blood lost and blood replaced indicate that after gasdispersion oxygenation there is a need for blood replacement without measurable bleeding (striped area in fig. 7).

Figure 8 shows the haemoglobin levels (mean and standard deviation) of the two patient groups. There is a more rapid regeneration of haemoglobin in patients after membrane oxygenation as compared with those after gasdispersion oxygenation. In no case blood was transfused after day 4.

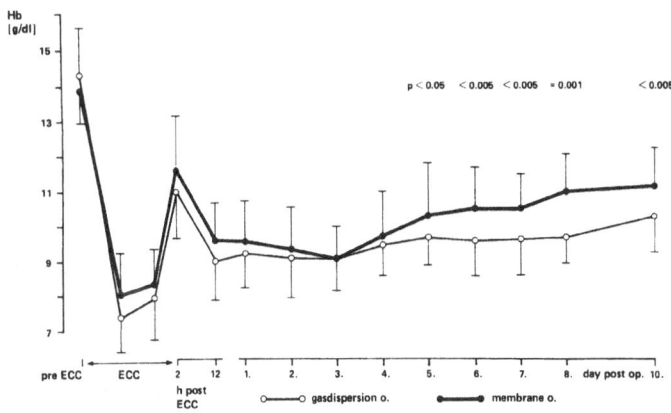

Fig. 8: Haemoglobin levels of patients under gasdispersion
(n = 76) and membrane oxygenation (n = 67).

## 4. DISCUSSION

The comprehension of <u>sublethal</u> damage of red blood cells became of important interest in medicine with the increasing request for foreign material being exposed to blood. Abnormalities of red blood cells after their circulation through ECC systems or exposure to shear forces in metabolic, functional and morphologic regard were described (3, 11, 22, 19). Of special interest are the changes of the intraerythrocytar sodium concentration (15), the presence of cell wall molecules (lipids) (14) and intraerythrocytar enzymes in the plasma (2) following the traumatisation of red cell suspension. ADP release was described as well (4).

The deviation of the MCV under ECC is considered due to a damage of the cell wall structures. Subsequently a main function of the cell membrane to maintain ion transportation and gradients becomes deteriorated by either derangement of the metabolic activity or break off or regroupment of structural units of the wall molecular

287

complexes with a final increase of the membrane porosity; an increased passive efflux of intracellular potassium plus water leads to shrinkage of the cells in both cases.

The loss of blood following an open heart surgical procedure represents an essential part of the postperfusional morbidity. While immediately postoperatively the local, even diffuse, bleeding tendency expresses disturbances of coagulation, the late postoperative anaemia is not well understood. Shortened half live time of red cells following ECC has been described (20). It is supposed that alteration of the volume of the red cells enhances biomorphosis in the sense of ageing of the cells; with other words: enhances accelerated sequestration. Sublethal damage therefore does not necessarily cause a detectable increase of the free plasma haemoglobin (in our patients plasma haemoglobin levels were not different between the two groups and never exceeded 70 mg%, but might be responsible for late post-cardiosurgical anaemia.

## 5. CONCLUSION

5. 1. A method is described for evaluation of alterations of the volume distribution of red blood cells as occuring under shear stress.

5. 2. Red blood cells of patients under gasdispersion oxygenation show a slight decrease of their volume, while under membrane oxygenation the volume remained constant.

5. 3. This parameter is very sensitive to detect subhaemolytic red cell damage as it may occur under extracorporeal circulation.

5. 4. After an open heart operation with the gasdispersion oxygenator patients need more transfusion blood and show a more pronounced late cardiosurgical anaemia than those with the membrane oxygenator. It is supposed that volume altered red cells are subjected to enhanced sequestration.

288

1.  Allen, J. G. , Extracorporeal circulation. Thomas Publ. ,
    Springfield/Ill. 1958

2.  Bernstein, E. F. , R. A. Indeglia, M. A. Shea, R. L. Varco,
    Sublethal damage to the red blood cell from pumping, Circu-
    lation Suppl. I, 35, 226 - 229 (1967)

3.  Bernstein, E. F. , Erythrocyte metabolism following surface
    induced injury. Trans. Amer. Soc. Artif. Int. Organs 17, 386 -
    391 (1971)

4.  Bernstein, E. F. , U. M. Marzec, Effect of wall interaction,
    shear stress and osmotic injury on erythrocyte adenosine
    triphosphate concentration 2, 3 diphosphoglycerate concentra-
    tion, and the oxyhemoglobin dissociation curve. Trans. Amer.
    Soc. Artif. Int. Organs 20, 47 - 56 (1974)

5.  Birnbaum, D. , R. Eisele, R. Thom, Kriterien zur Auswahl
    eines Membranoxygenators für die Langzeitoxygenierung.
    Langenbecks Arch. Chir. Suppl. 1976, 152 - 156

6.  Birnbaum, D. , R. Thom, E. S. Bücherl, The corpuscular vo-
    lume distribution of erythrocytes during ECMO and after
    exposure to shear forces (Strathclyde Bioengineering Semi-
    nar Glasgow Aug. 1976), p. 89; in: Artificial organs, ed. by
    R. M. Kenedi, J. M. Courtney, Macmillan Press, London
    1977

7.  Birnbaum, D. , Unpublished observations 1977

8.  Birnbaum, D. , Über die Wertigkeit der Hämolyse beim extra-
    corporalen Kreislauf. Kardiotechnik 3, 3 - 7 (1977)

9.  Dawids, S. G. , H. C. Engell, Physiological and clinical aspects
    of oxygenator design. Elsevier, Amsterdam 1976

10. Galetti, P. M. , G. A. Brecher, Heart lung bypass: principle
    and techniques of extracorporeal circulation. Grune &
    Stratton, New York 1962

11. Hochmuth, R. M. , N. Mohandas, E. E. Spaeth, J. R. Williamson, P. L. Blackshear, jr. , D. W. Johnson, Surface adhesion, deformation and detachment at low shear of red cells and white cells. Trans. Amer. Soc. Artif. Int. Organs 18, 325 - 332 (1972)

12. International Committee for Standardization in Hematology : Recommendations for hemoglobinometry in human blood. Brit. J. Haematol. 13 (Suppl. ), 71 - 75 (1967)

13. Lambert, J. , A. Naumann, Haemolysis caused by high, short duration laminar shear stress. Proc. Europ. Soc. Artif. Organs 3(1977), 686 - 688 (1978)

14. Langley, G. R. , M. Axell, Changes in erythrocyte membrane and autohaemolysis during in vitro incubation. Brit. J. Haemat. 14, 593 - 601 (1968)

15. Lubowitz, H. , F. Harris, M. H. Mehrjardi, S. P. Sutera, Shear-induced changes in permeability of human RBC to sodium. Trans. Amer. Soc. Artif. Int. Organs 20, 470 - 473 (1974)

16. Nanjappa, B. N. , H. -K. Chang, Ch. A. Glomski, Trauma of the erythrocyte membrane associated with low shear stress. Biophys. J. 13, 1212 - 1218 (1973)

17. Nosé, Y. , Manual on artificial organs, Vol. II:The oxygenator. Mosby & Co. , St. Louis 1973

18. Pierce, C. E. , Extracorporeal circulation for open-heart surgery. Thomas Publ. , Springfield/Ill. 1969

19. Schlick, S. , H. Schmidt-Schönbein, Measurement of single red cell deformability. Preliminary report. Blood Cells 1, 333 - 338 (1975)

20. Schmidt-Mende, M. , K. W. Frey, F. Sebening, Bestimmung der Erythrozytenüberlebenszeit nach Anwendung der Herz-Lungen-Maschine. Thoraxchir. 10, 685 - 693 (1963)

21. Schulz, J. , R. Thom, Electrical sizing and counting of platelets in whole blood. Med. Biol. Eng. 11, 447 - 454 (1973)

22. Sutera, S. P. , M. H. Mehrjardi, Deformation and fragmentation of human red blood cells in turbulent shear flow. Biophys. J. 15, 1 - 18 (1975)

23. Thom, R., A. Hampe, G. Sauerbrey, Electronic blood cell volume determination and its sources of error. Z. ges. exp. Med. 151, 331 - 349 (1969)

24. Thom, R., Methods and results by improved electronic blood-cell sizing, pp 191. In: G. Izak, S. M. Lewis, Modern concepts in hematology. Academic Press, New York 1972

25. Zapol, W. M., J. Qvist, Artificial lungs for acute respiratory failure. Academic Press, Washington 1976

Moderator: Williams

Williams:                  Thank you very much Dr. Birnbaum. That was
                           very interesting. I am afraid I do have some
                           comments to make regarding your technique for
                           measuring changes in cell volume. Our results
                           show that you do not get changes in red cell
                           volume while under shear and I am afraid that
                           I would most humbly suggest that our disagree-
                           ment is simply in that the device you are
                           using to assess changes in red cell volume
                           is not adequate for that job. If cells entering
                           the orifice all had the same shape, then the
                           Coulter Counter with hydrodynamic focussing de-
                           vice can be used to measure changes in cell
                           volume. However, it is known that hydrodynamic
                           shear stress changes the shape of the red cells.
                           Therefore, the changes that you measure could
                           well be explained by changes in the distribu-
                           tion of shapes of the cells going through the
                           orifice as in the case of platelets as we heard
                           yesterday. This would result in an apparent
                           change in cell volume but you have no way of
                           knowing if your device is estimating change of
                           cell volume or changes in cell distribution.

Birnbaum:                  We discussed this problem of methodology yester-
                           day already. I agree, that you may call what I
                           measured as you want it. If you want, call it
                           the parameter X. I learned for myself to re-
                           port on the fluid dynamics within the measuring
                           channel of the particle analyser.

Williams:                  I just want to hold on record for the other
                           people here.

Schmid-Schönbein:          There have been reports about photographs of
                           cells passing a "Coulter"channel, (e.g. by
                           KACHEL  et al., Methoden zur Analyse und Korrek-
                           tur apparativ bedingter Meßfehler beim elektro-

nischen Verfahren zur Teilchengrößenbestimmung nach Coulter, Berlin 1972 , D 83). This procedure allows one to see each single cell while it is passing and so the actual shape can be correlated to the signal. I am afraid that both Dr. Wenzel and you are trapped by an instrument with an inborn error which has been well analyzed.

Birnbaum:    During my presentation of our study I stated very clearly and I am going to repeat it, that the volume distribution of the red cells was analyzed by means of the PARTICLE ANALYSER TELEFUNKEN/AEG, which was distinguished from the original COULTER arrangement by the work of the hematologist Prof. R. Thom, as you certainly know. All data presented here were obtained under the supervision of this man. This analytical device has been approved for many years scientifically and clinically as a reliable and accepted apparatus if in proper use. Hydrodynamic focusing is not even the only difference to the Coulter Counter.

Wenzel:      Well, I agree fully with your critical remarks on the Coulter principle. However, I think we should keep those arguments separate and only take into consideration the theoretical side from those that are considered only on the clinical side. We have used both methods in our department, the Coulter principle and hydrodynamic focusing and our findings do not show any difference in the quality of interpreting the volume distribution curves of platelets.

By the way, the company that sells the Coulter Counter also sells the hydrodynamic focusing apparatus. Why isn't it possible for them to

perfect this apparatus? Perhaps this company
is just reluctant to do any extensive research
in the field of measurement, particularly hydrodynamic focusing.

Birnbaum:  I would like to make a proposition not to mix up
things more. If we talk about the focusing
method, call this apparatus the particle volume
analyser and call the other one the Coulter
Counter. We used the particle volume analyser.

Williams:  I think we are getting somewhat off the point.
I do not want to go into the merits of one
particular device against another device. Evi-
dently there are points for discussion there.
The basic points is that when you measure a
change in the volume distribution as displayed
by any Coulter Counter type machine then you
cannot be certain that it is a real volume
change until you know the shape distribution.
What you measure is a change in platelet or
red cell shape unless the particles going
through the orifice all have exactly the same
shape factor. Then you can start saying, yes,
it is a volume change. If there is any possibility of a change in this shape factor, particularly for platelets or red cells, then you
cannot claim that you are measuring changes in
cell volume. Is there any shape change in the
cells going through the orifice of your apparatus?

Birnbaum:  I repeat myself; in proper use the particle
analyser cannot size at the same time red cells
and thrombocytes. Shape changes are excluded
to get into the record of the impulses computer.

Schmid-Schönbein:  I am afraid there is another trap we have to
be careful about and that is the conductivity

of the membrane which could be altered and which could be also subject to alterations during the extreme deformation that red cells undergo during the passage through a Coulter pore. So there is another point to be concerned about.

Van den Dungen: As a comment on the differences Dr. Birnbaum measured between bubble- and membrane oxygenator, I would like to show some results we obtained during our clinical comparison of the Polystan VT 5000 bubble oxygenator with the Travenol Teflo membrane oxygenator. Because all cases were coronary artery bypass grafts with an about equal perfusion time (120 minutes), the two groups are strictly comparable. No differences could be measured in packed cell volume, erythrocyte number or plasma hemoglobin. However, platelet numbers and function were significantly better maintained during membrane oxygenator perfusion than during bubble oxygenator perfusion. But at the end of perfusion when increased cardiotomy suction is used and heparin is neutralized with protamin these good results are undone. Consequently no differences in blood transfusions or blood losses could be measured between the two groups.

Tillmanns: Did you ever test the influence of the roller pump which you are using on your data? Is there any influence by the pump on your volumes?

Birnbaum: I showed slides where we evaluated extracorporeal systems in dogs. We had a control group in there, where the oxygenator was avoided. There was just the pump in the system and we didn't see any alteration of the erythrocyte volume distribution.

Wildevuur: We have done experiments in dogs in which the conventional roller-pump (set non-occlusive) was compared to two other blood pumps. The centrifugal pump hematologically appears to be about the same as the roller pump. The Rhône-Poulenc pump was definitely better than these two pumps, although the differences are not very large.

Now I would like to add to what my co-worker Dr. Van den Dungen presented, that during clinical perfusion you do see better maintained platelet functions in the membrane oxygenator (MO) as compared to the bubble oxygenator (BO). However, at the end of the MO perfusion platelet function decreased rapidly to the same level as the BO group which coincided with the release of aortic crossclamping. At that moment bleeding is started from the incisions in the heart and consequently increased cardiotomy suction is needed. This finding corresponds with our dog experiments in which we have proved that everything that is gained by the use of a membrane oxygenator is destroyed by the use of high vacuum suction. A second point is that after protamin chloride is given to neutralize the anticlotting by heparin, again a substantial decrease of platelet function is observed. Altogether, platelet function in the clinical MO group reached the same low level as in the BO group after perfusion, just when optimal hemostasis is needed. It will be of no surprise that postoperatively no differences were seen in blood loss and blood transfusions in the BO and MO group.

|   |   |
|---|---|
| Agostoni: | Dr. Wildevuur what do you think about the possibility of improving the preservation of blood, using solutions different from ACD? For instance, adding inosine and phosphate? |
| Wildevuur: | I cannot give a direct answer, because nowadays |

the patients are operated with hemodilution. We
take several units of blood from the patient
himself just preoperatively and give it back
to him after the perfusion is terminated. So in
the immediate postperfusion period he doesn't
get donor blood. And if donor blood is used to
prime the heartlung machine, in most centres
fresh heparinized donor blood is used.

Schmid-Schönbein:  One question to Dr. Wildevuur: When you test
platelet function, do you take a platelet aggregation test? What do you use as a control? The
amplitude of the change in light transmission
following the ADP induced aggregation depends
greatly on the absolute number of the platelet
present. Therefore, I think in tests like this
it is necessary to preserve a platelet containing
plasma and dilute it so that you have a control
with the same platelet number. Has this been
done in these studies?

Wildevuur:  We have tested the influence of the platelet
number in relation to platelet function and
made a dilution curve. From this we obtained
a nomogram by which we correct the function
according to the numbers (J.C.F. de Jong,
C.Th. Smit  Sibinga and Ch.R.H. Wildevuur:
Platelet behaviour in extracorporeal circulation (ECC), Artificial Organs, p. 27, 1977).

Van den Dungen:  As shown the platelet numbers at 5, 15, 30 and
120 minutes bypass were about equal in both
groups while the platelet function was already
worse in the bubble oxygenator group. On the
other hand, the differences in platelet number,
measured at 60 and 90 minutes perfusion, are
not big enough to account for the great differences measured in platelet function.

Laurant:  Coming back to Dr. Birnbaum's paper, what about
maintaining the plasmatic osmolarity during

|  |  |
|---|---|
|  | extracorporeal circulation? Could you guarantee some constancy in this respect? Would you be able to comment on that aspect, because the test you are working on is very sensitive to osmolar environment? |
| Birnbaum: | The prime volume of the heart-lung machine is iso-osmolar. |
| Laurant: | When you run the extracorporeal circulation it will be necessary to check, with your approach in mind, the possibility of changes in plasmatic osmolarity all along the full run. It is known that there are strong changes. |
| Williams: | Could you give us an idea what sort of osmotic changes you observed? |
| Laurant: | Quantitative changes amounting to at least 5 % could be observed in the blood osmolarity during the extracorporeal runs. |
| Schmid-Schönbein: | Dr. Laurent, I think it is a very important point but, of course, in the Coulter Counter the so-called "isotonic" solution is used and the response of the cells is so quick and even if you had them coming out of the boddy totally hypotonic or hypertonic they would immediately adjust. |
| Williams: | Another point is, does the osmotic strength dedrease during the extracorporeal rund or does it increase? |
| Laurant: | The variations in osmolarity during extracorporeal circulation are depending on the actual protocole of the anaesthesiological team. More generally the tendency is a progressive decrease. |
| Olijslager: | I have a question to Dr. Birnbaum. Perhaps he said it already but I want a confirmation. You said that your results on the red cell volume |

depended on the blood flow through the oxygenator you used. Is that also for one type of
oxygenators and can you correlate that with the
shear in that group of oxygenators?

Birnbaum:          I don't know the shear force in the blood path
                   of the oxygenator. I didn't measure it. The
                   slides I showed here concerend the TEMPTROL-
                   oxygenator which is a prototype bubble oxyge-
                   nator and the DUALUNG, a machine which inci-
                   dentally, is no longer in use.

Olijslager:        When you use a membrane oxygenator, and when
                   you increase the flow, you can also say you
                   increase the shear stresses in the oxygenator.

Birnbaum:          The experiments did not include this aspect,
                   however, you have to adapt the flow to the
                   hemodynamic condition of the patients or
                   the animals. Otherwise you couldn't run the
                   experiment.

# 14.
## MECHANICAL RED CELL DISRUPTION

J.Lambert[+] , Aerodynamisches Institut der RWTH-Aachen

[+] present address: DFVLR

Bereich für Projektträger schaften

Abt. NT-1, Postfach 906058

5 Köln 90 (Porz-Wahn, Linder Höhe)

# INTRODUCTION

The destruction of red blood cells (RBC's) is regularly observed during extra-corporeal circulation with heart-lung-machines and haemodialysers ( 1 ). Even in some patients with artificial heart valves the life time of RBCs was unusually shortened ( 5 ). It was often suggested that in all these cases, besides the contact of the blood cells with nonphysiological surfaces, fluid mechanical effects, such as elevated shear stresses may play an important role ( 1 ). Earlier investigations on the effect of laminar shear stress on haemolysis were often carried out in rotational viscometer-like systems ( 8 ) ; they clearly demonstrated that shear stress in the order of 100 - 200 $N/m^2$ , applied to the cells for some minutes, caused erythrocytes to lyse. In a recent study, Th. Fischer was able to visualize, that RBC's under these conditions disintegrate into small spherical droplets ( 3 ).

The effect of high shear stresses applied to the RBC's only for very short time intervalls, but in a repetitive way was investigated by W.J.Williams by means of an oscillating wire system ( 11 ). In those experiments it was shown that with decreasing time of exposure the critical shear stress, at which RBC's become haemolysed, increases. Similar results were obtained with the "jet-test" by R. Forstrom et al. ( 4 ). The haemolysing effect of high laminar shear stresses applied to RBC's only once and only for fractions of a second, was hardly investigated at all and there was nothing known about the mechanism of haemolysis under these conditions. This range of high level shear stress and short exposure time is of some interest with respect to haemolysis in artificial devices. Fluid mechanicel estimations have shown that in roller pumps under severe pressure conditions laminar shear stresses in the order of

1000 - 3000 N/m$^2$ are reached, whereas the time of exposure of RBC's to these high shear stresses is in the order of milliseconds ( 7 ).

The aim of this study was to investigate the effect of very high, laminar shear stresses applied only once for milliseconds to erythrocytes, and to get some information about the "break-down"-mechanism of the cells under these conditions.

## METHOD

To produce a flow field with a well defined shear stress distribution, a narrow channel with rectangular crossection was used in this study. The velocity distribution in the channel, except a small region near the side walls and at the inlet of the channel, was parabolic, which means, that the shear stress was linearly distributed. The flow through the channel was produced by a pressure difference between the fluid reservoir and the separator trap (fig.1).

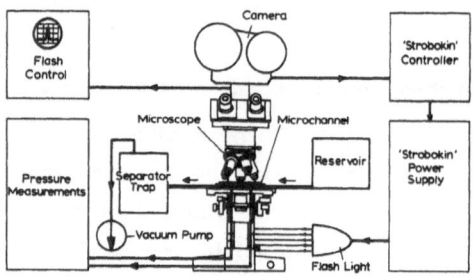

Fig. 1    Test device

The flow rate, velocities and shear stress gradient in the channel were linearly dependent on the measured pressure drop along the microchannel. Thus it was possible to calculate, from the measured pressure drop, the known viscosity of the fluid, and the geometrical parameters of the microchannel, the shear stress and the time of exposure for an erythrocyte flowing along a defined stream line.

The microchannel was cast in transparent resin and covered by a microscope cover glass. The mould for the channel was prepared by means of a photochemical technique, described earlier ( 6 ). The microchannel was mounted on the stage of a light microscope, which was illuminated by a flash light with a flash duration of about $1 \mu s$. During the experiment, the microscope was focused on a stream line near the upper cover glass and pictures of the RBC's during their passage through the high shear area were taken by means of the flash light.

The experiments were performed with a solution of Dextran (MW 40 000) in saline, in which fresh human RBC's were suspended. The suspension was dilute enough to ensure that it was still transparent. On the other hand there were enough RBC's per volume to see at least one erythrocyte at a time in the microscope. The viscosity of the suspension could be varied in a wide range. For the experiments viscosities between 55 cP and 120 cP were used to minimize errors due to the nonparabolic velocity profile at the inlet of the channel and due to the Carnot-pressure-losses behind the channel outlet. Under the conditions the experiments were carried out, the overall error in estimating the shear stress on a certain stream line was of the order of 20 % and the error in calculating the exposure time of the order of 3 %.

The flash light was used to take pictures of the RBC's during their exposure to the shear stress and allowed to analyze the shape change of the cells due to shear forces. To study the shape of the RBC's immediately after their passage through the high shear region, the light microscope was focused on a stream line downstream from the channel and the fluid flow was suddenly stopped by clamping the outlet tube. When the cells came to rest, they could be observed in continuous bright field illumination.

For a more detailed study of the shape of RBC's after shear stress loading, a small amount of the suspension was sucked out of a downstream port during the perfusion of the channel. These cells were collected in glutaraldehyde for

303

fixation and then prepared for scanning electron microscopy.

## RESULTS

The described system allowed to observe the deformation of RBC's exposed to
laminar shear stresses in the order of up to 8000 $N/m^2$ for exposure times in
the range from $10^{-4}$ to $10^{-2}$ s. Fig. 2 shows a photomicrograph of a RBC
taken during its exposure to shear stresses of approximately 5000 $N/m^2$.

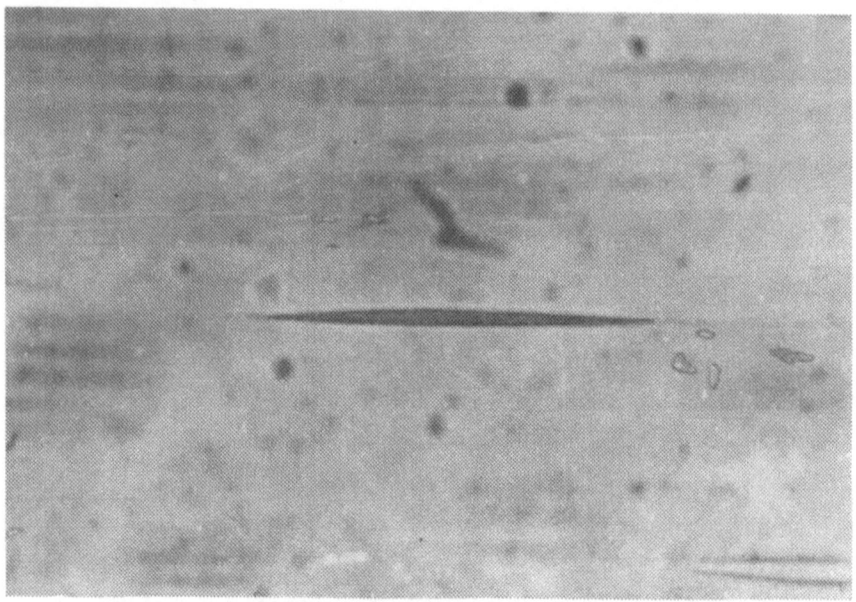

Fig. 2    Light micrograph of a red blood cell deformed
under laminar shear stress
$$\tau \approx 5000 \ N/m^2$$

The cell is stretched to a long, spindle-like body. In another series of experiments, which allowed the observation at a plane perpendicular to the plane
in Fig. 2, it could be shown   that the highly deformed erythrocyte is symmetric
with respect to its long axis ( 7 ).

Fig. 3 shows a light micrograph of RBC's, taken downstreams from the channel immediately after stopping the flow.

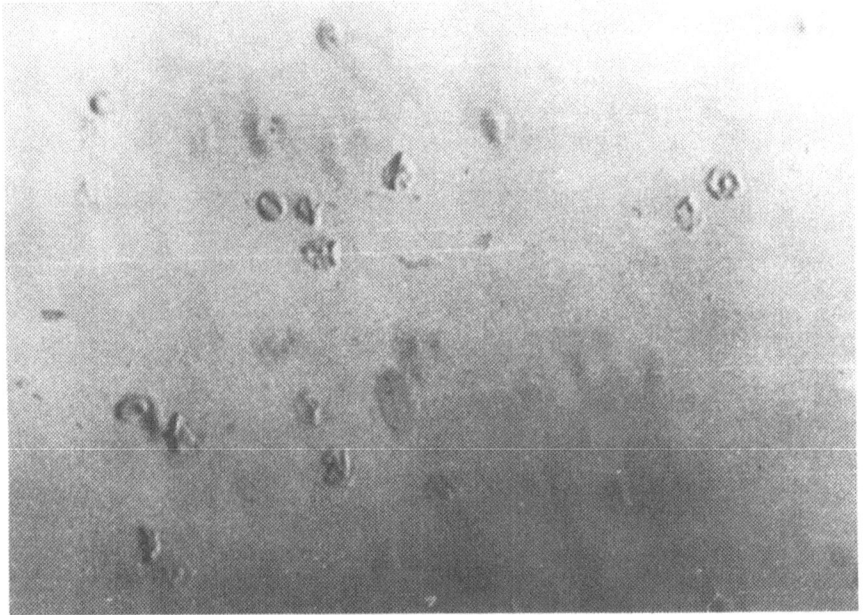

Fig. 3    Light micrograph of red blood cells immediately
after exposure to laminar shear stress
$\tau \approx 8000$ N/m$^2$, exposure time $t_B \approx 10^{-4}$ sec.

In this case, the shear stress was approximately 8000 N/m$^2$ , and the time of exposure to the shear stress was about $10^{-4}$ s. Most of the cells in focus have a characteristically crenated shape;  only a few cells exhibit the almost un-altered biconcave shape of erythrocytes. Assuming  that all cells in focus were exposed approximately for the same time to the same shear stress, this picture indicates, that RBC's have a fairly wide variation in their ability to resist a certain shear stress. During the experiments it was regularly observed that especially highly crenated RBC's in a time course of about 1 min. after their shear stress loading, lost their opacity and were finally only to be seen in phase contrast. This indicates  that the membrane of the cells had been changed in a way  that haemoglobin could leak out of the cell, even in the relaxed state after shear stress loading. It was never observed  that crenated

305

erythrocytes first became spherical before they began to lyse.

Fig. 4 shows a scanning electronmicrograph of a crenated RBC besides three erythrocytes with a fairly normal appearance.

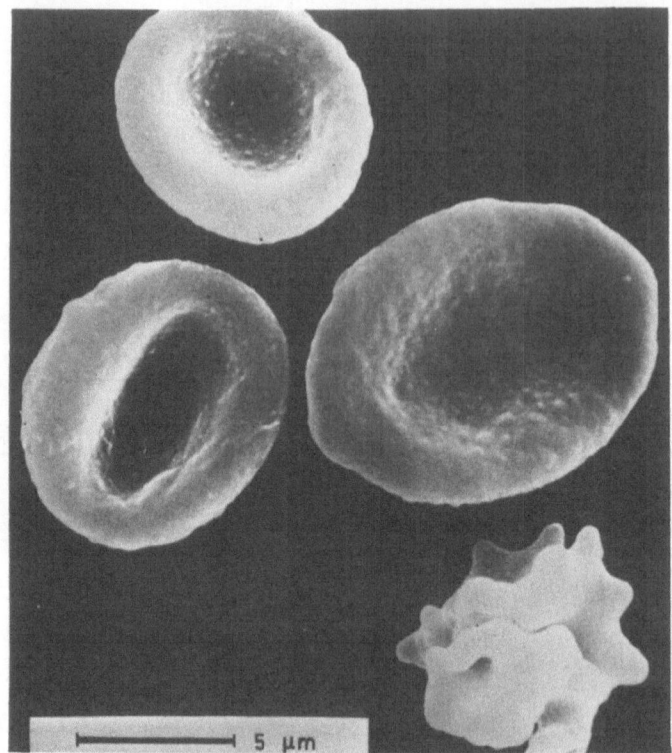

Fig. 4    Due to exposure to shear stress
crenated red blood cell, besides
unaltered cells

The crenated cells observed in this experiment are comparable with crenated cells, produced in hypertonic saline, but they are very different from echino-cytes, which result from physico-chemical changes in the cell membrane e.g. due to contact with glass surfaces. The fact that the crenated cells observed after shear stress loading have some similarity with cells suspended in hyperto-nic saline indicates that RBC´s during exposure to high shear stresses for a very short time interval loose irreversibly some of their cell contents.

To confirm this qualitative observation, in serial experiments pictures were taken from deformed erythrocytes exposed to different shear stresses at different viscosities. The length and the maximal thickness of the deformed cells were measured and under the assumption that the contour of the deformed cell could be approximated by a sinusoidal function, the surface area ( SA ) and the cell volume ( CV ) were calculated. For highly deformed erythrocytes a sinusoidal function describes the cell contour better than an elliptical function ( 7 ). The calculated cell volume showed a highly significant linear dependance on the product of shear stress $\tau$ and the square root of the exposure time $t_B^{1/2}$. Fig. 5 shows the relationship between cell volume CV $\pm$ SEM and $\tau \, t_B^{1/2}$ for different viscosities.

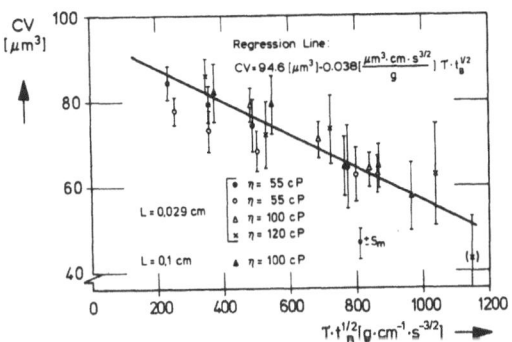

Fig. 5    Cell volume CV as a function of $\tau t_B^{1/2}$ for erythrocytes exposed to laminar shear stresses. $\tau$ = shear stress, $t_B$ = exposure time

This plott reflects the fact that with increasing shear stress and exposure time the volume of the RBC´s decreases.

In the range of shear stresses and exposure time investigated, there is only a small, but statistically insignificant change in surface area with increasing $\tau \, t_B^{1/2}$ ( 7 ).

## DISCUSSION

The light microscopic observation of the deformed RBC's during high shear loading suggests a comparison with G.I. Taylor's ( 9 ) experiments with droplets suspended in a shear field. In both cases very long, spindle-like bodies with pointed ends are produced. In Taylor's experiments the droplets broke into smaller ones presumably because of instabilities in the surface ( 10 ). Comparable results for RBC's suspended in a highly viscous Dextran solution recently have been obtained by Th.Fischer and H.Schmid-Schönbein ( 3 ), who exposed the cells to an uniform shear field in a counter rotating cone-plate-viscometer. In these experiments it was demonstrated that RBC's exposed for relatively long periods to low shear stresses, compared with the present study, disintegrate into small droplet-like fragments.

Results, which are more similar to those obtained in the present study were recently published by W.T.Caakley et al. ( 2 ), who found almost no microspheres in blood, which was extensively haemolysed by laminar shear stresses in capillaries of variing size. In these experiments the exposure time and shear stresses were in the range of those of the present study.

From these different observations it is concluded that at least two mechanisms exist for haemolysis induced by bulk shear stress:

For long exposures to low level shear stress, the mechanism of haemolysis is very similar to that observed for the break down of droplets.

For short exposures to high level shear stress, the cells loose contents without formation of microspheres. Presumably due to very high, but shortly acting tensions in the membrane microholes are formed in the cell membrane allowing larger molecules to penetrate the membrane. It may be that these microholes are resealed after relaxation, but it is as well possible that especially larger holes will not be resealed and the diffusion of haemoglobine molecules out of the relaxed cell may continue. This would explain our observations that the opacity of highly crenated cells is fading out during the first minutes after relaxation.

# ACKNOWLEDGEMENTS

This study was supported by grants from the Deutsche Forschungsgemeinschaft in the SFB 109. The author is grateful to Professor Dr.med.H.Buss and Dr.rer.nat.H.G.Hollweg for their kind support in the electronmicroscopic investigations and to Mrs. B. Mellwig for expert assistance.

( 1 )     Blackshear,P.L.Jr.,Mechanical Hemolysis in flowing Blood.
          In: Fung, Perrone, Anliker: Biomechanics, its Foundations and
          Objectives. p.p. 501, Prentice Hall, Inc Englewood Cliffs,
          N.J. (1972)


( 2 )     Coakley, W.T., C.J.James, I.J.C. Macintosh,Haemolysis of human
          Erythrocytes in Dextran Solution during rapid Flow in Capillaries.
          Biorheology 14, 91 (1977)


( 3 )     Fischer, Th., H.Schmid-Schönbein, Micromechanics of the red Cell
          in viscometric Flow. Presented Workshop Symposion on: Basic As-
          pects of Blood Trauma in extracorpreal Oxygenation, Stolberg
          (1978)


( 4 )     Forstrom,R., P.L.Blackshear, P.Keshaviah, F.Dorman, Fluid Dynamic
          Lysis of red Cells. Presented  3rd. Joint Meeting AICHE, San
          Juan, Puerto Rico


( 5 )     Gehrmann, G., W.Bleifeld, F.Loogen, Mechanische Hämolyse nach
          Implantation künstlicher Herzklappen. Zs.f.Kreislaufforschung 55 ,
          25 (1966)


( 6 )     Lambert,J., Eine neue Versuchsanordnung für die direkte mikrosko-
          pische Beobachtung des Fließverhaltens von Blut in Modellen na-
          türlicher und künstlicher Gefäßsysteme. Biomedizinische Technik
          20 ,139 (1975)

310

( 7 )   Lambert, J.,Die hämolysierende Wirkung hoher, kurzzeitiger lami-
        narer Schubspannungen. Dissertation RWTH-Aachen (1976)

( 8 )   Leverett,L.B., J.D.Hellums, C.P.Alfrey, E.C.Lynch, Red Blood
        Cell Damage by Shear Stress. Biophys.J. $\underline{12}$, 257 (1972)

( 9 )   Taylor,G.I., The Formation of Emulsion in definable Fields of
        Flow. Proc. Roy.Soc. (London) $\underline{146}$ A, 501 (1934)

( 10 )  Tomotika,S., On the Instability of a Cylindrical Thread of a vis-
        cous Liquid, surrounded by another viscous Fluid. Proc.Roy.Soc.
        (London) $\underline{150}$ A, 322 (1935)

( 11 )  Williams,W.J., D.E.Hughes, W.L.Nyborg, Hemolysis near a trans-
        versely oscillating Wire. Science 169, 871 (1970)

Williams:

A lot of the shapes that you see, we also found using our oscillating wire system, which can produce velocity gradients of the order of about $10^6$ to $10^7$ reciprocal seconds, again having very short exposure times per cycle. We did, in fact, see just the same sort of thing, namely the crumpled cells which were very similar to yours. I think, with regard to the point raised earlier by Dr. Fischer, that one would certainly expect this to be the case that the mechanism of membrane rupture will be different for a very short exposure time to that operating during a long exposure time at a lower stress. This is a qualitative difference, simply because of the viscoelasticity of the membrane. Anything which has a high viscosity component will be expected to behave in some way like a bar of toffee. If this is subjected to a small strain for a long period of time it will bend and deform (i.e. undergo plastic deformation). Yet, if you hit that same bar of toffee with a hammer, it will behave like a solid and shatter. The red cell membrane behaves (I believe) in some ways like this. If it is subjected to a very short, i.e. explosive, impact or stress it will behave as a solid entity and shatter or form cracks which may seal up or may not. Under lower shear stress conditions where there is a longer time of exposure the membrane would undergo re-arrangement and one would get fatigue mechanisms dominating. But there is probably no sharp demarcation between these two regions, they probably fuse one into the other.

Fischer:

Principally, I agree to what Dr. Williams said, but as a matter of fact in Dr. Lambert's film the red cells don't behave like a solid hit by a hammer because we don't see fragments. We see that the volume may have changed and we see ghosts. So these cells are not destroyed. The ghosts just opened their pores for a short time but their membrane was not des-integrated and the crumpled cells although they were echinocytes, looked better than the cells I showed in the movie.

Williams:     I totally agree. But I was just using the ana-logy of the bar of toffee to distinguish, for someone who is not familiar with rheological concepts, the difference between the impulse exposure to shear stress and a slow continuous deformation.

In response to these very high shear stresses our cells do appear to be crenated and if you have them in contact with glass under the mi-croscope you will find these cells suddenly losing their hemoglobin and becoming much paler, becoming less opaque and forming "ghosts". There seems to be a distribution of times in that you can shear a cell suspension, take the cells out and put them under the microscope and look at them, and you find out that one cell will suddenly lose its hemoglobin. It doesn't do it continuously, but suddenly. As you watch one cell it will suddenly become transparent and several seconds later another cell will become transparent, and so on. We believe that this effect is at least partly the result of being in contact with the glass.

Fischer:      Could you please say what is sudden, seconds or tenths of a second?

Williams:     That depends on the time resolution of the eye. All I can say is that you will see that

from a point we first could detect a change in
absorbance to the point it was completely transparent the time of the order of about a second.

Schmid-Schönbein:    This may look like a confusing situation. There
is increasing red cell volume as described by
Dr. Birnbaum but decreasing red cell volume
during the actual shear deformation, i.e. when
the stress is still acting on the cell. Hope-
fully, some kind of story evolves from this
confusion. Dr. Lambert's results are similar
to those of Jay et  al. (A.W.L. JAY, P.B. CANHAM,
Viscoelastic Properties of the Human Red Blood
Cell Membrane, Biophysical J., Vol. 17,
(1977)). These authors showed that the volume
is reduced when the red cell passes a glass capillary of 2,9 μm diameter which does not acco-
modate the red cell deformed into a cylinder
with two hemispherical caps (a sausage) which
has the same volume and the same surface area
as the biconcave red cells. And so it looks as
if possibly both under your experimental condition and those of JAY there is a cytoplasmatic increase in pressure due to the extreme
deformation. This might press off the cytoplasmatic electrolyte solution, presumably mostly
with potassium ions.Later, after the release of
the shear-stress and extreme deformation this
pressure might be released as well, initially
producing a high hypovolumic red cell.
Obviously, at the same time something seems to
have happened to the membrane. The membrane
might have lost or altered its selective permeability characteristics; such a change is
indicated by the results from Mehrardy
(M.H. MEHRARDY, DSC Dissertation, University
of Washington, St. Louis College, 1975). He
has shown that red cells subjected to high shear

stresses take up sodium from the extracellular space. One might speculate that during shearing a mechanically induced loss of cytoplasmatic potassium solution occurs, while following the exposure extracellular fluid containing high sodium concentration is taken up by the cell. At any rate, Dr. Birnbaum's results suggest that the active and/or passive membrane transport mechanisms for ions is so much deteriorated that the cell starts to swell. This may be an important aspect of the so-called "subhemolytic damage" of the red cells.

Williams:      I agree. This is what I also believe to happen under these particular conditions, that is, under extremely high shear stress. Does anyone have any special comments on this before we move on?

Lambert:       I should like to make a comment on the differences that are observed in experiments, where erythrocytes have been exposed to high shear stresses for a short time interval in comparison to those experiments with long times of exposure at a lower shear stress level: In 1977 W.T. Coakley and coworkers from the University College of Cardiff (U.K.) published some results from experiments, where suspended erythrocytes were forced through capillary tubes by means of a high pressure gradient. In those experiments again some of the erythrocytes were exposed to high shear stresses for relatively short times, comparable to our own experiments. And the Cardiff group again measured high degrees of hemolysis, but they hardly found any spherical cell elements. This indicates as well as our results, that the "breakdown" mechanism for erythrocytes must be different in the "high shear short exposure case" from what we have seen in Dr. Fischer's

film, which clearly demonstrated  that the exposition of erythrocytes to lower shear stresses
for a time in the order of minutes results in
numerous microspheres due to the disintegration
of the erythrocytes.

Williams:          Well, I don't see that these concepts are completely incompatible. Because, if you have the
situation where a cell is subjected to high
pressure you have caused perhaps the release
of potassium solution. Now, on the removal of
the pressure it takes in a sodium solution.
This will so disturb the internal biochemistry
of the cell that it will be non-viable, and a
finite time later, depending on the amount of
material which has left and been resorbed, the
cell will in essence self-destruct. Perhaps
in the experiments which Terry Coakley did, the
time interval between subjecting the cells to
the pressure and examining the cell suspension
could have prevented them from detecting
spherical cells.

Lambert:           I think that this hypothesis includes a step
where osmotic swelling of the cells finally
leads to hemolysis. But in our own experiments,
when we suddenly stopped the flow and observed
the crenated cells behind the gap in a resting
state, we saw that especially those cells which
were very much wrinkled kept their wrinkled
shape and suddenly got pale. This release reaction happened in about half a minute or so,
I can't tell the exact time. But we never observed the cells to become spherical first and
then to loose their hemoglobin.

Schmid-Schönbein:  Dr. Lambert's results may be influenced by the
dextran solutions he used. These solutions are
not only extremely viscous but also have an
extremely high colloid osmotic pressure; there-

fore, you might counteract colloid osmotic hemolysing effect of the intracellular hemoglobin. In "natural" situations "cell fragmentation" and formation of "schizocytes" really occurs, it is seen in all artificial organs (artificial heart valves and heart lung machines).

Williams: Another one point on this topic. We were doing our oscillating wire experiments in saline or in blood plasma so that we had no dextran present. We saw that our crumpled cells also "faded out" without going through a spherical stage. They did not sphere and then lyse. The hemoglobin just disappeared in a very short time.

Engell: Is the cell losing potassium or losing hemoglobin? Have you any idea of size of those losses?

Lambert: I am sorry to say, that we didn't have the opportunity to measure the release of anions and cations in our laboratories. We only observed the mechanical effects of shear stress loading on erythrocytes.

Agostoni: I think that the measurement of intracellular pH is essential. In fact, in case of a leakage of potassium ions from red cells, the hydrogen ion activity of the interior of the red cells is increased and the shape of the cell is changed (stomatocytosis).

Fischer: I would like to comment on the late hemolysis of the cells which were only shortly in the area of high shear stress. It is known from biochemistry: If you produce a ghost the membrane pores do not close immediately. The resealing process takes a finite time. So it could be that during the shear that even though

317

the pores are open no hemoglobin loss occurs
because the hemoglobin exchange is a slow process. The pores are not too many and since
they don't close immediately it takes time especially at room temperature for resealing.
Resealing is faster at $37^{\circ}C$ under certain special conditions.

Dawids:                  I am a little confused concerning the colloid-
osmotic pressure within the cell. Because the
hemoglobin has such a high molecular weight
that it is difficult for me to see that the
hemoglobin can induce a considerably higher
colloid-osmotic pressure than the extracellular
plasma. We know that hemoglobin is nearly saturated and if one were to reduce the amount of
water one would induce oversaturation. You would
therefore produce a crystallisation of the hemoglobin without much change in the oncotic
pressure.

Schmid-Schönbein:        You are right, but mind you we have a low mo-
larity of the hemoglobin at a very pronounced
deviation from Van't Hoff's law in all concentrated protein solutions including hemoglobin
solution. Together with Dr. Mendler (Deutsches
Herzzentrum in Munich), I measured the colloid-
osmotic pressure of physiologic concentrations
of 350 g/l and we found it in the order of one
atmosphere. Deviation from Van't Hoff's law in
concentrated protein solutions was recently corro-
borated for hemoglobin by SCHOLANDER's group
(HARGENS et al., Microvasc. Res. 15, 265
(abstr.) (1978 )) and results from protein-water
interactions in such a concentrated system. Consequently, the actual colloid-osmotic pressure
of the normal hydrated red cells may amount to
as much as 15 % of the total osmotic pressure,
rising quickly after slight dehydration. Let me

318

come back to the problem of subhemolytic damage
and subsequent cell destruction. The normal
fluidity of the red cells not only optimizes
traffic in the microcirculation   but the very
same property is equally essential for the survival of the red cells. Fluidity - or flexi-
bility in conventional terms - might be disturbed following the sequence of events drawn
up above. Red cell fluidity can be jeopardized
both by cell shrinking and by cell swelling.
The so-called late hemolysis that has been observed following the exposure of red cells to
artificial organs of various kinds might therefore be caused either by *dehydration* or by *over-
hydration* of the red cells. And, of course, any
other mechanism that disturbs red cell deformability or membrane deformability is known to
reduce the half life of the affected cells and
therefore produces "late" anemia.  When seeing
pictures of so-called schizocytes and knowing
about reduced half life of red cells after extracorporeal oxygenation in bubble oxygenators
a rheologist is forced to conclude that the damage inflicted on the red cells leaves them
with less than an optimal deformability (as it
was demonstrated recently by Velker et al.
(VELKER et al., Trans. Am. Soc. Artif. Intern.
Organs, 23, 723, (1977)). It is now generally
accepted by hematologists that "red cell rigi-
dification" is usually responsible for their
untimely sequestration in the spleen or in
any other restricted microcirculation of the
body - this mechanism is being blamed for most
of hemolytic anemias. .

Agostoni:          I just would like to add a point on Dr. Fischer's
comment. We are familiar with the technique of
loading enzymes inside the red cells and I am
quite sure that it does not take such a long

time to close the pores of the erythrocyte ghosts (ghosts produced by a short exposition to hypotonic solutions). The sealing of red cells is a very quick process.

Williams: One point I would like to bring out from this work is that erythrocytes are not only ruptured by a single passage through this very high shear stress region. Even though cells can survive this high stress trauma, they are not normal. The work of Dr. Larry McIntire in Houston has shown that cells subjected to sublethal shear stresses appear to be normal biconcave discs. If you now filter these sheared cells through Nucleopore filters you find that their filterability is seriously reduced, i.e. they are much more rigid or less flexible entities, even though they are apparently biochemically and morphologically normal. So, exposure to high shear stresses for short times does, in fact, produce significant amounts of "sub-lethal" fatigue within the membrane. That is, the membrane has been altered by its exposure to the shear stress.

Tillmann: With the roller pump situation you estimated very high shear stesses. Do you have any idea how high ther percentage of these cells is which experience these high shear stresses? I am asking because from the two previous papers I learned that the roller pump is not doing too much damage to the red cells.

Lambert: An estimate of the percentage of erythrocytes subjected to these high shear stresses is very difficult. Firstly, it depends on the capacitance of the tube-system inside and outside the roller pump. For this capacitance limits the time interval during which blood is forced back through the opening gap due to the high pressure

320

difference and therefore determines the number of cells passing through the high shear stress area as well as the maximal shear stress that is reached in the gap. Secondly, erythrocytes flowing through the gap on different stream-lines are exposed for different times to different shear stresses. Therefore, it is not possible to give a precise answer to your question.

# 15.

H. Schmid-Schönbein[1], G.V.R. Born[2], P.D. Richardson,
J. Rohling-Winkel[3], P. Blasberg, N. Cusack, A. Wehmeyer
and E. Jüngling
Department of Physiology, RWTH Aachen, Department of Pharmacology University of London, Kings College and Division
of Engineering, Brown University, Providence, Rhode Island

## 1. INTRODUCTION

The deposition of thrombotic material (primarily platelets) upon the surfaces of natural but damaged surfaces
(e.g. BAUMGARTNER et al.), as well as onto any artificial
surfaces (e.g. LEONARD  et al., GRABOWSKI et al.) requires
continuous blood flow rather than blood "stasis". For the
simple reason that the material to be deposited comprises
only a few percent of the volume of the blood, it can thus
be only derived from a very much larger volume of blood
than a volume of a deposit. This absolute flow requirement
makes it necessary to reconsider many current biochemical
theories about the mechanisms governing thrombotic processes - since the "essential" blood stream not only supplies
the reaction partners but also carries   away activating
species (e.g. released mediators, activated enzymes, as
elaborated elsewhere: SCHMID-SCHÖNBEIN 1977). This notwithstanding, it is well established that thrombotic processes
are much enhanced by rapid flow, especially in the presence
of red cells. The reason for the enhancement of platelet
"reactivity" in the presence of flowing red cells has not
been established. Applying mass transport principles

---

1  Supported by Sonderforschungsbereich 109 (Künstliche Organe) of the Deutsche Forschungsgemeinschaft at RWTH
   Aachen, Project $C_2$

2  Supported by Thyssen Foundation, Cologne

3  In partial fulfillment of the requirements of a doctoral
   dissertation (RWTH Aachen)

customary in engineering sciences, BLACKSHEAR et al.,
LEONARD et al. and TURRITO et al. have often explained the
phenomenon by the assumption of an enhanced "platelet dif-
fusivity" (diffusion coefficient), i.e. an acceleration of
spontaneous platelet motions towards the vessel wall by
directed convective motion induced by "swirling" red cells
that "mix" the platelets and move them towards the thrombotic deposit. In life sciences (see text-book of General
Physiology), and especially in circulatory physiology, a
more strict differentiation between processes governed by
diffusion (motion of dissolved species along a concentration gradient) and convection (motion of the solute or continuous phase) is customary. GOLDSMITH et al. have therefore recently used the term "radial dispersion coefficient".

Irrespective of these semantic ambiguities, it appears
problematic to relate an increased rate of thrombus formation during flow of red cell-thrombocyte suspensions simply
to a diffusion process. Firstly, it is not established
that the platelets deposited onto a thrombus move down an
existing concentration gradient, since platelet density
in the plasma layer near the wall cannot only decrease
through deposition but might also increase through the rapid axial motion of red cells away from the vessel wall and
the deposited thrombi (as shown by WIEDEMAN), resulting in
a skimming of platelet rich plasma. Secondly, the actual
deposition process is governed by complex fluid dynamic
interactions between the fluid and the wall and between
platelets in the fluid and platelets already deposited
(as shown by MÜLLER-MOHNSSEN and KRATZER, s. p. 101).
Thirdly, the blood cells themselves are involved, since
the fluid dynamic forces generated in flow act upon them,
provoking cell specific responses which are a function of
the incident local shear stress (e.g. platelet activation
as shown by FORST, RIEGER and SCHMID-SCHÖNBEIN, see page
46 ) or passive red cell disruption (as shown by FISCHER
et al., see page 244). Platelets are biologically much
more active than red cells, they can respond to specific
as well as unspecific stimuli which trigger their contractile and secretory apparatus and transform the platelets

from their resting to their adhesive state ("viscous or sticky metamorphosis" in the sense of EBERTH and SCHIMMEL-BUSCH, or "shape change"). As originally shown by GAARDER red cells contain one of the most potent specific stimuli (adenosine-diphosphate); however, the mechanism by which ADP traverses the erythrocyte membrane, which is normally impermeable to adenine nucleotides (see text books of Biochemistry) is unsettled. The well established deformation and/or disruption of erythrocytes in shear opened the possibility that specific changes in the membranes of red cells under strain, and/or overt mechanical hemolysis might liberate sufficient ADP to stimulate platelets. We attempted, therefore, to design an experiment in which red cells are exposed for short periods to shear stresses above $50 \text{ N/m}^2$. The advent of hollow fibers with truly semi-permeable membrane as wall (Amicon-XM-50) allowed us to use a tube-rheometer apparatus for these experiments. In such a device, ultrafiltrate stemming from the marginal fluid layers subjected to high shear stresses in flow can be obtained and collected for further chemical analysis. It was hoped to analyse in more detail rapidly occurring, strictly localized rheological and biochemical events taking place during red cell deformation and/or disruption.


2. Methods and Materials

The experiments were executed by pumping a blood sample only once through a capillary of known dimensions under controlled driving pressure and thus controlled transmural (filtering) pressure. The experiments were designed so that the diameter (500 µm), the permeability to plasma ultrafiltrate ($3 \text{ µl} = 3 \cdot 10^{-3} \text{ ml/min/mmHg}$) and the flow rates were matched to allow the perfusion rate of the unit with a total volume of blood (about 300 - 500 ml) to produce a wall shear stress of 50 to 200 $\text{N/m}^2$ while obtaining an ultrafiltrate of 500 - 2000 µl for chemical analysis. These requirements were met when we contructed a capillary of 18 cm length, perfused under a driving pressure of 1-4 bar for 200 $\text{N/m}^2$ for 10 min. Previous studies in our labora-

tory and other (HEUSER) had shown that high pressure as
such did not produce any measurable hemolysis in the blood.

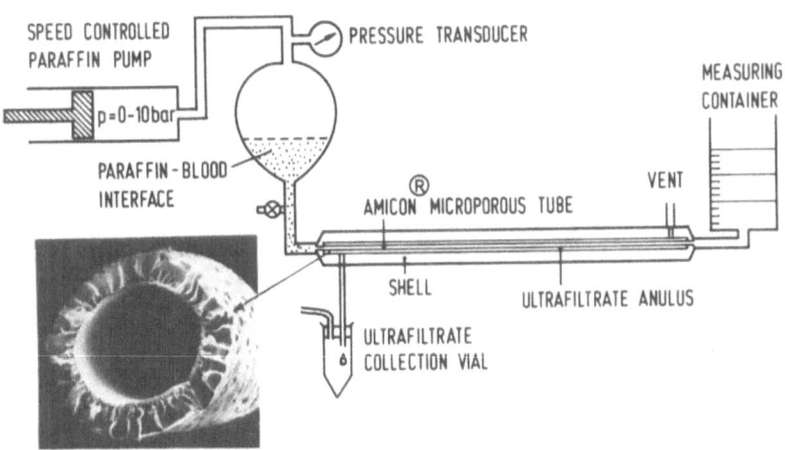

Fig. 1: Schematic representation of the ultrafilter-tube-
        rheometer. A micoporous tube (insert showing scan-
        ning-electron-microsope picture of tube produced by
        GEMEINSCHAFTSLABOR FÜR ELEKTRONENMIKROSPIE, RWTH
        AACHEN, Dr. Burchard) is fixed into a groove of a
        plastic shell. The tube is perfused with blood or
        red cell suspensions pressurized by a pump using
        paraffin as a driving fluid. The blood is pumped
        only once through the unit. The ultrafiltrate pro-
        duced is collected by vents and drains of the groo-
        ve. (Design: Mr. H. Myrenne)

The apparatus used is shown s ematically in Fig. 1. A red
blood cell suspension was pumped through the hollow fiber
tubing using paraffin as the driving fluid. A semipermeable Amicon hollow fiber membrane of 0.5 mm internal diameter and a length of 18 cm, permeable to molecules up to
a molecular weight of 50.000 was employed (Amicon XM 50,
supplied by Amicon Corporation, Lexington/Mass.). The wall
shear stresses in the tube (50 and 200 $N/m^2$) were obtained

325

by continuously measuring the pressure difference between
the upstream and the downstream of the unit using a National Semiconductor pressure transducer Model LX 1720 A, the
amplified signal was recorded on a DC compensation recorder
(SERVOGOR Model 502). As a control of the hydrodynamic conductivity of the hollow fiber, the driving pressure for a
given flow rate was measured continuously. The permeability was tested daily by measuring the transmural
flux of distilled water at a pressure of 0.15 bar. The
reflection coefficient for human serum albumin was tested
by measuring the protein concentration in the ultrafiltrate
obtained during perfusion with 1% Albumin. Units permitting
Albumin (or Hemoglobin) passage were discarded, thus in-
suring that there was no leak of cells or macromolecules
through the walls of the hollow fiber.

500 ml of blood were drawn from an apparently healthy
donor with heparin as anticoagulant. After gentle centrifugation, removing the plasma and the buffy coat, the RBC's
were washed twice with 500 ml of phosphate buffered isotonic saline containing 0.1 g% glucose, and were resuspended
in the same medium with 5 g/l human serum albumin added.
Two suspensions were prepared with hematocrits of 40 and
60%. In other experiments, the cells were resuspended in
their native plasma at a hematocrit value of 40 and 60% by
the appropriate admixture of platelet poor plasma filtered
after high g-centrifugation. One half of each suspension
was sheared with 50 N/m$^2$ the other with 200 N/m$^2$. A very
small amount from each suspension was kept unsheared as
controls. Samples were taken from both the sheared and the
unsheared red cell suspension and from the ultrafiltrate.

Processing of the samples was carried out immediately
in the cold. After centrifugation of the blood samples,
1 ml of the supernatant and 1 ml of the ultrafiltrate was
added to 50 µl of icecold 6n perchloric acid for precipi-
tating the proteins (where present). The precipitate was
spun down and the supernatant titrated to neutrality with
6n KOH. The dilution factor was estimated by weighing.

The nucleotides were separated on the HPLC (Waters
Associates, Model 440) followed by photometric detection on

a U.V. spectrophotometer (254 nm). In other experiments, nucleotides were analysed after synthesizing strongly fluorescent derivatives by detection on a spectrofluorometer (Jobin Yvon, Model JY3, excitation 280 nm, fluorescence 424 nm). In either case, peak areas were integrated by a Spectra-Physics Autolab Minigrator. Derivatives were synthesized as described by YOSHIOKA with 100 µl of acetate buffer and 10 µl of 4m chloroacetaldehyde per 500 µl of sample. The tubes were immersed for 20 min at $80^{\circ}$C, controls with gravimetrically determined adenine nucleotide concentration were treated and measured identically to correct for nucleotide dephosphorylation during the heating procedure. For the measurement of the hemoglobin concentration, the cyanmethemoglobin-method was employed. Extinction was measured at 540 nm and 680 nm on a Zeiss spectrophotometer Model PMQII. Potassium concentrations in the supernatant and the ultrafiltrate were measured on an Eppendorf flamephotometer after appropriate calibration.

## 3. RESULTS

### 3.1. Spontaneous hemolysis

Despite very careful preparation of the blood samples, there was considerable spontaneous hemolysis. Spontaneous hemolysis at the beginning of the experiments was minimal in the red cell suspension using albuminated isotonic saline as a continuous phase. Here, however, spontaneous hemolysis continued in samples not subjected to flow. In all samples, the spontaneous hemolysis varied greatly from donor to donor. In plasma samples adjusted 60% hematocrit, the hemolysis was lower (computed as percent of the cells in the sample) than in the 40% samples, because less of the already slightly hemolytic plasma was added to the sample after cell washing.

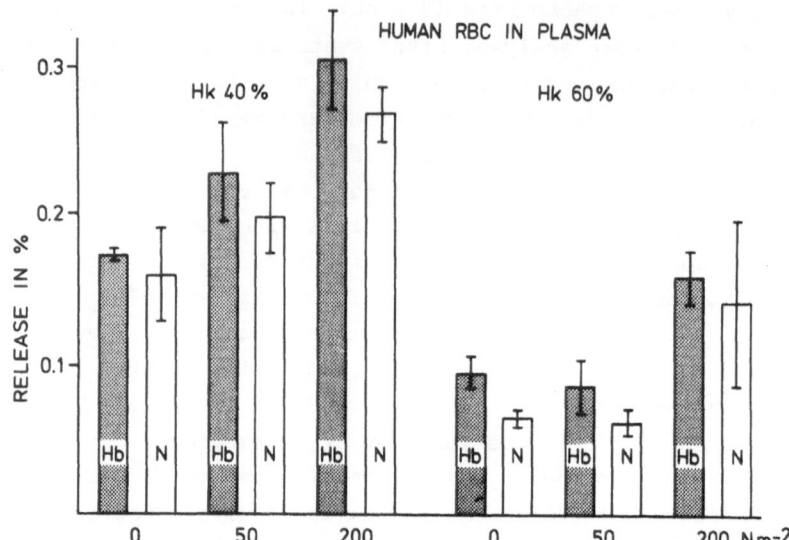

Fig. 2: Release of hemoglobin (dotted colums, Hb) and total adenine nucleotides (open colums, N) from human RBC in isologous citrated plasma calculated as fraction of total nucleotides present in the supernatant after rest (0), after one single passage with a wall shear stress of 50 and 200 $N/m^2$ respectively. The fractional release of hemoglobin and nucleotides is not significantly increased by perfusing with 50 $N/m^2$, but significantly increased at 200 $N/m^2$. (n = 3, $\bar{x} \pm$ S.E.M.)

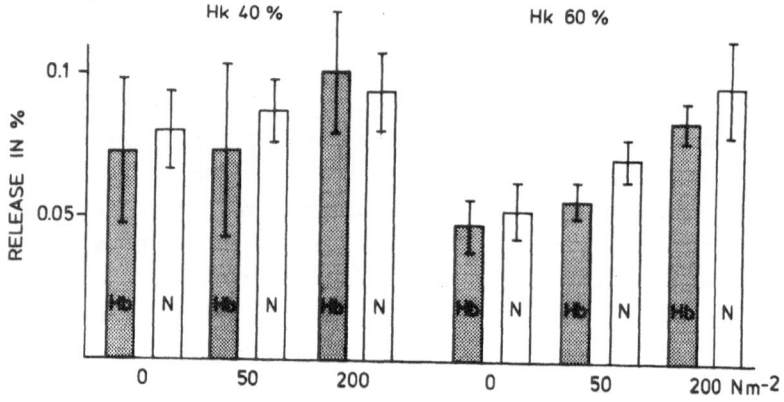

Fig. 3: Data as in Fig. 2, obtained in human RBC suspended in buffered, isotonic, albuminated saline. Note significant increase in hemoglobin and nucleotides only at 200 $N/m^2$. (n = 4 at 40% HK, n = 5 at 60% HK, $\bar{x} \pm$ S.E.M.)

## 3.2. Low flow effects on hemolysis at $\tau_w$ = 50 N/m$^2$

As shown in Fig. 2 and 3, a single passage of red cells through the capillary at a wall shear stress of 50 N/m$^2$ did not increase the hemolysis, neither at 40 nor at 60% hematocrit. To account for the total hemolysis occurring the hemoglobin concentrations in the supernatant were transformed by computing the percentage of the total hemoglobin contained in all red cells of the sample. Nucleotide concentrations were computed similarly (v.i.) There was a considerable scatter of data. In some cases (especially with red cells in plasma), we did notice an increased hemolysis, in others we found no increase.

Pending further clarification, we tend to attribute the elevated hemolysis at 50 N/m$^2$ to individual sensitivity or technical reasons (see below). When all experiments are taken together, the absolute hemoglobin concentration in the 40% control samples (in albuminated saline 0.049±0.025 in plasma 0.137±0.034) are not different from those after a single passage through the unit (in albuminated saline 0.058±0.032, in plasma 0.148±0.039). From this we conclude, that the apparatus as such, the contact of blood to the AMICON tubing and the filtration through the tube wall did not cause a significant additional hemolysis, i.e. the procedure and apparatus is compatible to the blood. The same trend was seen in all 60% Hct samples. This assumption is born out by the similar measurements of the total nucleotides, the distribution of nucleotides and the potassium concentration in the supernatant and the ultrafiltrate (v.i.).

## 3.3. High flow effects on hemolysis ($\tau_w$ = 200 N/m$^2$)

When flow was accelerated, resulting in a wall shear stress of 200 N/m$^2$, the single passage of the red cell suspensions through the capillary did produce a significant increase in hemolysis rate in the 40% hematocrit samples, with plasma or albuminated saline as a control. As can be seen from figures 2 and 3, the hemoglobin released rose from 0.049% to 0.101% (in albuminated saline) and from 0.137 to 0.242% in plasma; this is a highly significant effect. In other words; about $5 \times 10^{-4}$ and $10^{-3}$ respectively of all erythrocytes passing through the AMICON tube released their hemoglobin. The same trend was seen at 60% hematocrit - but numerically the increase is more significant.

3.4. Release of total adenine nucleotide

In either red cell suspensions and at both hematocrit levels, the sums of the ATP, ADP and AMP concentrations in the supernatant, calculated as a fraction of the sum of the same adenine nucleotides in the red cells were practically identical to the fraction of hemoglobin released from red cells. In the experiments with red cells in plasma, the percent total adenine nucleotide release is slightly lower, in albuminated saline it is slightly higher than the percent hemoglobin release. In all samples, the percent nucleotide release increased when wall shear stress was elevated from 50 to 200 $N/m^2$.

Table I

Percent release of total adenine nucleotides (based on total nucleotide control of red cell suspension pumped, n = 4)

| RBC in | Hct 0.4o | | Hct 0.60 | |
|---|---|---|---|---|
| Plasma | Supernatant | Exsudate | Supernatant | Exsudate |
| Control | $0.161 \pm 0.046$ | - | $0.065 \pm 0.011$ | - |
| 50 $N/m^2$ | $0.199 \pm 0.084$ | $0.077 \pm 0.015$ | $0.062 \pm 0.013$ | $0.046 \pm 0.005$ |
| 200 $N/m^2$ | $0.269 \pm 0.019$ | 0.099 | $0.084 \pm 0.030$ | $0.045 \pm 0.009$ |
| RBC in alb. Saline | | | | |
| Control | $0.0926 \pm 0.033$ | - | $0.053 \pm 0.021$ | - |
| 50 $N/m^2$ | $0.097 \pm 0.028$ | $0.051 \pm 0.022$ | $0.072 \pm 0.015$ | $0.045 \pm 0.013$ |
| 200 $N/m^2$ | $0.097 \pm 0.0232$ | $0.072 \pm 0.020$ | $0.093 \pm 0.034$ | $0.074 \pm 0.052$ |

3.5. Concentration and distribution of adenine nucleotides in the supernatant and the ultrafiltrate

In the presence of plasma or hemolysed red cells, nucleotides released from the intracellular compartment

of cells are likely to be dephosphorylated in a time dependent fashion from ATP to ADP or AMP by plasmatic myokinases
or cytoplasmatic ATPases released into the continuous phase. In an attempt to gain information on the relative concentration of ADP (a platelet activating substance) compared to ATP and AMP (which inhibit platelets) the nucleotide
concentrations of the ultrafiltrate were compared to those
of the supernatant before and after shearing. As can be
seen from Table II, the total concentration of nucleotides in the supernatant and the ultrafiltrate was between
1 and 5 x $10^{-6}$ Moles/L, the fractional release of the
nucleotides was equivalent to the fractional release of
hemoglobin (Figure 2 and 3). These findings indicate that
1) in the control samples the total extracellular nucleotides are the consequence of spontaneous hemolysis, and
that 2) in the samples exposed to 50 and especially
200 N/m$^2$ wall shear stress, the additional nucleotides are
likewise the consequence of a total disruption of a fraction of red cells (shear induced mechanical hemolysis).

Table II

Content and Composition of Adenine-Nucleotides in Supernatant und Ultrafiltrate (μMol/l)

| | HK 40% | | | | HK 60% | | | |
|---|---|---|---|---|---|---|---|---|
| | [ATP] | [ADP] | [AMP] | total | [ATP] | [ADP] | [AMP] | total |
| RBC in Plasma | Supernatant | | | | Supernatant | | | |
| RBC (x10$^3$) | 10.27 | 0.63 | 0.0 | 10.90 | 17.19 | 0.87 | 0.06 | 18.12 |
| Supernatant Control | 0.35 | 0.17 | 2.28 | 2.80 | 0.32 | 0.27 | 2.44 | 3.03 |
| Supernatant 50 N/m$^2$ | 1.09 | 0.31 | 2.23 | 3.63 | 0.40 | 0.28 | 1.90 | 2.58 |
| Supernatant 200 N/m$^2$ | 1.57 | 0.28 | 2.72 | 4.57 | 1.11 | 0.25 | 2.20 | 3.56 |
| RBC in alb. Saline | Supernatant | | | | Supernatant | | | |
| RBC | 9.99 | 0.87 | 0.02 | 10.88 | 16.51 | 0.93 | 0.05 | 17.49 |
| Supernatant Control | 0.73 | 0.45 | 0.63 | 1.81 | 0.71 | 0.40 | 1.12 | 2.23 |
| Supernatant 50 N/m$^2$ | 1.00 | 0.53 | 0.85 | 2.38 | 1.33 | 0.48 | 1.53 | 3.34 |
| Supernatant 200 N/m$^2$ | 0.86 | 0.33 | 0.74 | 1.93 | 1.79 | 0.75 | 1.84 | 4.38 |
| | Exsudate | | | | Exsudate | | | |
| RBC in plasma 50 N/m$^2$ | 0.10 | 0.14 | 1.03 | 1.27 | 0.19 | 0.16 | 1.43 | 1.78 |
| RBC in plasma 200 N/m$^2$ | 0.45 | 0.15 | 1.20 | 1.80 | - | - | 1.46 | - |
| RBC in alb.Sal. 50 N/m$^2$ | 0.23 | 0.28 | 0.46 | 0.97 | 0.24 | 0.37 | 1.46 | 2.07 |
| RBC in alb.Sal. 200 N/m$^2$ | 0.48 | 0.31 | 0.67 | 1.46 | 0.62 | 0.22 | 1.41 | 2.25 |

When comparing the absolute amount of adenine-nucleotides released - and the absolute amount of hemolysis in the 40 and 60% Hct sample, there were no significant differences in the values for identical shear stresses. (The apparent reduction in fractional release at 60% is a result of the computation on the basis of all red cells pumped). These findings suggest that for a <u>constant</u> shear stress up to 200 N/m$^2$, the hematocrit as such is not significant. It remains to be clarified in the future whether or not under natural conditions the same relationship holds: here, a higher hematocrit and thence higher viscosity produces <u>higher shear stresses</u> for any given flow (or cardiac output).

When compared to the distribution found in intact red cells, the concentrations of ATP, ADP and AMP in the supernatant and the ultrafiltrate markedly differs. There is a pronounced relative and absolute increase of AMP. The concentration of the ADP varied between $10^{-7}$ and $10^{-6}$ mol/L, i.e. both in the supernatant and in the ultrafiltrate ADP is found in sufficient concentrations to activate

platelets - which was indeed found in separate experiments (v.i.).

According to hydrodynamic theory, in a perfused tube the highest shear stresses occur in the layer immediately adjacent to the tube wall, i.e. in the region likely to provide the fluid ultrafiltered in our experiments. Therefore, the assumption that only the high shear stresses near the tube wall give rise to mechanical hemolysis would include the expectation that the compounds released there should be more concentrated in the ultrafiltrate than in the supernatant (which is a mixture of a small amount of plasma exposed to high and a large amount of plasma exposed to lower shear stresses). Contrary to expectation, the concentrations are even lower. Nucleotide absorption to the AMICON-material is the most likely reason for this relative decrease in ultrafiltrate nucleotide concentration - such adsorption was indeed measured in perfusion experiments using dissolved nucleotides of known concentration (ROHLING-WINKEL, in preparation).

332

## 3.6. $K^+$-concentration in ultrafiltrate and supernatant of plasma

The $K^+$-concentration, on the other hand, was regularly found higher in the ultrafiltrate than in the supernatant - a finding supporting the basic hypothesis of the present experiments. At both 40 and 60 % Hct $K^+$ was higher in the sheared supernatant than in the control, and in the ultrafiltrate higher than in the respective supernatant. While basically these data support the idea of a preferential $K^+$ release near the wall (from which the supernatant is obtained), the data are extremely difficult to evaluate quantitatively at the moment. Neither the dead space in the AMICON tubing, nor the depth of the layer from which the ultrafiltrate originates can be determined at present. Whether or not a preferential release of $K^+$ from sheared red cells occurs can only be determined after further experiments in which total nucleotides (including the adsorbed adenine nucleotides)are recovered by desorbtion. Experiments to this end are in progress.

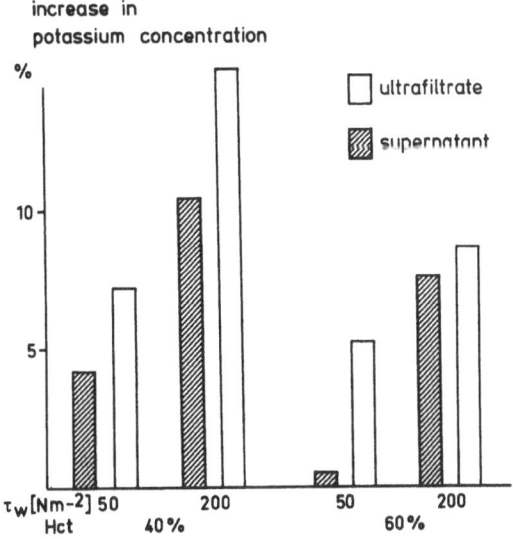

Fig. 4: Influence of the wall shear stress (50 and 200 N/m$^2$) on the potassium content (% increase) of supernatant and ultrafiltrate at 50 and 200 N/m$^2$ (n = 6)

333

## 4.   Discussion

### 4.1. Technical comments

To our knowledge, the present experiments are the first attempt to analyse the biochemical consequences of mechanical red cell destruction in   t u b e    flow. In some respects, the ultrafiltering capillaries used proved helpful: it is possible to gain access to the low molecular weight chemical species produced by mechanical red cell destruction and to analyse them qualitatively. Furthermore, their action on platelets can be monitored. On the other hand, these experiments are difficult to interpret quantitatively. First, the depth of the layer from which the ultrafiltrate is stemming cannot be determined. Consequently, even though one can calculate the wall shear stress distribution in the entire tube, it is not possible to calculate the shear stress acting on those cells that are actually destroyed or damaged. However, when calculating the transmural flux (e.g. 500 µl/min at $\tau_w$= 200 N/m$^2$) in a tube of about 300 mm$^2$ total inner surface as a funtion of filtration  area ($\sim$ 28 nl/sec mm$^2$), the mean of the velocity component towards the wall is 1.6 mm/min or 28 µm/sec. This velocity component towards the wall is small in comparison to the flow velocity. At a distance of 2.5 µm (= 0.99 R) the velocity parallel to the wall is 7.0 cm/sec, at 25 µm (0.90 R) it is even 67.1 cm/sec. The mean flow velocity is about 1.77 m/sec. Thus, it is unlikely that layers far away from the wall contribute much to the ultrafiltrate.

On the other hand, the requirements of large filtrate volumes for chemical analysis made it necessary to use a long tube. Consequently, the exposure times of the red cells near the wall (= 0.99 R) are quite high (6 - 10 sec at 50 N/m$^2$, 1.7 - 2.6 sec at 200 N/m$^2$). In light of the well established time dependency of red cell destruction (see OLIJSLAGER, SUTERA), these long exposure times are a serious disadvantage of the present experiments. Clearly, experiments with better time resolution are mandatory to further clarify the shear dependent interaction of red cells and thrombocytes in tube and/or COUETTE flow.

The obvious advantage of having a semipermeable tube wall is reduced by the tendency of nucleotides to adsorb to the AMICON tubing. The adsorption is not surprising in light of the spongy structure of the AMICON tubing (see Fig. 1), specific desorption experiments are therefore necessary for a more quantitative analysis.

## 4.2. Experimental results

Irrespective of the technical limitations of the apparatus, a number of significant results were obtained which can be summarized as follows:

1. following a single passage of red cells suspensions in either a native plasma or in an artificial potassium-free continuous medium at shear stresses of 50 $N/m^2$ there is no significant hemolysis over that present in the control cell suspension, whereas at 200 $N/m^2$ there is an overt hemolysis equivalent to the destruction of 0.055 - 0.1% of all cells perfused through the apparatus.

2. In the supernatant, the adenine nucleotides and the hemoglobin appear in the same relative molar concentration. Thence, when calculated in percent of the total amount pumped, the fraction of hemoglobin and the fraction of nucleotides released is not different. In other words, in the present experiments there is no indication of a preferential release of either ATP, ADP or AMP.

3. The distribution of adenine nucleotides in the supernatant and the exsudate differs significantly from that found in freeze-thaw hemolysate of intact red cells.

4. The ultrafiltrate obtained from the marginal fluid layers contains consistently higher potassium concentrations than the supernatant.

5. The adenosine-diphosphate concentration (0.2 - 0.5 μmolar) both in the supernatant and in the exsudate is certainly sufficient to activate platelets. It is well known that the affinity of the adenosine-diphosphate to its

receptor on the platelets is by several orders of magnitude higher than that of ATP and AMP, which can only inhibit the ADP-response at much higher concentrations (mMol, BORN 19  ).

In all experiments, a very high relative concentration of adenosine-monophosphate and a relatively low concentration of adenosine-triphosphate was found. This is explainable, however, since there are a number of possible mechanisms leading to a change in the distribution of energy-rich phosphates. There may be a breakdown of adenosine-triphosphate before, during and after rupture of red cells. Since, especially in the experiments with citrated plasma as a continuous phase, an ATPase from the plasma and from lysed red cells was functional, a rapid breakdown of ATP to ADP and of ADP to AMP and even a complete dephosphorylation of AMP to adenosine is quite likely.

Therefore, the platelet aggregating activity of the "hemolysate" produced by the mechanical rupture of a red cell in shear is probably much higher than can be extrapolated from the mere concentration of ADP at the end of an experiment.[+)]
A very pronounced activation of platelets by the ultrafiltrate was actually observed in separate experiments using the same apparatus. In these experiments, the isologous platelet rich plasma was perfused through the "extravascular compartment" immediately adjacent to the ultrafiltering semipermeable AMICON-tubing. When passing through the extravascular space, the platelets were only activated (i.e. "shape changed" and aggregated) when red cell suspensions were driven through the unit with shear stresses

─────────────

+) Since the completion of these experiments, we found that a hemolysate (produced by osmotic red cell destruction) is indeed more potent in producing platelet aggregation, 5-HT and β-thrombo-globulin release than an equimolar amount of ADP added to PRP (WURZINGER and BLASBERG , Proc. World Congress Thrombosis, London 1979).

above 50 N/m$^2$ (BLASBERG, ROHLING-WINKEL and WEYER
to be published). These results are especially significant
in light of the fact that a major part of the adenine-nucleotides is likely to be adsorbed onto the AMICON-material
in these experiments as well. On the other hand, the activation is not surprising in light of the well established
susceptibility of platelets to ADP doses as low as
$10^{-8}$ mol/L in the presence of Ca$^{++}$ (see paper WURZINGER
et al., p. 80 ).


Summary and conclusions

1) The present experiments have shown that mechanical rupture of the fluid-drop-like red cells in shear can lead to
release of adenosine-diphosphate. This mechanism may well
be an essential step in the natural activation of platelets.
Our findings may explain

a) the mechanism of transport of ADP from the intracellular to the extracellular space of red cells - and thus
   in the vicinity of platelets,

b) the mechanism by which a platelet activator meets its
   target well before the platelet reaches the wall onto
   which it is to be deposited following activation("shape
   change" or viscous metamorphosis). Previous assumptions
   about the wall as the origin of the activator are  in
   conflict with some of the most elementary fluid dynamic
   facts. As detailed elsewhere (SCHMID-SCHÖNBEIN 1977),
   an upstream diffusion of activator from the wall against
   a rapid downstream convection is extremely unlikely.


2) The experiments provide a microrheological and biochemical explanation for the well known fact that platelet
deposition and platelet aggregation is markedly enhanced
by
a) the presence of red cells,
b) any increase in shear rate and/or shear stress


3) The experiments emphasize the significance of hemolysis,
which should no longer be considered as a mere threat to

the red cell mass, the hemoglobin metabolism and oxygen
transport, but rather as a triggering event in natural and
pathological hemostatic reactions involving platelets.
A more general discussion of the physiological significance of red cell-thrombocyte interactions in natural hemostasis is given elsewhere   (SCHMID-SCHÖNBEIN et al. 1979).
In the context of blood trauma, the results underscore the
call for an even better control of hemolysis in order to
improve "non-thrombogenicity" of biomaterials and entire
artificial internal organs.

# REFERENCES

1 BAUMGARTNER, H.R.: The rôle of blood flow in platelet adhesion, fibrin deposition, and formation or mural thrombi. Microvasc.Res. 5, 167-179 (1973)

2 LEONARD, E.F.: The role of flow in thrombogenesis. Bull.N.Y.Acad.Med. 48, 273-280 (1972)

3 TURITTO, V.T., and H.R. BAUMGARTNER: Platelet deposition on subendothelium exposed to flowing blood: mathematical analysis of physical parameters. Trans.Amer.Soc.Artif. Organs 21, 593-601 (1975)

4 SCHMID-SCHÖNBEIN, H.: Microrheology of Erythrocytes and Thrombocytes Blood Viscosity and the Distribution of Blood Flow in the Microcirculation. Handbuch der allgemeinen Pathologie III/7 Mikrozirkulation. H. Meessen (ed.) Springer-Verlag Berlin, Heidelberg 1977, p. 289-384

5 GRABOWSKI, E.F., L.I. FRIEDMAN, E.F. LEONARD: Effects of shear rate on the diffusion and adhesion of blood platelets to a foreign surface. Ind.Eng.Chem.Fund 11, 224 (1972)

6 BLACKSHEAR, P.L., K.W. BARTELT, R.J. FORSTROM: Fluid dynamic factors affecting particle capture and retention. Ann.N.Y. Acad.Sci. 283, 270-279 (1977)

7 GOLDSMITH, H.L.: Platlet motions and interactions in tube flow. Proceedings Third Intern. Congress of Biorheology, La Jolla, Calif. 1978. Biorheology (in press)

8 WIEDEMAN, M.P., E.H. MARGULIES: Factors affecting production of platelet aggregates and motion picture documents shown during 7th European Conference Microcirculation, Aberdeen 1972

9 MÜLLER-MOHNSSEN, H., M. KRATZER, and W. BALDAUF: Microthrombus formation in models of coronary arteries caused by stagnation point flow arising at the predilection sites of atherosclerosis and thrombosis. In:The role of fluid mechanics in atherogenesis (R.M. Nerem and J.F. Cornhill, Eds.), Ohio State Univ., Ohio, p. 12 (1978)

10 FORST, R., H. RIEGER, H. SCHMID-SCHÖNBEIN: Stimulation of human platelets under the influence of high shear stresses in tube flow. This volume.

11 FISCHER, T.M., M. STÖHR-LIESEN, and H.SCHMID-SCHÖNBEIN: Micromechanics of the red cell in viscometric flow. This volume.

12 EBERTH, C.J. and C. SCHIMMELBUSCH: Die Thrombose nach Versuchen und Leichenbefunden. Stuttgart, Verlag von Ferdinand Enke (1888)

13 GAARDER, A., J. JONSON, S. LALAND, A. HELLEM, P.A. OWREN: Adenosine diphosphate in red cells as a factor in the adhesiveness of human blood platelets. Nature (London) 192, 531 (1961)

14 HEUSER, G., Aerodynamisches Institut der RWTH Aachen. Personal communication.

15 YOSHIOKA, M.: Fluorimetric determination of adenine and adenosine and its nucleotides by HPLC. J.Chrom. 123, 220-224 (1976)

16 OLIJSLAGER, J., J. FEIJEN, J.C.F. DE JONG, and Ch.R.H. WILDEVUUR: Cellular blood damage caused by foreign materials: An engineers view of the problem. This volume.

17 SUTERA, S.; Flow-induced trauma to blood cells Circ. Res. 41, 2 - 8 (1977)

| DISCUSSION | Moderator: Born |
|---|---|
| Born: | Thank you for that summary of the present situation and our collaboration. Can I open this for discussion? |
| Kratzer: | We heard a very interesting experiment about the behaviour of red cells under the influence of extreme flow conditions. I don't think that such flow conditions will be observed in any human being. You applied a very high pressure up to 10 Atü, did I get it, or 3-10 Atü? - This is a one hundred meter water column. This is nearly the height of a sky-scraper. I tried to calculate the velocities in your experiment. You got about 8 m/second centre line velocity for the erythrocytes. This is more than Armin Hary in his well-known olympic record - and that for erythrocytes. Well, but I will come to the point. You concluded from your experiment that the rupture of the red cell membrane is caused by the high shear-stress generated in the marginal layer of the tube flow. However, there may be an important second hemolysing factor: the so-called red cell tether as observed by BLACKSHEAR. Fast flowing red cells come into contact with the rough tube wall and will be torn. BLACKSHEAR made a consideration about fluid forces acting on an isolated particle flowing near a filtering wall. If the filtration velocity which is directed towards the wall overcomes the axial, migration which is directed away from the wall the cell will be pressed towards the wall. Still having a calculated velocity of about 9 cm/second, which is very fast, this phenomenon can be observed in a reflective interference microscope. We observed destruction of red cell membranes even at relatively low wall shear stresses. When red cells are attached to a glass wall, tethers form which rupture at a shear stress of about 7 $dyn/cm^2$. |

A similar attachment could occur in your experiment, did you consider that possibility? Since you
have filtration, you must expect that red cells
are carried towards the wall. Interaction of cells
with the wall will occur if viscosity and filtration rate exceed a certain value, which also depends on the square of the particle radius and
wall shear rate. You'll have interaction if:

$$\frac{V^{\frac{1}{2}} \cdot U}{R^2 \cdot S^{\frac{3}{2}}} > 0.11$$

V = kinetic viscosity
U = filtration rate
R = particle radius
S = wall shear-rate

Born:           Thank you. To the best of my knowledge this does
                not happen in vivo. The only evidence I know of
                red cells being disturbed like this is by FLOREY
                who saw red cells caught temporarily on some
                curious obstacle like a spike sticking out from
                the endothelial surface into the circulating
                blood. Red cells were caught for a few seconds
                but never broken up. You may say that is not re-
                levant to that what is done *in vitro*. I have not
                done a calculation but I would have thought that
                the filtration effect is negligible in relation
                to the other flow effects in the system.

Schmid-Schönbein:   It is certainly important to talk about actual
                values here. Pressure up to 10 bar as such has
                no effect on red cells as has been shown by a
                number of groups (e.g. LAMBERT et al.). This
                is not surprising because the red cell under
                pressure behaves like a water pillow which trans-
                mits the pressure from the extracellular to the
                intracellular space, therefore no membrane strains

occur other than a compression of a lipid film . The latter is a fluid itself which is incompressible to normal stresses. However, shear-stresses have very strong effects. In our system, we had to find a compromize between several requirements. We were interested in high shear-stress levels we conjecture to occur in the disturbed circulation (not in the intact one). Under the situation of arteriolar incision these high shear stresses exist; they are, of course, a function of the driving pressure $^{\Delta p}/l$. Now we had one other problem. We wanted to have as much filtrate as possible, therefore, we had to make long tubes and an apparatus which allowed us to pump the blood at very high pressure. Actually 500 ml blood were pumped in one run at 3 atm. of pressure. Our main problem was to obtain sufficient filtrate through the hollow fibers. The amicon filters we use are quite a-thrombogenic and are constructed in such a way that even macromolecules do not clot the filter. Thus, we are not too much concerned about the possible adhesion of the red cells. We expect red cell trauma at the entrance region; however, the manner by which these tubes are glued into our flow chamber makes us rather certain that the entrances do not attract red cells. This is substantiated by the fact that with low flow we see no effects. Last, regarding the question of filtration polarization, we do not consider this important in our experiment as we get less than 0.01 % filtration. So I think it's fair to say radial motion of red cells are negligible. We do not press the red cells towards the wall, furthermore, we have a coat of proteins which prevents red cell adhesion even to glass.

Williams: The problem is what speeds and velocities are developed during flow through the tubes. Surely,

343

the Reynolds number is high and so it is not
fair to talk with us of radial migration and flow
separation of the cells coming away from the wall.
In fact, you may have turbulent flow within that
capillary. I see, it is 800, thank you.

Schmid-Schönbein:     But again we are concerned about it but we don't
know much about it. We are now planing to in-
vestigate this but for this purpose we have to
destroy these precious units.

Williams:             We refer to Dr. Schmid-Schönbein's excellent paper entiteld "The first evidence of induced ADP-
release from red cells subjected to high shear-
stress". I would like to go on record with our
experiments which describe the second evidence
of induced ADP-release from red cell by shear-
stress. My other research field is the investigation of the possible biological effects of ultrasound. And so ultra sound keeps creeping into my
shear-stress work. Because, if you take gas
bubbles and subject them to an ultrasonic field,
they undergo radial pulsation and generate a second order acoustic microstreaming field, e.g.
a high local shear-stress field. If you now have
platelets in plasma but mixed with an extract of
firefly tails (Luciferase, which can detect minute quantities of ATP by emmitting visible light)
then, ultrasonic exposure causes the emission of
light. If red cells are also present then much
more light is emitted even though the red cells
are not ruptured.

Born:                 That is interesting because it takes us back to
the original question, whether nucleotides can
escape from red cells without loss of hemoglobin,
i.e. without classical hemolysis. That and your
observations seem to provide some evidence for it.
Could I ask one or two questions? The experiment
is done with ultrasound, right? And then you measure free hemoglobin and free adenin-nucleotides

344

mainly as ATP?

Williams:           We use the Luciferase system because it is an
                    exceptionally sensitive system for the detection
                    of ATP release. With it we can detect nanogram
                    quantities of ATP. And it does so even in blood
                    plasma where any released ATP will otherwise be
                    rapidly broken down. So that in using the firefly
                    extract one can have an exceptionally sensitive
                    system. And we then subject platelets to a small
                    amount of hydrodynamic trauma using ultrasound
                    as a convenient way of producing small scale
                    shear-forces within the suspension of platelets.
                    But if you subject these platelets to shear-
                    stresses greater than 300 dyn/cm$^2$ for exposure
                    times of the order of milliseconds one can get
                    predictable amounts of ATP coming out. And this
                    amount is vastly increased if red cells are
                    present.

Born:               Could it be that red cells which are an enormous
                    reservoir of myokinase turn any ADP from released
                    platelets into ATP.

Williams:           The only preparation of Luciferase that we had
                    was already contaminated with myokinase. Conse-
                    quently, any ADP doming out from the platelets
                    or red cells would itself be seen as ATP.

Müller-Mohnssen:    I beg your pardon, if I direct the discussion
                    again to the results of BLACKSHEAR. The reason is,
                    that your argumentation is based, in my opinion
                    too exclusevely on the shear-stress neglecting
                    other hydrodynamic forces which might be involved.
                    The old experiment of BLACKSHEAR can be compared
                    in its details with yours and it is more trans-
                    parent with respect to the parameter, Dr. Kratzer
                    had in mind when discussing the particle-wall
                    collision. The driving forces of both flow com-
                    ponents in BLACKSHEAR's apparatus are different.
                    First he induces a COUETTE flow tangential to the

surface plane by a rotating cylinder. Secondly
he superimposed a pressure gradient normal to the
plane of surface. Because the wall of the cylinder
is porous, an ultrafiltration flow through the
wall is induced. Whereas the driving forces of
both flow components can easily be separated in
his experiment, the driving force for the ultrafiltration flow and the tube-flow is the same in
your experiment.
Not only the tube-flow velocity and the shear-
stress depend on the pressure gradient but also
the rate of ultrafiltration flow which antagoni-
zes axial migration and may presumably cause the
RBC to contact the surface of the porous wall
mechanically. These collisions may lead to a
rupture of RBC as in the experiment of BLACKSHEAR.
Because the driving force for ultrafiltration
flow is not separated in your experiment one may
overlook, that there may be a dependency of hemolysis rate not only on the shear stress, but also on the rate of ultrafiltration flow as a consequence of a pressure component perpendicular
to the wall (as it is the case in the experiment
of BLACKSHEAR).
This way I interpret the discussion remark of
Dr. Kratzer about the influence of pressure on
the hemolysis rate. We don't think that the
higher pressure itself acts directly on the RBC
but that the it acts rather indirectly via higher
rates of ultrafiltration flow and thus higher
rates of collision between RBC and the wall. Direct experimental evidence (microscopical observation) is necessary if you adhere to the assumption, that interaction between particles and wall
can be neglected in your experiment.
In response to Dr. BORN: I maintain that porous
walls are relevant for in vivo conditions. In the
Department of Pathology at the University of

Düsseldorf, Dr. MEESSEN showed that by scanning electron micrographs of the inner surface of arteries in animals which have an artificial hypertension that large pores are found in the intima and that the inner arterial surface tends to become very rough. Alterations like these may also be a cause for rupture in vivo, where velocity components perpendicular to and towards the wall lead to a collision of RBC and the wall (at curvatures, branchings etc.).

Schmid-Schönbein: In response to this comment, let me again repeat that we are working with the Amicon-material. This Amicon-material is really unique (see Fig. 1, page 325), it is not comparable to those filters that BLACKSHEAR and FORSTROM used. This material is so constructed that the inner surface repels albumin. And as any chemist, who works with the same material as a flat filter will tell you, very gentle swirling motion will prevent a filtration polarisation. In other words not only does albumin not enter the filter, it does not even polarize on the surface. The filtration limit of our filters is about 50.000 Dalton and the pores are two or three orders of magnitudes smaller than the particles which are known to be reflected a hundred percent from the surface we use in our experiment. So, with due respect, I don't think that this argument is valid. Furthermore, there are many electronemicroscope pictures of the same material after use in vivo, and very few platelet adhere to it. Hardly any red cells adhere to it after very much longer exposure times.

Müller-Mohnssen: Did you measure the dependency of your ultrafiltration volume flow through the porous walls on the pressure gradient?

Schmid-Schönbein: This is done every day as a check of the units for hydraulic conductance and permeability (ml of fluid filtered per unit pressure, area and time).

Müller-Mohnssen:     Did you compare the pressure dependency of hemo-
                     lysis rate with that of ultrafiltration flow rate?

Schmid-Schönbein:    This is done every day.

# 6.

## EFFECTS OF CARDIAC SURGERY AND CARDIO-PULMONARY BYPASS ON HUMAN IMMUNE SYSTEM

J. HAKIM, M.-A. GOUGEROT-POCIDALO
and Y. LECOMPTE

From the Laboratoire Central d'Immunologie
et d'Hématologie - Université Paris 7 and
Hôpital Bichat - 170 boulevard Ney -
75877 PARIS CEDEX 18 - F R A N C E .

## 1. INTRODUCTION

Rates of postoperative bacterial infections are high in
patients undergoing cardiac surgery with cardiopulmonary
bypass (CPB) (1,2). These data suggest that host defence
mechanisms may be impaired in the postoperative period. The
purpose of this study is a reappraisal of the postoperative
immune status in these patients since several investigations
have reported its deficiency (3-5) while others found it
normal (6,7).

The parameters we measured, were the serum concentrations of immunoglobulins, total hemolytic complement (CH50),
C3, C4 and C3-proactivator and granulocyte's functions. They
were measured before and after surgery. In this occurrence
each patient  is his own control, and any observed difference can be assigned to the surgical procedure taken as whole,
i.e. including surgical trauma, CPB, anesthesia and other
unknown components included in the surgical period. Our
only purpose was thus, to know if host defence mechanisms
are impaired in this peculiar clinical situtation, and not
to recognize which component of the surgical procedure is
responsible of the postoperative abnormalities observed.

## 2. PATIENTS AND METHODS

### 2.1. Patients

Thirteen patients (5 female and 8 male ; aged 21-67 years)

undergoing cardiac surgery for interauricular communication, aortic or mitral insufficiency, or coronary insufficiency (aorto-coronary bypass), were studied. None of the patients had other pathological manifestations than those related to the heart disease. Blood was drawn preoperatively (1 to 8 days before surgery), 14 to 20 hours after termination of the operation and CPB (J1), and 7 days latter (J8). No drugs were given for at least two weeks before the preoperative blood examination. The drugs used immediately before surgery and during operation (sodium phenobarbital, diazepam, pancuronium bromide, phenoperidine, diperidol, hydrocortisone and epsilon amino-caproic acid) were similar in all patients. Whole blood (250-1500 ml), washed red blood cells (200-400 ml), and plasma (0-400 ml) perfused during surgery were adapted to blood loss and hemodynamic status during surgery. All patients received penicilline G during the two first postoperative days. Penicilline V or lincocine were then administered for the subsequent days. Some of the patients received calciparine and/or digoxin postoperatively. It was tested that the postoperative given drugs had no effect on the parameters of the immune status which we studied.


## 2.2. Methods

### 2.2.1. Preparation of serum
Venous blood samples were allowed to clot at room temperature for 2 hours, and serum separated by centrifugation. A fraction of each serum was immediately used and the remainder was stored in 1 ml aliquots at -80°C, until further testing. Ten control AB sera were pooled and stored in 1 ml aliquots at -80°C. Storage did not modify the activities measured.

### 2.2.2. Serum immunoglobulins and complement
Serum immunoglobulins (IgG, IgA, and IgM) were measured by radial immunodiffusion . Commercially prepared plates

(Behring) were used. Total serum hemolytic complement (CH50) was determined according to Kabat and Meyer (8). Complement components (C3, C4 and C3 proactivator) were measured by radial immunodiffusion (Behring plates).

### 2.2.3. Preparation of granulocytes suspension
Granulocytes from patients and controls were isolated as described previously (9) from heparinized venous blood. The final cell suspension was adjusted to $10^7$ granulocytes/ml. It contained more than 80 % granulocytes and contaminating cells were mainly lymphocytes.

### 2.2.4. Granulocyte function tests
The following tests were performed in either autologous serum or pooled AB serum (control serum) as described previously (10). Ingestion rate was measured with heat-killed non-virulent $^{14}$C-labelled klebsiella in the presence of 10 % serum. Results expressed in terms of microorganisms-associated per granulocyte in 10 min, are the means of triplicate experiments. Cyanide-insensitive $O_2$-consumption of resting and zymosan-stimulated granulocytes, and $H_2O_2$-production were measured polarographically. Results are expressed in nanoatoms of $O_2$ consumed and in nanomoles of $H_2O_2$ produced per min and per $10^6$ granulocytes. Zymosan-stimulated superoxide anion $(O_2^-)$ production was measured by the superoxide-dismutase (SOD)-inhibitable reduction of cytochrome c. Results expressed in nanomoles of reduced cytochrome c per min per $10^6$ granulocytes are the mean of triplicate experiments. Iodination tests were performed in the presence of either 20 or 100 µM iodide. Results expressed in nanomoles of iodide converted to a trichloro-acetic precipitable form per hour, per $10^7$ granulocytes are the means of triplicate experiments. Resting and zymosan-stimulated quantitative nitroblue tetrazolium (NBT) reduction were performed in the absence of serum. Results expressed in nanomoles of NBT reduced per min per $10^6$ granulocytes are the means of triplicate experiments. Myeloperoxidase (MPO)

| | IMMUNOGLOBULINS mg/100 ml | | | CH$_{50}$* | COMPLEMENT SYSTEM mg/100 ml | | C3 proactivator |
|---|---|---|---|---|---|---|---|
| | IgG | IgA | IgM | | C3 | C4 | |
| **PATIENTS** | | | | | | | |
| Mean | 1270 | 270 | 179 | 102 | 77 | 47 | 19 |
| $\pm$ 1 SD | 247 | 72 | 48 | 19 | 11 | 16 | 4 |
| Range | 930-1800 | 124-404 | 118-250 | 72-131 | 72-146 | 23-68 | 11-24 |
| **CONTROLS** | | | | | | | |
| Mean | 1240 | 254 | 162 | 100 | 73 | 46 | 20 |
| $\pm$ 1 SD | 225 | 56 | 36 | 20 | 11 | 12 | 4 |
| Range | 800-1800 | 90-450 | 80-280 | 70-125 | 55-120 | 20-50 | 10-45 |

TABLE I : Immunoglobulins and Complement system before surgery.

* CH$_{50}$ : Total hemolytic complement expressed in % of the day controls.

|  | INGESTION RATE (1) | | Q. NBT RED (2) | | CYT.c RED. (3) | | SP.O2 (4) | | STIM. O2 (5) | | H2O2 (6) | | IODINATION 20 µM (7) | | IODINATION 100 µM (8) | | MPO (9) |
|---|---|---|---|---|---|---|---|---|---|---|---|---|---|---|---|---|---|
|  | AB | Auto | Sp. | Prov. | AB | Auto | AB | Auto | AB | Auto | AB | Auto | AB | Auto | AB | Auto |  |
| **PATIENTS** | | | | | | | | | | | | | | | | | |
| Mean | 7,2 | 7,4 | 0,60 | 1,64 | 3,4 | 3,6 | 1,0 | 1,1 | 8,6 | 9,1 | 3,3 | 3,5 | 0,25 | 0,26 | 0,48 | 0,51 | 186 |
| ± 1 SD | 2,1 | 2,2 | 0,14 | 0,32 | 0,8 | 0,7 | 0,5 | 0,4 | 1,6 | 1,8 | 0,7 | 0,8 | 0,7 | 0,8 | 0,12 | 0,14 | 44 |
| **CONTROLS** | | | | | | | | | | | | | | | | | |
| Mean | 7,6 | | 0,58 | 1,61 | 3,5 | | 0,8 | | 8,0 | | 3,1 | | 0,27 | | 0,53 | | 197 |
| ± 1 SD | 2,0 | | 0,12 | 0,29 | 0,6 | | 0,3 | | 1,3 | | 0,5 | | 0,05 | | 0,09 | | 34 |

TABLE II : Granulocyte functions before surgery.

See Methods for units used in the results. Tests were performed in control AB serum (AB) or in autologous serum (Auto). SP. = resting granulocytes ; STIM. = zymosan stimulated granulocytes.

(1) Number of ingested Klebsiella ; (2) Amount of nitroblue tetrazolium (NBT) reduced ; (3) Amount of cyto-chrome c reduced ; (4) and (5) $O_2$ taken-up ; (6) $H_2O_2$ produced ; (7) and (8) Iodination with 20 or 100 µM iodide ; (9) Myeloperoxidase activity (MPO) in nanomoles x 106 granulocytes x $min^{-1}$

activity in the granulocytes was measured in the homogenate
of a purified population of granulocytes prepared as
described previously (11).

## 2.2.5 Statistical calculations

Comparison of the results observed before and after (J1 or
J8) surgery were done by the Student t-test for paired data.
Comparison between the results observed in the patients
before surgery, and in the control group were done by the
Student t-test.


# 3. RESULTS AND DISCUSSION


## 3.1. Immune status before surgery and CPB

The results observed in the patients before surgery, were
not different from those of a control population (Table I
and II). This shows that the heart disease of the patients
was not associated with measurable modifications of their
immune status. Moreover, granulocyte functions were similar
when studied in autologous serum or in control AB serum
(Table II). These results clearly allowed to use preoperative data in each patient as a control of the effects of
surgical procedure on its immune system, since underlying
illness was not responsible for additional variables.


## 3.2. Immune status after surgery and CPB

### 3.2.1. Humoral factors

On J1, all serum immunoglobulins (Fig 1) as well as (Fig 2)
total hemolytic complement CH50, C3, C4 and C5 proactivaor
were lower (p < 0.001) than preoperatively. On J8, serum
IgA concentration was not different from its preoperative
level, while IgG remained slightly lower (p < 0.01) and IgM

Fig.1 : Serum levels
of immunoglobulins.
Results observed
on first (J1) and
eighth (J8) post-
operative days are
expressed in % of
preoperative values
x    p < 0.05
xx   p < 0.01

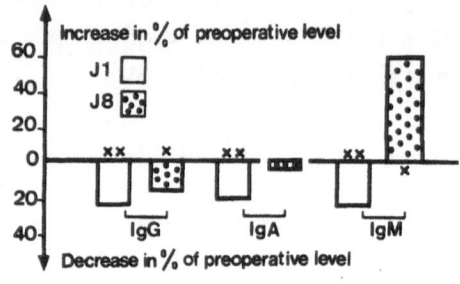

Fig.2 : Complement
system.
Same legends as
under Fig.1.
CH50 : total hemo-
lytic complement,
C3PA : C3 pro-
activator

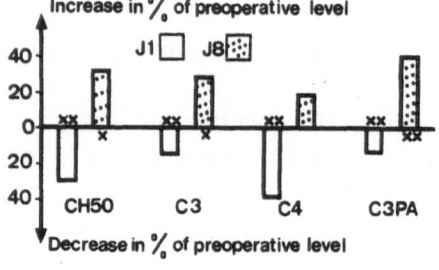

was much higher (p < 0.01). CH50, C3, C4 and C3 proactivator
were higher than preoperatively.

The observed mofidications in serum immunoglobulins
are quite similar to those previously reported in patients
undergoing major surgery with (12) or without CPB (13-19).
The decrease in CH50, C3 and C4 are also in agreement with
previously reported results in patients undergoing surgery
(19). C3 proactivator which, to our knowledge, have not

been measured in these patients, seems to follow the same
pattern as other complement components.

In conclusion, all the humoral modifications observed
in patients undergoing cardiac surgery and CPB, are probably
mainly related to surgery and not to the associated CPB. It
is however possible that CPB could have slightly increased
the effect of surgery, since long term CPB have been
reported to induce plasma protein denaturation (20,21).

### 3.2.2. Granulocyte functions

On J1, no abnormalities were observed for $O_2$-stimulated
uptake, $H_2O_2$ stimulated formation, quantitative NBT-
stimulated reduction and cytochrome c-stimulated reduction
while spontaneous quantitative NBT reduction (Fig 3) and

Fig.3 : Granulocytes
function. Spontaneous
NBT reduction.
Same legends as under
Fig.1

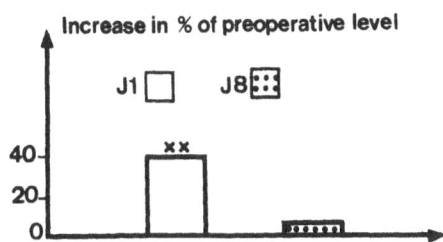

Ingestion rate (Fig.4) were higher than preoperatively. In

Fig. 4 : Granulocytes
function. Ingestion
rate.
Same legends as under
Fig.1.

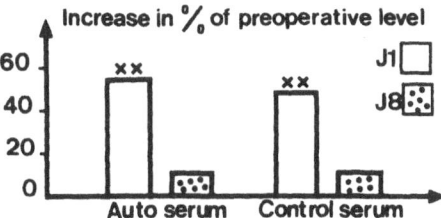

contrast iodination and MPO activities (Fig 5 ) were very

Fig.5 : Granulocytes
function. Iodination
and myeloperoxidase
(MPO).

Same legends as under
Fig.1

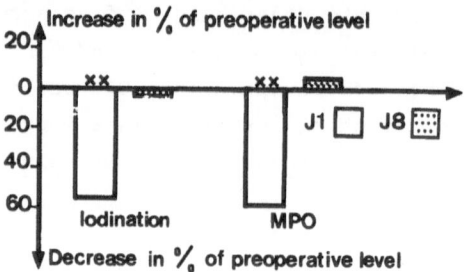

much lower than preoperatively. All granulocytes function
tests, whether measured in autologous or in control AB
serum, were similar. This suggests that the primary lesion
involves the granulocyte itself (22). The modifications
observed in granulocyte function tests, need to be discussed
in the framework of our current knowledge on granulocyte
functions.

Granulocytes are potent cellular agents for aspecific
defence (23,24). They assume their bactericidal functions
through mobilization (25), and ingestion (26) followed by
intraleukocytic killing of bacteria (27). The most potent
bactericidal system of the granulocytes is $O_2$-dependent (28,
29). $O_2$ metabolism, leading to bactericidal forms $O_2$ is the
following (28,29) : upon granulocyte-membrane stimulation $O_2$
is taken up by the granulocyte. The $O_2$-taken up is reduced
into $O_2^-$ and $H_2O_2$. $O_2^-$ generation can be measured by the SOD-
inhibitable reduction of ferricytochrome c or by NBT
reduction. $H_2O_2$ generated will, in the presence of MPO and a
halide, halogenate the bacteria (30). This $H_2O_2$-MPO-halide
system, a very potent bactericidal system, can be evaluated
by the iodination test (9).

The only deficiency observed in the granulocytes of
patients which had undergone cardiac surgery and CPB is on
the lattest step of the $O_2$-dependent bactericidal events i.e.

iodination. This deficiency may be related to various
mechanisms (11) among which is a MPO deficiency. Since MPO
activity was decreased it is highly probable that it was
the cause of the iodination defect. Both iodination and MPO
deficiencies were not found (31) in patients undergoing
surgery not associated with CPB. We thus suggest that CPB
may be, by some way, responsible for the defect. This,
however, needs to be more directly demonstrated.

On the other hand, ingestion rate was enhanced on J1.
This was not reported by other investigators (3,4,6,7).
None of them really measured ingestion rate (26). Enhancement of spontaneous NBT reduction suggest that our patients
had subclinical bacterial infections (32).

On J8, all the abnormalities of granulocytes functions
disappeared suggesting that the granulocyte lesion was
transitory. It is worthy to note that none of the patients
studied had patent postoperative bacterial infection. Thus
the reported decrease in the immune system are not
sufficient for inducing bacterial infections, and environmental opportunistic bacteria may be important for that.

### 3.2.3. Conclusion

In conclusion, patients with abnormalities of their immune
systems, have after cardiac surgery and CPB 1) a decrease
in serum immunoglobulins (IgG, IgA and IgM) concentrations ;
2) a decrease in total hemolytic complement C3, C4 and
C3 proactivator ; 3) a decrease in granulocyte MPO activity
which is reponsible for an iodination defect. All these
deficiencies may be, in part, responsible for the high
susceptibility towards bacterial infections in patients
undergoing cardiac surgery and CPB.

Aknowledgements : The authors wish to thank Miss M. Dumont
for her skilled secreterial help.
This work was supported by Inserm grant AT N°55.

## REFERENCES

1 . Goodman, J.S., W., Schaffner, H.A., Collins, E.J., Battersby, M.G., Koenig, Infection after cardiovascular surgery : clinical study involving examination of antimicrobial prophylaxis. N. Engl. J. Med. 278:117 (1968).

2 . Iribarren, C.O.I., S., Ekeström, The causes of death after open heart surgery. J. thorac. cardiovasc. Surg. 47:725 (1964).

3 . Bowers, T.K., J., O'Flaherty, R.L., Simmons, H.S., Jacobs, Postsurgical granulocyte dysfunction : studies in healthy kidney donors. J. Lab. clin. Med. 90:720 (1977).

4 . Lundström, M., P., Olsson, P., Unger, S., Ekeström, Effect of extracorporeal circulation on hematopoiesis and phagocytosis. J. cardiovasc. Surg. 4:664 (1963).

5 . Silva, J. Jr. , H., Hoedsema, F.R. Jr., Fekety, Transient defects in phagocytosis functions during cardiopulmonary bypass. J. thorac. cardiovasc. Surg. 67:175 (1974).

6 . Kaplan, E.L., A.R., Castaneda, E.M., Ayoub, P.G., Quie, Effects of cardiopulmonary bypass on the phagocytic and bactericidal capacities of polymorphonuclear leukocytes. Circulation 37 (Suppl.II):158 (1968).

7 . Ros , A., M.E., Reverdy, J., Fleurette, P., Mikaeloff, Activité phagocytaire et bactéricide des polynucléaires sanguins chez des malades cardiaques opérés sous circulation extracorporelle. Nouv. Presse méd. 5:1490 (1976).

8 . Kabat, E.A., M.M., Mayer, Experimental immunochemistry. 2nd Ed., Ch.C., Thomas, Springfield, pp 135-139 (1964).

9 . Hakim, J., E., Cramer, P., Boivin, H., Troube, J., Boucherot, Quantitative iodination of human blood polymorphonuclear leukocytes. Europ. J. clin. Invest. 5:215 (1975).

10. Feliu, E., M.A., Gougerot, J., Hakim , E., Cramer, C., Auclair, B., Rueff, P., Boivin, Blood polymorphonuclear dysfunction in patients with alcoholic cirrhosis. Europ. J. clin. Invest. 7:571 (1977).

11. Cramer, E., C., Auclair, J., Hakim, E., Feliu, J., Boucherot, H., Troube, J.F., Bernard, E., Bergogne, P., Boivin, Metabolic activity of phagocytosing granulocytes in chronic granulocytic leukemia : ultrastructural observation of a degranulation defect. Blood 50:93 (1977).

12. Hairston, P., J.P., Manos, C.D., Graber, W.H.Jr., Lee, Depression of immunological surveillance by pump-oxygenation perfusion. J. surg. Res. $\underline{9}$:587 (1969).

13. Cohnen, G., Changes in immunoglobulin levels after surgical trauma. J. Trauma. $\underline{12}$:249 (1972).

14. Fuller, J.M., J.W., Keyser, Serum immunoglobulins after surgical operation. Clin. Chem. $\underline{21}$:667 (1975).

15. Gierhake, F.W., K., Ebert, P., Hagen, N., Papastravrou, L., Rickmeyer, R., Stocker, H.U., Valk, K., Zimmermann, Gerinnugsphysiologische und immunologische Moglichkeiten und Perspektiven zur Prophylaxe postoperativer Wundheilungsstorungen und Infektionen. Zbl. Chir. $\underline{100}$: 797 (1975).

16. Klein, W., G., Klein, Verhalten der Immunoglobuline IgA, IgG und IgM nach operativen Eingriffen am Herzen. Wien. med. Wschr., $\underline{120}$:298 (1970).

17. Lackner, F., Untersuchung von Parametern der zellulären und humoralen Abwehr gegen bakterielle Infektion während Herzoperationen mit der Hrzlungmaschine. Acta Chir. austr. $\underline{16}$ (Suppl.):1 (1975).

18. Parker, D.J., J.W., Cantrell, R.B., Karp, R.M., Stroud, S.B., Digerness, Changes in serum complement and immunoglobulins following cardiopulmonary bypass. Surgery $\underline{71}$:824 (1972).

19. Vermesse, G., D., Camus, P., Wattre, A., Capron, C., Gautier-Benoit, Modifications immunitaires dans les suites opératoires immédiates. Nouv. Presse méd. $\underline{7}$:529 (1978).

20. Brinsfield, D.E., M.A., Hopf, R.B., Geering, Hematological changes in long-term perfusion. J. appl. Physiol. $\underline{17}$:531 (1962).

21. Lee, W.H.Jr., D., Krumhaar, E.W., Fonkalsrud, O.A., Schjeide, J.V.Jr., Maloney, Denaturation of plasma proteins as a cause of morbidity and death after intracardiac operations. Surgery $\underline{50}$:29 (1961).

22. Hakim, J., E., Cramer, C., Auclair, M.A., Gougerot, E., Feliu, P., Boivin, Acquired functional defect of human blood polymorphonuclear. In : Movement, metabolism and bactericidal mechanisms of phagocytes, Rossi, F., Patriarca, P.L., D., Romeo, Eds, Piccin Medical Books, Padua-London, pp 375-383 (1977).

23. Hakim, J., E., Cramer, M.A., Gougerot, Le polynucléaire neutrophile : système de défense de l'organisme. In : Le sang en anésthésie et réanimation, Conseiller, C., J.M., Desmonts, Eds, Arnette, Paris, pp 507-570 (1976).

24. Stossel, T.P., Phagocytosis (3 parts). New Engl. J. Med. 290:717,774,833 (1974).

25. Gallin, J.I., S.M., Wolff, Leukocyte chemotaxis : physiological considerations and abnormalities. Clin. Haemat. 4:567 (1975).

26. Stossel, T.P., Phagocytosis : a recognition and ingestion. Semin. Hemat. 12:83 (1975).

27. Klebanoff, S.J., Intraleukocytic microbicidal defects. Annu. Rev. Med. 22:39 (1971).

28. Babior, B.M., Oxygen-dependent microbial killing by phagocytes (firts of two parts). New Engl. J. Med. 298: 659 (1978).

29. Klebanoff, S.J., Antimicrobial mechanisms in neutrophilic polymorphonuclear leukocytes. Semin. Hemat. 12:117 (1975).

30. Klebanoff, S.J., C.B., Hamon, Role of myeloperoxidase-mediated antimicrobial systems in intact leukocytes. J. Reticuloendothel. Soc. 12:170 (1972).

31. Bröte, L., O., Stendahl, The function of polymorphonu-clear leukocytes after surgical trauma. Acta chir. scand. 141:565 (1975).

32. Park, B.H., S.M., Fikrig, E.M., Smithwick, Infection and nitroblue-tetrazolium reduction by neutrophils. A diagnostic aid. Lancet 2:532 (1968).

DISCUSSION        Moderator: Laurant

Agostoni:

First, I want to congratulate on Dr. Hakim's presentation which is quite up-to-date. If you permit, I have two comments on your presentation:

1. I was a little surprised that you have not found a decrease in CH 50. It has been shown by CRADDOCK that dialyzer cellophane membranes induce a decrement in serum total hemolytic complement through alternative complement activation. $C_{5a}$ seems to be a critical effector of this phenomenon. Perhaps, you have to take blood samples earlier then you have done at your point $Y_1$.

2. Concerning superoxyde dismutase, our preliminary data indicated that the activity of this enzyme is reduced in erythrocytes of patients with chronic hypoxemia. Thus, in these subjects the superoxide effects could be more pronounced.

Hakim:

I do fully agree with your first comment since our studies on J1 were done at least 16 hours after termination of the CPB. It is thus possible that the observed decrease in total hemolytic complement was only the tail of a more pronounced decrease.

Concerning your second comment, I want to point out that we should be very cautious when we extrapolate to the leukocytes, results observed with red blood cells. As you know the superoxide dismutase found in the red blood cells is the copper-zinc form of the enzyme while in the granulocytes two different forms of the enzyme are found: the copper-zinc one and mainly the manganese one (C. Auclair et al.: Febs Letts 79, 390, 1977). We, however, also know from the work of Rister and Baehner (J. Clin. Invest., 58, 1174, 1976) that superoxide dismutase activities of the granulocytes increase under hyperbaric oxygen.

363

To my knowledge, no data are available on the effect of a hypoxemic state. On the other hand, our patients had no symptoms of chronic hypoxemia.

Birnbaum: Concerning to the immune-globulins and complement do you have any idea what does anesthesia itself or any surgical proceedure? In other words, do you have a control group?

Hakim: As stated in my talk, all the results reported are, for the moment, ascribed to surgery + anesthesia + CPB. In this preliminary study we did not try to recognize the precise cause of the abnormalities but only to show that they do exist. Our control group was thus chosen for this purpose.

Birnbaum: This is not a specific finding in cardiac surgery as much more of surgery in general.

Hakim: Just as we do not know if the abnormalities observed are related to CPB, we do not know whether it is a problem of surgery in general or anesthesia only. Referring to the literature, I, however, think that the humoral abnormalities are a problem of general major surgery while granulocyte function abnormalities i.e. iodination and myeloperoxidase deficiencies are a problem of CPB. We aim to test these hypothesis.

# 7. SUSCEPTIBILITY TO INFECTIONS RELATED TO EXTRACORPOREAL CIRCULATION: SOURCES OF INFECTION, GRANULOCYTE FUNCTION AND IMMUNOGLOBULINS

K. Deggeller, J.J.A.M. van den Dungen, J. Dankert, J. Marrink,
M.R. Halie, G.F. Karliczek and Ch.R.H. Wildevuur

Central Laboratory for Clinical Chemistry,
Department of Hospital Infection,
Department of Immunochemistry,
Department of Hematology,
Department of Anesthesiology,
Department of Experimental Surgery,
University Hospital Groningen, The Netherlands

## 1. INTRODUCTION

In open heart surgery airborne infection has been identified as one of the main sources of a relatively high incidence of clinically manifest postoperative infections (1). The coronary suction line, through which air is constantly drawn, was considered to be the main source of infection. This was substantiated by the fact that in 75% of the cases the extracorporeal circuit became contaminated during operation. This could be confirmed in our hospital: in 119 open heart operations 79% of the oxygenators proved to be contaminated at the end of bypass (2). The airborne contamination was demonstrated by the fact that this high rate of contamination could be reduced to 17% if a cross-flow ventilation system was used. It could be shown in an experimental set-up that the air flow through the suction lines was mainly responsible for this contamination. (3).

In dog experiments evidence was obtained that phagocytosis by granulocytes was reduced as a result of extracorporeal circulation (4) and this could be related to the occurrence of postoperative sepsis (5). The question whether a diminished number and/or function of white blood cells of patients undergoing open heart surgery contributes to the increased infection rate of these patients prompted us to investigate granulocyte functions.

The purpose of this study is to provide more data concerning the risk factors of infection as related to extracorporeal circulation.

2. MATERIALS AND METHODS

2.1. Experimental studies

2.1.1. Evaluation of the route and the effect of bacterial contamination (3)

These experiments were performed on mongrel dogs. The effect of aspiration of air through the suction lines was studied by comparing the conventional method (uncontrolled suction) with an automated suction device (6) which prevents aspiration of air with the blood (controlled suction). A Bentley autotransfusion system was used in the abdominal cavity of a heparinized dog during bleeding of the cannulated femoral artery into the peritoneal cavity at a rate of 400 ml/min during 1 hour. The overall level of air contamination in the operation theatre was about 180 micro-organisms/$mm^3$. In addition an indicator micro-organism was sprayed every 15 minutes to achieve a mean contamination of 50 Staphylococcus aureus per $m^3$. The dogs did not receive any antibiotics.

2.1.2. Evaluation of the effect of extracorporeal circulation on granulocyte function

Extracorporeal circulation was accomplished in mongrel dogs in a 2 hours total bypass using a bubble oxygenator (Temptrol Q-110). Carbonyl-iron phagocytosis was determined in whole blood according to Woltjes (4) with some modifications. Briefly, 0,8 ml of heparinized blood was diluted with 1,2 ml dextran solution and 10 mg carbonyl-iron added. After continuously tumbling in a water bath at $37^{\circ}C$ during 30 minutes, the carbonyl-iron particles were removed with a magnet. In the supernatant, leucocytes were counted with an electronic cell counter.

2.2. Clinical studies

Heparinized blood samples were taken from patients undergoing open heart surgery, just before the start of the extracorporeal circulation and two hours later. In six patients plasmaprotein concentrations were also followed daily up to day seven postoperatively. Isolation of granulocytes: Heparinized blood was diluted with an equal volume of Gey's solution. The diluted blood was layered over Lymphoprep (Nyegaard & Co.) and the erythrocytes allowed to sediment during 35 minutes at room temperature. The supernatant was centrifuged over a small layer of Lymphoprep. The following steps were performed at $0^{\circ}C$. The precipitate was washed once with Gey's solution. Erythrocytes in the preparation were lysed with 155 mmol/l $NH_4Cl$, 10 mmol/l $KHCO_3$ , 0,1 mmol/l $K_2$ EDTA, the granulocytes were collected by centrifugation. The precipitate was washed twice with Gey's solution and finally suspended to obtain $10 \times 10^6$ cells/ml in Gey's solution. Chemotaxis was measured in a Boyden chamber (7) with a millipore filter with 8 μ pores and casein as attractant. Superoxide radical formation was measured with cytochrome C as indicator (8). Iodination of proteins was measured with zymosan as substrate according to Hakim (9). Killing of bacteria was measured as described by Solberg (10). Plasmaproteins were measured immunochemically with an Auto-Analyser.

## 3. RESULTS

### 3.1. Experimental study

#### 3.1.1. The effect of airborne contamination

The effect of controlled suction, which eliminates aspiration of air, gives a substantial reduction of contamination with bacteria (table I).

Table I Contamination with microorganisms of dogs during extracorporeal circulation.

| CONTAMINATION | SUCTION | |
|---|---|---|
| | UNCONTROLLED | CONTROLLED |
| WOUND AREA | 80% | 49% |
| BLOOD (PEROP.) | 61% | 36% |
| BLOOD (POSTOP.) | 60% | 25% |

Elimination of an air stream to the wound area reduced the overall contamination by about half. This reduction was mainly caused by a decrease of micro-organisms (m.o.) from exogenous sources. The blood also became proportionally less contaminated by m.o.. Postoperatively, 4 out of 13 dogs in the uncontrolled suction group had a bacteraemia with m.o. of exogenous sources, whereas no dogs in the controlled series were infected. In this latter group only m.o. from endogenous sources could be detected in the blood samples postoperatively.

#### 3.1.2. The effect of extracorporeal circulation (ECC) on granulocyte function

The leucocyte phagocytosis during and after ECC is given in figure 1.

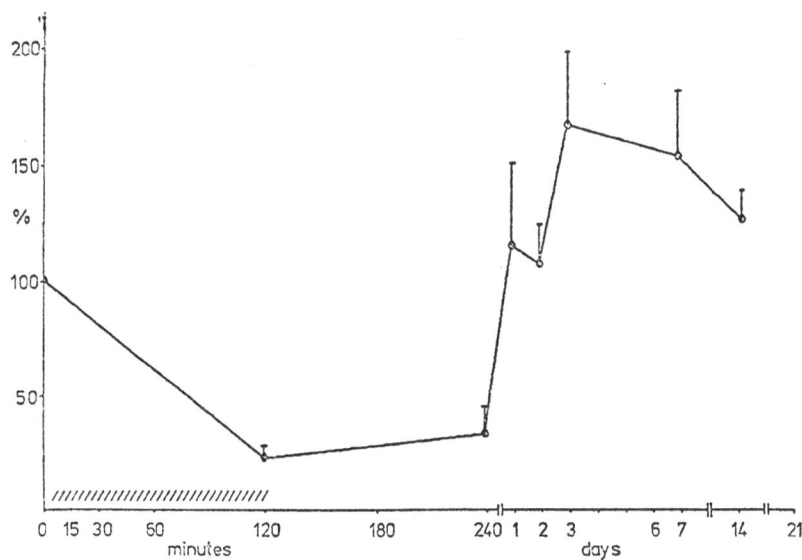

Fig. 1.Phagocytosis of carbonyl-iron by leucocytes of dogs. Mean values
of 6 dogs undergoing extracorporeal circulation with a bubble
oxygenator.

Phagocytosis, given as percentages of the preoperative values, decreased to about 20% by the end of ECC. Complete recovery was seen on the
first postoperative day.

### 3.2. Clinical study

Chemotaxis was increased after two hours exposure to extracorporeal
oxygenation. The stimulus of casein increased the distance of granulocytes moving into the filter (n = 4): before ECC: 27 $\pm$ 10 $\mu$m

after ECC: 53 $\pm$ 20 $\mu$m.

Superoxide radical formation did not change during extracorporeal
circulation (n = 6): before ECC: 480 $\pm$ 100 $\mu$mol/10$^{10}$ cells hr

after ECC: 510 $\pm$ 100 $\mu$mol/10$^{10}$ cells hr.

Iodination of proteins by granulocytes was measured, but the results
were not reproducible in duplicate tests yet, so no data are reported. Killing of E. coli was decreased under influence of extracorporeal
circulation (n = 4): before ECC: 99,1 $\pm$ 1.3%

after ECC: 94 $\pm$ 3%.

369

A representative example of the results obtained in an individual patient is given in table II.

Table II  Granulocyte functions of a patient during extracorporeal circulation.

| FUNCTION | BEFORE ECC | AFTER ECC |
|---|---|---|
| CHEMOTAXIS | 21 µm | 80 µm |
| $O_2^-$  RADICALFORMATION ($\mu$mol/hr $10^{10}$ cells) | 492 | 550 |
| KILLING | 99.6% | 93.6% |
| LEUCOCYTE COUNT | 3.5 | 4.2 |
| DIFFERENTIAL COUNT | | |
| − LYMPHOCYTES | 13% | 14% |
| − NEUTROPHILS | 72% | 72% |
| − BAND NEUTROPHILS | − | 8% |
| − MONOCYTES | 11% | 6% |
| − EOSINOPHILS | 4% | − |

Plasmaprotein: the measurement of concentration of plasmaproteins was performed on the immunoglobulins G, A and M, on $\alpha$-antitrypsin (AT) and transferrin (TF) (Table III). The concentrations of the proteins in the pre-perfusion sample are below the normal values, mainly while the samples are taken after anaesthesia started and infusions were already given. The hematocrit decreased from 45% to 38% on average. The decrease after 2 hrs ECC was related to dilution of the plasma volume, by a factor 2-2.5. IgG and TF increased to normal levels after 7 days. IgM, IgA and AT after 4, 2 and 1 day respectively. In this regard it has to be taken into account that the extracorporeal circuit was primed with 5 liters of albumin solution. Between the end of ECC and the first measured value on day 1 , 1.5 liter  of blood was infused, on average.

Table III. Mean concentrations of plasmaproteïns of 6 patients during and after extracorporeal circulation (g/l).

|  |  | IgG | IgA | IgM | AT | TF |
|---|---|---|---|---|---|---|
| Before | ECC | 8.0 | 1.52 | 0.82 | 2.5 | 1.9 |
| After | ECC | 3.9 | 0.67 | 0.32 | 1.2 | 0.8 |
| Day | 1 | 6.2 | 1.19 | 0.69 | 2.7 | 1.7 |
|  | 2 | 6.2 | 1.26 | 0.74 | 4.6 | 1.5 |
|  | 3 | 7.3 | 1.52 | 0.74 | 5.9 | 1.6 |
|  | 4 | 7.4 | 1.67 | 0.97 | 6.6 | 1.7 |
|  | 5 | 7.9 | 1.79 | 1.12 | 5.6 | 1.7 |
|  | 6 | 8.5 | 1.95 | 1.70 | 5.9 | 1.8 |
|  | 7 | 10.0 | 2.25 | 2.33 | 5.8 | 1.9 |
| Normal range | | 10-18 | 1.2-4.0 | 0.8-1.7 | 1.6-3.5 | 2.0-4.0 |

# 4. DISCUSSION

Our investigations were performed to study three aspects of bacterial infections, which occur with high incidence after extracorporeal oxygenation: the sources of infection, the granulocyte function and the immunoglobulinconcentrations.

Bacterial infections are caused by microorganisms of exogenous or endogenous sources. Dankert and coworkers (2) demonstrated that a decrease of contamination by exogenous microorganisms could be attained if a laminar air flow was used. Reduction of bacterial contamination from exogenous source can be achieved too by eliminating the aspiration of air through the lines of the cardiotomy suction, as demonstrated in our experimental studies (3).

The role of a diminished number and/or function of the white blood cells, as a contribution to the increased infection rate, of patients undergoing open heart surgery, has not been investigated in depth yet. The function of the several classes of leucocytes i.e. the granulocytes the monocytes-macrophages and the lymphocyte subpopulations have to be examined separately.

In several studies a temporary decrease in the number of the leukocytes, after start of extracorporeal circulation (ECC),is seen, depending amongst others on the materials used in the system (4, 11-16). During, or shortly after perfusion a leucocytosis is seen in most cases (4). This was also seen in our clinical study (table II). The increase in the total number of leucocytes is more pronounced than the figure indicates, if we take into account the hemodilution. The appearance of band neutrophils (table II) supports the conclusion that leucocytes are entering the circulation during ECC.

The function of granulocytes appears to be impaired too (13-15). Studies on dogs taught us that phagocytosis by granulocytes (fig. 1) is decreased during and shortly after ECC (4-6). In our clinical study we found decreased killing of E. coli by granulocytes, isolated from blood samples taken after 2 hrs ECC. Our biochemical measurements did not allow us to locate the defective reaction, that could be responsible for the decreased function, as demonstrated in the overall test: the killing of bacteria. This aspect needs further study.

The concentrations of IgA, IgM and IgG decreased during ECC and steadily returned to normal values in the following days. The interpretation of this effect is possible if we take into account the effects of hemodilution and blood transfusion. For this reason we also measured transferrin levels as an indicator of these effects. The decrease of all proteïns after ECC can be explained by the hemodilution. The concentrations of IgG on the days after ECC follows the same procentual changes as the concentrations of transferrin. IgA returns to normal levels on day 2; IgM on day 4 and increases to levels above normal on day 7. IgM is the first immunoglobulin to appear after immunisation and the question arises against which antigen this IgM antibody is formed. From the data in table III it cannot be substantiated that specific denaturation of immunoglobulins occurs. However,the actual values point to the fact that the concentration of immunoglobulins is considerably lower than normal during ECC and for the first day thereafter. These low levels, the reduced killing by granulocytes,and high risk for airborne contamination of the extracorporeal circulating blood cell contribute to an increased susceptibility to infection.

## REFERENCES

1. Blakemore, W.S. et al., Surgery 70: 830, 1971.

2. Dankert, J. and A. Eijgelaar, Ant. v. Leeuwenhoek, 44, 247, 1978.

3. Zijlstra, J.B., E. Logher, J. Dankert, A.G.M. van Asseldonk, Ch.R.H. Wildevuur, Proc. ESAO 5: 222, 1978.

4. Woltjes, J., H.J. ten Duis, J.C.F. de Jong and Ch.R.H. Wildevuur, Proc. ESAO 3: 89, 1976.

5. De Jong, J.C.F., J. Woltjes, R.H.L. Paping and Ch.R.H. Wildevuur, Proc. ESAO 4: 523, 1977.

6. Ten Duis, H.J., J.C.F. de Jong, A.G.M. van Asseldonk, C.Th. Smit Sibinga and Ch.R.H. Wildevuur, Trans. Am. Soc. Artif. Intern. Organs 24: 656, 1978.

7. Boyden, S., J. Exp. Med. 115: 453, 1962.

8. Weening, R.S., D. Roos and J.A. Loos, J. Lab. Clin. Med. 83: 570, 1974.

9. Hakim, J., E. Cramer, P. Boivin, H. Troube and J. Boucherot, Europ. J. Clin. Invest. 5: 215, 1975.

10. Solberg, C.O., Acta Pathol. Microbiol. Scand. (B) 80, 559, 1972.

11. Brinsfield, D.E., M.A. Hopf, R.B. Geering, P.M. Galetti, J. Appl. Physiol. 17: 531, 1962.

12. Galetti, P.M., J. Surg. Res. V, 97, 1965.

13. Kusserow, B.K., R. Larnow, J. Nichols, Fed. Proc. 30: 1516, 1971.

14. Lundström, M., P. Olsson, P. Unger, S. Ekeström, J. Cardiovasc.Surg. 4: 664, 1963.

15. Silva, J., H. Hoeksema, F.R. Fekety, J. Thorac. Cardiovasc. Surg. 67: 175, 1974.

16. Wildevuur-van Hamersveld, C., J.C.F. de Jong, M.R. Halie, et al., in: Physiological and clinical aspects of oxygenator design, eds. S.G. Dawids and H.C. Engell/North Holland Biomedical Press, Amsterdam, 1976.

Moderator: Laurant

Laurant:              Do you think that the RBC fractions are preserved
                      since commonly in extracorporeal circulations
                      stored bank blood is used?

Deggeler:             We have not done measurements on that function on
                      blood bank blood. Perhaps Dr. Wildevuur can tell
                      us something about the length of time when the
                      blood is stored.

Van den Dungen:       Granulocyte function measurements were made be-
                      fore and after 120 minutes perfusion and for the
                      oxygenator a bloodless prime was used, so there
                      was no stored blood used at the moments the func-
                      tions were measured.

Schmid-Schönbein:     Is there any indication from your work what could
                      be the reason for the initial disappearance of
                      P.M.N.'s from the circulation. Is it a shift from
                      the circulating to the residual population, in
                      other words, are they moving to the venular walls
                      in the whole circulation, or in the pulmonary
                      circulation?

Wildevuur:            I would like to refer to the acute event in the very
                      first minutes of the extracorporeal circulation.
                      The initial dip for platelets has been elaborated
                      upon already yesterday, but leucocytes are affec-
                      ted in the same way (C. Wildevuur - van Hamersveld,
                      J.C.F. de Jong, M.R. Halie, C.Th. Smit Sibinga
                      and Ch.R.H. Wildevuur: Hematologic abnormalities
                      in extracorporeal circuits (ECC) in: Clinical
                      Aspects of Oxygenator Design, p. 197 (eds. Dawids
                      and Engell), Elsevier, Luxemburg, 1976). To my
                      knowledge it has not been studied in these cir-
                      cumstances where the leucocyte aggregates are
                      settling. As shown by Mielke (Drug influence on
                      platelet loss during extracorporeal circulation,
                      J. Thorac. Cardiovasc. Surg. 66: 845, 1973),
                      platelet aggregates are more located in the liver

375

than in the lung. But it might be possible that
the leucocyte aggregates are more located in the
lung, where they are quite often observed histo-
logically. However, the initial dip of the leucocytes is more quickly compensated by the release
of the marginating pool into the circulation
and compensate for the momentary massive disappearance of leucocytes from the circulation.
As a consequence even leucocytosis is seen often
already during perfusion in clinical as well as
in experimental circumstances. After the initial
leucocytosis we do see most often a second leucocytosis peak around day 4-5, probably as a
response of the bone marrow to stimulating agents
during the perfusion.

Schmid-Schönbein:  The topic of this symposion is "blood trauma".
Do you consider the initial dip as symptom of
blood trauma?

Wildevuur:  I think that you can better answer this question
than I can do. I believe that the initial dip can
only be explained by a release of bioamines from
damaged blood cells after their first contact with
the non-physiological surfaces. To study the
mechanism of what happens in these very first
minutes by the basic scientists seems to me
very appropriate. Even more if they could find a
way to prevent this phenomenon.

Schmid-Schönbein:  We have to keep in mind that the leucocytes also
have interesting flow properties and I think the
work of Dr. Ulf Bagge (Advances in Microcircul.,
7, 29-48, 1977, J. Clin. invest. 52, 350, 1973)
in Dr. Brånemarks laboratory in Göteborg has un-
covered important differences between white cells
and red cells. Both have to be deformed to pass
through the microcirculation and they are being
deformed, but only provided that there are sufficient forces. The forces required to deform white

cells are much higher, and, of course, if one has any sort of circulatory insufficiency it is very likely that these forces may be missing. And I would therefore suggest that leucocytosis in a patient with a disturbed circulation could develop into a risk factor. If patients have "microcirculatory deficiency" following artificial organ exposure they may have possibly even "stifened" white cells, and the blood flow be quite severely affected.

Wildevuur: If I may react on that briefly, I fully agree with your considerations which actually have brought us to the next step of our investigation and that is that we try to correlate the hematological changes in dogs with tissue perfusion. This study is now under way in a "concerted action" with Dr. Lübbers from Dortmund and we are looking to see how hematological changes might be reflected in the tissue perfusion as measured with the $pO_2$ histogram. The practical relevance of studying this is the clinical observation that patients after a longer perfusion regularly have icecold extremities, demonstrating an impaired peripheral circulation.

Agostoni: Coming back to the granulocytes, it has been shown that the granulocytes are activated by the properdin system. Successively, they are trapped into the lung. Again, this is a consequence of the activation of the properdin system. I think, Dr. Schmid-Schönbein, that the activation of the properdin system is one of the first consequences of blood trauma during ECC.

Hakim: I would like to comment on the provocative suggestion of Dr. Schmid-Schönbein stating that the granulocytes may leave the vessels by means of an increased blood pressure. I think we have to keep in mind that the granulocytes are actively mobile cells.

They are distributed in the vessels into two
pools: one is in circulation and the other is
marginating. These two pools are in permanent
exchange. There is general agreement that the
granulocytes leave the vessels actively after
margination. Epinephrine, a drug which has the
ability to demarginate the granulocytes, inhi-
bits their extrusion from the vessels while increasing blood pressure. On the other hand, studies of granulocyte movements, in vitro with
the Boyden chamber or under agarose, showed
clearly that chemotaxis was under the influence
of chemical agents called cytotoxins. No studies, to my knowledge, have shown that pressure
may play a role in granulocyte movements.

Schmid-Schönbein:  Let me clarify: I am not talking about amoeboidal
motion, but about the simple fact that white
cells require deformation due to the fact that
the nutritive capillaries are about 3-4 μm in
diameter and the white cells are about 6-7 μm
in diameter. Consequently, there is a traffic
problem in the microcirculation. Thus, despite
the fact that the white cells are more rigid
they are being deformed to pass through the
narrow capillaries. But this happens only in the
presence of sufficient driving forces. If there
is not sufficient blood pressure these will
simply act as plugs of the microcirculation.
I am talking about flow through the capillary
during which the PMN's have to be deformed
*passively* or else they will block the microcirculation. In the case of PMN's there is at least
a hope that the blockade will be temporary,
because, as you said, there is a chance that the
granulocytes travel through the capillary walls
and therefore re-open the capillary lumen. This
is an active        event which has nothing to
do with the normal passive motion of flowing

378

blood cells.

Hakim: I until now, misunderstood that you were commenting on the cell flux along the axis of the vessel since in your first comment you said that an abnormality of the movement will induce leucocytosis. I now understand that you suggested that an excess of leucocytes in the capillaries could induce some kind of thrombosis and I do agree.

Schmid-Schönbein: Yes, that's an interesting suggestion. We know that leucocytes are lodged at the wall of the postcapillary venules. The extent of lodging and therefore the extent of liberation could also depend on the pressure gradient and therefore on the general condition of the circulation.

Laurant: We know, Dr. Hakim, that you are not going to win against the mechanistic people.

Williams: In response to the comments about white cells I would like to point to some work done in Dr. Nyborg's laboratory in Vermont, USA. They have been using the oscillating wire system to generate shear stresses and subjecting white cells to these shear forces and seeing that they are affected by quite low shear stresses of the order of 50-100 $dyn/cm^2$. These stresses affect the morphology, mobility and phagocytic index of various lymphocytes. They find this even after very short time exposures. First of all the very low shear stresses increase the phagocytic index. When one puts higher stresses on them, the reverse happens.

The white cells become less mobile and have a smaller phagocytic index to bacteria. And eventually, even though they are still intact, they are non-functional. They just sit there. This happens at very low shear stresses.

379

# 18. PROTEIN DENATURATION AND THE EFFECT OF HEPARIN DURING EXTRACORPOREAL CIRCULATION

J. S. Fleming

Department of Surgery

Royal Postgraduate Medical School

London W12 OHS.

## Introduction

The hypothesis of protein denaturation as a cause of morbidity and death resulting from extracorporeal circulation for intracardiac surgery was proposed by Lee et al (14) following the discovery of fat emboli in post-perfusion tissues by Owens et al (19). Protein denaturation was believed to be caused largely at the blood-gas interface in the bubble and disc oxygenators. Proteins, because of their high surface-active property could unfold from their native configuration to produce denatured species (16). If the concept was correct then the use of membrane oxygenators should reduce the rate of denaturation and decrease the incidence of morbidity. The concept provoked a series of experiments by different authors into various aspects of protein denaturation over the following two decades. These included comparisons between the bubble-type and membrane-type oxygenators (6,9,13,14,15,20,29,34,35,37), the conclusions of which are confusing and uncertain.

The findings may be divided into 3 main groups:

(1) Denaturation of lipoproteins with the production of embolic fat (2,14,15,19,20,35,37).

(2) Gammaglobulin and non-specified protein aggregation and complement alteration (7,15,21,22,23,28,29,32,34).

(3) Absence of any substantial denatured species or adverse reaction (1,10,11,13,25).

Whereas embolic fat has been assumed to be produced in the oxygenators, Ellison et al (5) found fat emboli in the lungs of patients prior to extracorporeal perfusion; and Hill (9) suggested that suction from

380

the chest cavity or donor blood was the source of the fat globules.

Furthermore anaphylactoid shock could be induced in dogs simply by exchange transfusion without extracorporeal perfusion (4). Gamma globulin can be readily aggregated by oxygenator systems but the presence of albumin in the solution substantially reduces the denaturation rate (23). Although the results of the various authors appear to be confusing, the gross denaturation obtained by Lee et al (14) has not been subsequently reproduced. It should be noted that minor surgical trauma without perfusion causes plasma protein changes (31). These discrepancies may be due in part to the wide variations in experimental design, animal models and the status of the blood at the time of the experiment. This could be especially relevent to the mode of anticoagulation used. Heparin is, at the moment, the only suitable anticoagulant for extracorporeal perfusion work, but has the ability to release lipases into the circulation in the form of heparin complexes (12,18,28) which remain active after the blood has been withdrawn (3). Thus there is a potentially gross difference between blood heparinised in vitro and blood withdrawn from a heparinised subject. Alterations in the protein species caused by heparin-induced lipolysis could, possibly, be mistaken for denaturation.

The term "denaturation" continues to be used without a clear definition, especially in the literature concerned with extracorporeal circulation. Unfortunately, since the term was introduced by Wu (36) to mean protein which had become insoluble, the meaning has become confused and, as stated by Lumry and Eyring (17) "has taken on so many different meanings as to become a virtually useless definition". Tanford (27) clarified the definition: "a large alteration in the conformation of a protein molecule but excluding peptide bond cleavage". Unfortunately this term is not a practical working definition especially for such complex protein solutions as plasma. It was therefore necessary to use model denaturants, i.e. heat, and detergent (sodium dodecyl sulphate - SDS) to determine the alterations to the plasma proteins and protein solutions which could possibly be classified as denaturation.

## Methods and Observations

To simulate the trauma occuring in bubble-type oxygenators, plasma obtained from human subjects undergoing cardiopulmonary perfusion was sealed into glass ampoules and shaken at $37^{\circ}$C on a horizontal shaker for up to 24 hours (7). Whereas heat denaturation and shaking causes readily detectable and quantifiable aggregation of some proteins, fibrinogen and gamma globulin are readily aggregated by heating but the rate of insoluble denaturation in plasma is surprisingly low (7, 29). However, it is reasonable to assume that soluble, non-aggregated denatured species exist in the solutions. Heat denatured albumin binds to protamine sulphate to produce insoluble precipitates (24), whereas native albumin is unreactive. The lipoproteins are also precipitated by protamine but the complex formation is altered by structural changes in the molecule (3).

Phosphate buffered (pH 7.6    0.25M) and Tris-Glycine buffered (pH 8.3 0.015M) solutions of protamine sulphate (0.5 mg/ml) were used to assess the presence of denatured protein species in the solutions and in plasma. Addition of 20 $\mu$l of plasma or 100 $\mu$l of 1% albumin to 2 ml of the protamine solutions was adequate to produce readily measurable turbidities at 700 nm. The turbidity is augmented in plasma by heat, SDS denaturation and by shaking. (See Table I). The apparent denaturation by shaking is very low when compared with heat and SDS denaturation. Electrophoretic analysis in agarose gels (pH 8.6) and location of the proteins with buffered protamine solutions demonstrated the influence of SDS on the lipoproteins, (See Figure 1), in pre and post heparin plasmas. Gross alteration of the lipoprotein molecule occurs in SDS and in the native post heparin sample.

Similar analysis during the course of cardiopulmonary perfusion demonstrated a shift in the lipoproteins after heparinisation (Figure 2). The effect decayed during the perfusion and as the heparin level fell and was eliminated after the protamine injection.

## Table I

## Protamine Induced Turbidity of Denatured Proteins

### O.D. at 700 nm

#### Heat Denaturation 60°C

| | | | | Time (mins.) | | | |
|---|---|---|---|---|---|---|---|
| | 0 | ½ | 1 | 2 | 4 | 8 | 10 |
| Albumin 1% | 0.02 | | 0.06 | 0.18 | 0.36 | 0.6 | 0.63 |
| Plasma | 0.1 | 0.13 | 0.17 | 0.20 | 0.21 | | 0.24 |

#### SDS Denaturation

| | | SDS mg/ml | | |
|---|---|---|---|---|
| | 0 | 0.5 | 1.0 | 2.0 |
| Plasma | 0.04 | 0.08 | 0.21 | 0.35 |

#### Shaking at 37°C

| | | Time (hours) | | | |
|---|---|---|---|---|---|
| | 0 | 2 | 5 | 9 | 24 |
| Plasma | 0.09 | 0.1 | 0.13 | 0.145 | 0.16 |

383

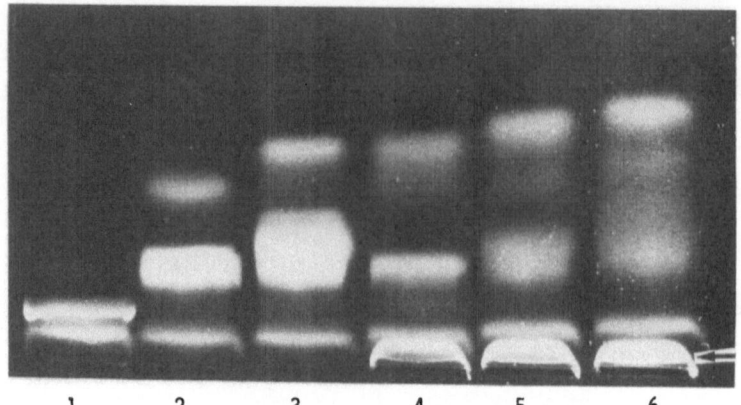

Fig. 1.    Influence of SDS on pre- and post-heparin plasma.
1, 2 and 3 pre-heparin;  4, 5 and 6 post-hpearin.
2 and 5 - 5mg/ml SDS,   3 and 6 - 10mg/ml SDS.
Note:  enhanced mobility of lipoproteins after heparin
induction (4) and after SDS (2, 3, 5, 6).

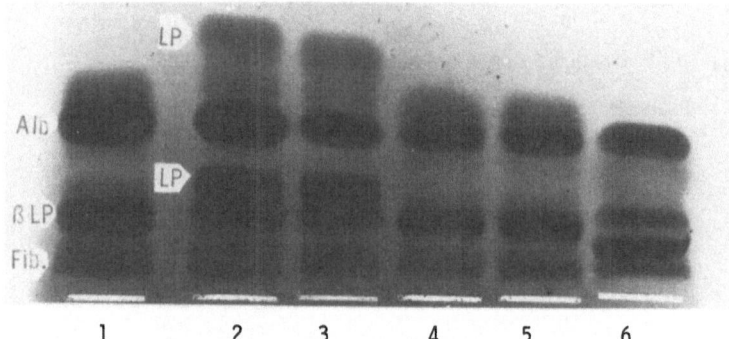

Fig. 2.    Electrophoresis of plasma proteins in samples taken
during perfusion.   Location of proteins with
protamine sulphate.
1) Pre-heparin     2) Post-heparin    3) 5min. perfusion
4) 90min. perfusion   5) Pre-protamine neutralisation
6) Post-protamine neutralisation

## Discussion

The effect seen in the post heparin samples is due to heparin-induced lipolysis, most of which probably occurs after the sample has been collected, and is also dependent upon the lipoprotein type of the subject. Fatty acids released from the lipoprotein accounts for most of the shifts seen, and are carried in the circulation bound to albumin. In the circulation they are transported through the vascular wall to the tissue cells but during perfusion if the lipolytic rate is high it is possible that lipoprotein alteration and fatty acid release will occur to a greater extent during the time that the blood is out of the body i.e. not in contact with the vascular bed.

Although lipolysis is apparently not an oxygenator induced form of denaturation, the possible influence on the other proteins and on the platelets (8,30) should not be overlooked. The formation of calcium soaps has been suggested (33) when the fatty acids are raised and insoluble calcium and phosphate containing precipitates do occasionally form in plasmas when excessive lypolysis is present (Figure 1 - arrowed).

## Conclusion

Production of denatured proteins in in vitro systems occurs at a surprisingly slowrate, most of the alterations in vitro and during perfusion appear to be due to circulating heparin-lipoprotein lipase (11).

References

1   Anderson, L.G., Selby, D.M. and Campbell, G.S.
    Absence of untoward reactions with prolonged disc oxygenator and
    partial perfusion of dog blood.
    TASAIO. 10. 89. 1964.

2   Belzer, E.O., Ashby, B.S., Huang, J.S. and Dunphy, J.E.
    Etiology of rising perfusion pressure in isolated organ perfusion.
    Ann. Surg. 168. 382. 1968.

3   Burstein, M. and Morfin, R.
    Detergents anioniques et lipoprotein seriques.
    N.R.F. Hematologie, 11. 2. 173. 1971.

4   Dow, J.W., Dickson, J.F., Hamer, N.A.J. and Gadboys, H.L.
    The effects of anaphylactoid shock from blood exchange in
    cardiopulmonary bypass.
    J. Thor. Cardiovasc. Surg. 39. 449. 1960.

5   Ellison, L.T., McPherson, J.C.Jr., Anabtawi, I.N. and Ellison, R.G.
    Incidence of free fat in the lung during open-heart surgery.
    Ann. Thor. Surg. 7. 509. 1969.

6   Fleming, J.S.
    Partial perfusion in awake neonatal lambs: a comparison of
    three methods.
    J. Cardiovasc. Surg. 18. 6. 611. 1977.

7   Fleming, J.S.
    Rate of protein denaturation in bubble and membrane oxygenators.
    Proc. ESAO. 4. 544. 1977.

8   Gjesdal, K.
    Platelet function and plasma free fatty acids during acute
    myocardial infarction and severe angina pectoris.
    Scand. J. Haematol. 17. 205. 1976.

9   Hill, J.D., Aquilar, M.J., Baranco, A., Lanerolle, P. and
    Gerbode, F.

    Determination of the incidence of microemboli in the brains of
    215 autopsies.

    Ann. Thor. Surg. 7. 5. 409. 1969.

10  Jeyasingham, K., Althous, U., Berg, E. and Albrechtsen, O.

    Alterations in the plasma proteins and lipids of human and
    canine blood in bubble and disc oxygenators.

    Scand. J. Thorac. Cardiovasc. Surg. 6. 172. 1972.

11  Kaspar, von F., Gillert, K.E. and Grunert, R.D.

    Untersuchungen uber Blutveranderigen bach Hypothermia and
    extrakorporalum kreislaf.

    Thoraxchirugie. 12. 475. 1965.

12  Korn, E.D.

    Clearing factor, A heparin-activated lipoprotein lipase.

    1. Isolation and characterisation of the enzyme from normal
    rat heart.

    J. Biol. Chem. 215. 1. 1955.

13  Larmi, T. K. and Karkola, P.

    Plasma protein electrophoresis during a three hour cardiopulmonary
    bypass in dogs.

    Scand. J. Thor. Cardiovasc. Surg. 8. 152. 1974.

14  Lee, W.H.Jr., Krumhaar, D., Fonkalsrud, E.W., Schjeide, O.A.
    and Maloney, J.V.Jr.

    Denaturation of plasma proteins as a cause of morbidity and death
    after intracardiac operations.

    Surg. 50. 29. 1961.

15  Lee, W.H.Jr., Krumhaar, D., Fonkalsrud, E.W., Schjeide, O.A.
    and Maloney, J.V.Jr.

    Comparison of the effects of membrane and non-membrane oxygenators
    of blood.

    Surg. Forum. 12. 200. 1961.

16  Lee, W.H.Jr. and Hairston, P.

    Structural effects on blood proteins at the gas-blood interface.

    Fed. Proc. 30. 5. 1615. 1971.

17  Lumry, R. and Eyring, H.

    Conformation changes of proteins.

    JACS. 58. 110. 1954.

18  Olivecrona, T., Bengtsson, G., Marklund, S-E., Lindahl, V. and
    Höök, M.

    Heparin-lipoprotein lipase interactions.

    Fed. Proc. 36. 1. 60. 1977.

19  Owens, G., Adams, J.E., McElhannon, F.M. and Youngblood, R.W.

    Experimental alterations of certain colloidol properties of blood
    during cardiopulmonary bypass.

    J. Appl. Physiol. 14. 947. 1959.

20  Owens, G., Adams, J.E. and Scott, H.W.Jr.

    Embolic fat as a measure of adequacy of various oxygenators.

    J. Appl. Physiol. 15. 999. 1960.

21  Parker, J., Cantrell, J.W., Karp, R.B., Stout, R.M. and
    Digermess, S.B.

    Changes in serum complement and immunoglobulins following
    cardiopulmonary bypass.

    Surg. 71. 824. 1972.

22  Pretty, H.M., Fundenberg, H.H., Perkins, H.A. and Gerbode, F.

    Anti gammaglobulin antibodies after open heart surgery.

    Blood. 32. 205. 1968.

23  Pruitt, K.M., Stroud, R.M. and Scott, J.W.

    Blood damage in the heart lung machine.

    Proc. Soc. Expt. Biol. Med. 137. 714. 1971.

24 Russ, V.

Hydrogen-ion activity and precipitation of bovine serum albumin
and β-lactoglobulin with salmine.

Arch. Biochem. Biophys. 50. 34. 1954.

25 Siltamen, P., Kekki, M., Merikallio, E., Myllyla, G., Somer, T.
and Tala, P.

Alterations of plasma proteins during extracorporeal circulation.
1. Experimental studies with [131]I-labelled plasma protein fractions.

Ann. Chir. Gynaec. Fenn. 57. 1. 1968.

26 Takano, K., Tsutsumi, E., Suzuki, H., Hwang, C., Ishikawa, M.,
Matoba, N. and Kasai, M.

Effect of denatured plasma on peripheral circulation.

Tohoku, J. Exp. Med. 101. 175. 1970.

27 Tanford, C.

Protein denaturation. In: Adv. in Protein Chemistry. 23. 121. 1968.

Publs: Academic Press. Eds: C.B. Anfinsen, M.L. Anson,
J.T. Edsall.

28 Trimble, A.S., Osborn, J.J. and Gerbode, F.

Lipoprotein lipase during extracorporeal circulation.

Surg. 58. 324. 1965.

29 Tsutsumi, E., Takano, K., Suzuki, H., Kwang, C.T., Ishikawa, M.,
Matoba, N. and Kasai, M.

Determination of denatured protein in plasma after long term
extracorporeal perfusion.

Tohoku, J. Exp. Med. 101. 215. 1970.

30 Wallace, H.W., Liquori, E.M., Stein, T.P. and Brooks, H.

Denatured plasma and platelet function.

TASAIO. 21. 450. 1975.

31 Wandall, J.H.

Concentrations of serum proteins during and immediately after surgical trauma.

Acta. Chir. Scand. 140. 171. 1974.

32 Wandall, H.H.

In: Physiological and Clinical Aspects of Oxygenator Design. 1976.

Publs: Elsevier. Eds: S.G. Dawids and H.C. Engell.

33 Whitsett, J. and Tsang, R.C.

In vitro effects of fatty acids on serum-ionised calcium.

J. Pediat. 91. py 2. 233. 1977.

34 Wright, E.S., Sarkozy, E., Harpur, E.R., Dobell, A.R.C. and Murphy, D.R.

Plasma protein denaturation in experimental circulation.

J. Thor. Cardiovasc. Surg. 44. 550. 1962.

35 Wright, E.S., Sarkozy, E., Dobell, A.R.C. and Murphy, D.R.

Fat globulemia in extracorporeal circulation.

Surg. 53. 500. 1963.

36 Wu, H., Tenbroek, C. and Li, C.P.

Antigenic character of denatured egg albumin.

Proc. Soc. Exp. Biol. Med. 24. 472. 1927.

37 Zapol, W.M., Levy, R.I., Kolobow, T., Spragg, R. and Bowman,R.L.

In vitro denaturation of plasma alpha lipoproteins by bubble oxygenation in the dog.

Current Topics in Surg. Res. v.i. 444. 1969.

Moderator: Laurant

Laurant:          One simple question: Could you summarize the
                  possible mechanisms involved?

Fleming:          This is a well documented mechanism which involves
                  the complexion of heparin with tissue bound lipo-
                  protein-lipases, which are released into the cir-
                  culation. So when you get a blood sample they are
                  cleaving the beta-lipoproteins (VLDL) to produce
                  the apoprotein, and releasing the free fatty acids.
                  The free fatty acids are then transported on the
                  albumin as they usually are. Thus, the basic me-
                  chanism is that FFA are first transported by the
                  beta-lipoproteins and then by the albumin. What
                  happens in vitro, when we get these heavy precipi-
                  tates in blood that has been stored and not secon-
                  darily anticoagulated is presumably displacement
                  of Ca and phosphate from the albumin by fatty acids
                  We see these precipitates quite often, but I do not
                  know whether this mechanism has any relevance to
                  what happens in vivo.

Birnbaum:         Did you ever try to eluate your plasma from the
                  fat particles?

Fleming:          No, I have not done that. But what I have done is
                  to take the protamine precipitate which I get.
                  I have recovered the complex of the lipoproteins
                  by redissolving it in KCl, which leaves behind
                  most of the other proteins, which are generally de-
                  natured. I have then reelectrophoresed them and
                  have demonstrated that they are indeed lipoproteins.
                  And they do have the same electrophoretic mobility
                  as it appears on the normal electrophoresis of
                  fresh blood after heparin is been given.

Wenzel:           Did you find in your protamin precipitates any
                  fibrin or fibrin degradation products?

Fleming:          Fibrinogen is always present. There are two condi-
                  tions in which I do find fibrinogen and fibrinogen
                  precipitates, one is phosphate buffered at pH 7.6

and the other is TRIS-buffered at pH 8.6. Normally in untreated plasma at pH 7.6, only fibrinogen precipitates are found, which cannot be recovered again. I do not know about fibrinogen degradation products. In the TRIS-buffer, fibrinogen and the lipoproteins co-precipitate, but after heparin activation or after S.D.S. denaturation, the lipoproteins never precipitate in the phosphate protamin, whereas normally they do. That appears to depend on the cleavage of the V.L.D.L. or the beta-lipoproteins, I do not know which one as yet. It could be the prebeta-or the beta-lipoproteins or both. But nevertheless, a precipitate occurs which is very distinctively lipoprotein in nature.

Birnbaum: What do you guess is the percentage of this fraction of the total electropherogram situated anodally?

Fleming: I do not know, I would guess about 3 %. But the precise estimation is difficult because there are both lipoprotein and fibrin components in this precipitate. It is therefore difficult to make a precise judgement. Judging by the protamine precipitate and by what remains in the supernatant, it seems to be a very small amount, 1 % or even less.

Agostoni: We have experience with long term oxygenation in human and sheep. We were looking at the fibrinogen degradation products and in our experience the production of fibrinogen degradation products with this type of oxygenator is practically irrelevant. I do not think that there is a large scale destruction of fibrinogen during long term oxygenation.

Fleming: I agree with that. I have not investigated this question as thoroughly as you have, but as far as we can say it looks as if fibrinogen remains essentially stable. I have one case only in which there was frank fibrinolysis occurring during extracorporeal oxygenation. But only just that one case.

Schmid-Schönbein:     Much of the concern about protein denaturation is derived from an old observation of LEE, quoted over and over in the literature. LEE observed in the conjunctival blood vessels of patients under extracorporeal oxygenation a severe intravascular red cell aggregation and flow retardation, the classical "sludging" phenomenon. "Sludging" is a pre-rheological term which was very popular in the late fifties and early sixties which has never been adequately defined. However, KNISELY and other proponents regarded it as the cause of disease or death. For various reasons the interest in sludging has died down almost completely; the loss of interest has methodological reasons but it may well be revived again when more is known about the true mechanisms of intravascular aggregation. At the time of its initial discovery sludging was essentially claimed to be a sign of severe illness and attributed to a hypothetical protein substance. It was thought that denatured proteins glue together red cells in an irreversible fashion, producing the so-called "charge aggregates"which were claimed to block the microcirculation by occluding the arterioles. The hypotheses of denaturated proteins coating the red cells and glueing them together ("sticky substance") has since been abundant. We now know that sludging can be either the cause or the consequence of flow retardation. Furthermore, it has no significance itself, but only as a consequence and complication of a general hemodynamic disturbance of the microcirculation. I believe that the early observers of a "disturbed microcirculation" saw an important phenomenon in red cell aggregation which we should still be concerned about. But we should not attribute it primarily to so-called coating but rather to a more general flow retardation of the microcirculation in patients under extracorporeal oxygenation.

393

The theory of sludging will probably be revived,
once the modern theory of blood as a non-Newtonian
fluid with structural viscosity due to cell aggregation has acquired a general acceptance in hemo-
dynamics. Structural viscosity of blood is caused
by red cell aggregates but it manifests itself if
the hematocrit is normal or even elevated.
"Structural viscosity" is a sort of "virtual
property", which manifests itself only in the
absence of adequate flow forces (Fig. 1)

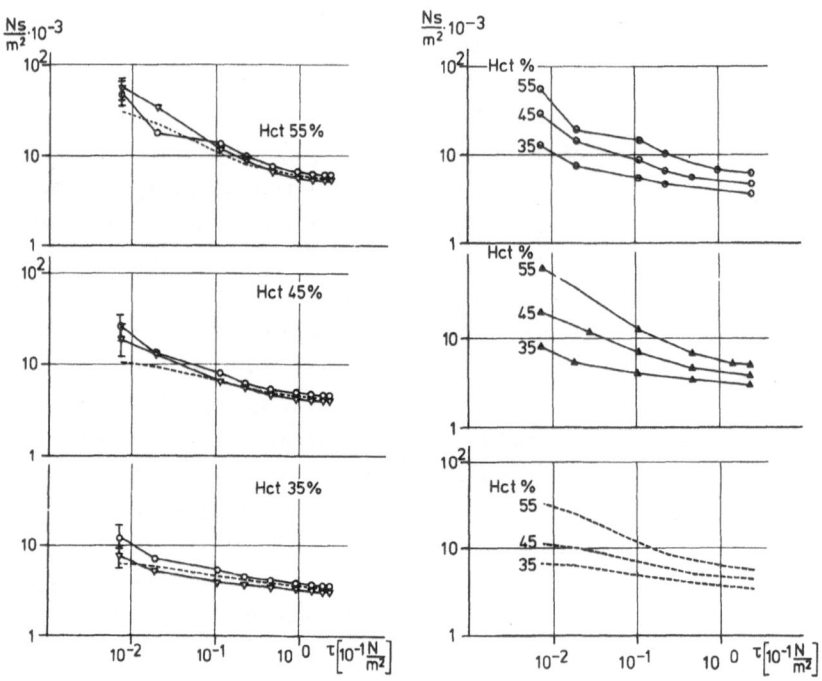

Fig. 1: Influence of shear stress, hematocrit and tendency
to aggregation on apparent blood viscosity
--- no aggretation ▲——▲ normal aggregation,
○——○ pathological aggregation

So sludging and its deleterious influence on the
microvascular flow can be avoided quite simply by
reducing the hematocrit (by hemodilution) or by
keeping up the flow forces in the microcirculation.
Fig. 2 shows normal and abnormal blood (as seen
in the rheoscope).

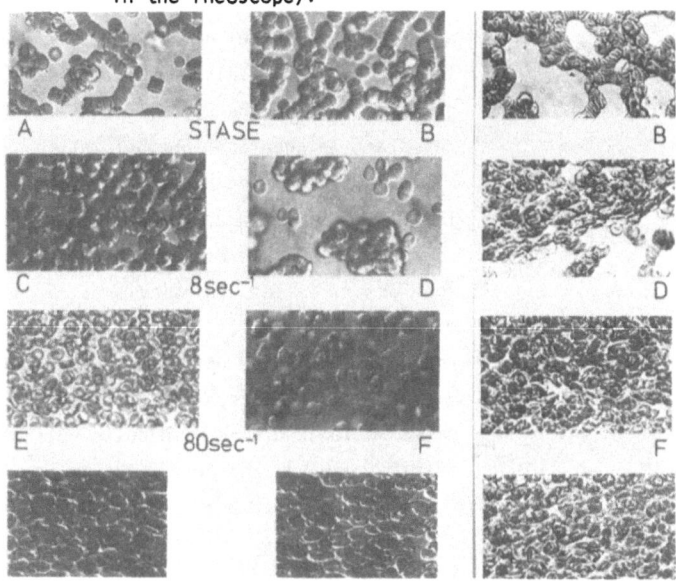

Fig. 2: Microrheology of normal blood (A,C,E) and
of pathological blood with enhanced red cell
aggregation. B, D, F: diabetes mellitus, B'D'F':
pregnancy at term. All three samples show pronounced aggregation in stasis (A, B and B').
At 8 $sec^{-1}$, normal blood is partly dispersed (C),
pathological blood is highly aggregated (D,D').
At 80 $sec^{-1}$ clump aggregates or strand aggregates
persist. At 1050 $sec^{-1}$ (lower pictures) all cells
are desaggregated, deformed and aligned in flow.
In the bottom row (high shear) red cells are desaggregated, deformed to ellipsoids and aligned
with their major axis parallel to the direction
of flow (this picture is part of Dr. Fischer's
film, which he showed earlier). Now, in all the
cases as soon as the shear rates are reduced, cell
aggregates of various forms appear. In normal blood
we see at about 80 $sec^{-1}$ the presence of more or

395

less dispersed cells, which are randomly oriented. In the diabetic blood we see typically spherical clumps containing two to three red cells. And these little clumps rotate in flow and are very difficult to disperse. In the heavily aggregating blood from the pregnant woman at term we see again dispersion but not quite as complete as in the normal blood. This means that under patholo-gical conditions the red cell aggregates are more resistant to shearing. Further reduction of the shear rates to about 8 sec$^{-1}$ produces aggregates in all three cases but the most severe ones, of course, are seen in diabetes and pregnancy, in the former, we see typical clumps, in the latter we see equally typical strands in which single red cells are being deformed under shear. The diabetic clump aggregation produces discontinuous dense rouleaux clumps with quite extensive plasma gaps between the aggregates, pregnancy leads to the continuous "strand" formation with the many plasma gaps within the aggregates.

Now, by changing the shear rates up and down between 8 and 1000 sec$^{-1}$, all of these can completely be dispersed. If first dispersed at 900 sec$^{-1}$ and then brought        to a complete stop, the aggregates reform spontaneously, as be seen in the upper row; here the rouleaux net-works in stasis look quite similar. The velocity of aggregate formation is 5 - 10 times faster in the pathological cases. So to summarize, we can now say sludging can be both normal and pathologi-cal, it can occur as a phenomenon in either cases in the absence of adequate flow forces;then being generally more pronounced in diseased states.

396

However, it must be stressed, that there the hemodynamic effects of aggregates are quite negligible as long as the hematocrit is between 30 and
35 % (or below) whereas in the higher (normal)
hematocrit range, the cell aggregates are responsible for the structural viscosity already mentioned. Again, only in the absence of adequate
flow forces, structural viscosity occurs. Thus,
hemodilution and the concommittant increase in
microvascular flow keeps the red cell aggregates
dispersed, even when sticky substances of any kind
should be circulating in the plasma. Let me just
add that in animal experiments (and in occasional
human cases) which we studied together with
Dr. R.E. Wells at the Peter Bent Brigham Hospital
in Boston, we found reduced or sometimes even totally absent red cell aggregation in blood taken
from the oxygenator. In preliminary experiments
then in our laboratory we find intravascular
sludging in the dog mesentery and in the conjunctival vessel whenever an animal is fixed to an
oxygenator and this can be easily oblivrated by
hemodiluting the animals and thereby increasing
the local flow velocity in the microcirculation.
Now, coming back to Dr. Fleming's paper: I would
like to pose a provocation question (which I
have asked him before): Is it justified to state
that the blood denaturation, as it occurs in present day extracorporeal oxygenation, does not
have the vital significance that was previously
attributed to it? Is it justified to ease our
mind about this problem? Is protein denaturation
a minor complication? I would like to go one step
further in stating taht the aggregation observed
in the microcirculation of diluted patients or
experimental animals is an "epiphenomenon" of
other hemodynamic disturbances there, upon which
we should centre our interest. Unless associated
with hemoconcentration "sludging" is not likely
to have any significance of its own.

Feijen:                    I think we have a different protein conformation
                           which interacts in another way with platelets
                           or with other cells. In the case of the hydro-
                           phobic surfaces compared to the hydrophilic sur-
                           faces. We have some evidence that binding on hy-
                           drophilic surfaces is more reversible. So this
                           might be a sign for a minor conformation change.

Hemker:                    We do not want to go into too many details but in
                           our experiments with an ellipsometer, which is
                           an apparatus in which you can registrate and
                           measure the thickness and the refractive index
                           of very thin layers (down to 1 $\overset{o}{A}$ range) we can
                           see what monomolecular layers adsorb onto a sur-
                           face from various solutions. I completely agree
                           with Dr. Feijen when he says that the adsorption
                           is not only determined by the species of mole-
                           cules but also by the kind of its interaction
                           with the wall. Because when in an ellipsometer
                           experiment you adsorb fibrinogen onto a hydrophi-
                           lic surface then you see it will grow to a mono-
                           molecular layer. The thickness of this layer is
                           the mean thickness of a fibrinogen molecule ; on
                           another scale you enter the refractive index and
                           you see that from the moment you can determine it
                           remains constant and equal to the refractive index
                           of a hydrated protein molecule. But then when
                           you do the same experiments with a hydrophobic
                           surface, you will see that the thickness of the
                           wall will grow and then decline again and fall
                           to an additional dimension which is smaller
                           than that of the hydrated fibrinogen molecule
                           whereas the refractive index goes up. This means
                           that on a hydrophobic surface the molecule is de-
                           hydrated and spread out whereas on a hydrophilic
                           surface it is more or less in the configuration
                           it has in solution. This may very well serve to
                           demonstrate that indeed the way in which the
                           fibrinogen molecule or any other molecule adsorbes
                           may change both its physical and its chemical
                           properties.

398

CONDENSATION OF THE GENERAL DISCUSSION
(by  H. Schmid-Schönbein)


The last afternoon of the meeting was devoted to a free-
lance discussion on practical applications of the basic
knowledge available. Very soon, it became obvious that a
considerable gap still exists between the needs of the
practicing surgeons trying to avoid complications and experimental workers trying to understand the very nature of
the problems involved. As Dr. HEMKER stated, the theoreti-
cian cannot help the surgeons without a clear formulation
of his problems ("what you want to do depends on what you
want to know"). The surgeons, on the other hand, are primarily concerned with the bleeding complications, for which
only massive confusion is available as a treatment. Therefore, prognostic tests indicating an iminent bleading tendency are urgently needed.

At this point it was agreed that the present state of the
open heart surgery only in exceptional cases confronted
the surgeons with the actual hemorraghe. Nevertheless, membrane as well as bubble oxygenation always still leads to
a severe disturbance of the coagulation system and the platelet function from which the patients have a chance to re-
cover. Since long term extracorporeal oxygenation is not
used presently, it was agreed that open heart surgery lend
itself as an ideal model for the investigation of procedures, apparatus and drugs preventing or at least dimini-
shing the trauma to the blood. In the attempt to focus on
the central issue of blood trauma from as many sides as
possible, many differing suggestions for future research
efforts were proposed.

The significance of foreign surfaces and abnormal flow conditions was stressed by Dr. MÜLLER-MOHNSSEN and the significance of overt or imminent disseminated intravascular
coagulation and consumption coagulopathy was stressed by
Dr. HEMKER and by Dr. WENZEL while observation of unspecific stimuli (hypothermia and hypocapnia) was stressed by
Dr. SCHMID-SCHÖNBEIN.

It was further agreed, that diagnostic testing procedures
are of very limited practical or theoretical value in patients with massive oozing from skinned incisions or other
forms of hemorraghe and that therefore all future efforts
should be directed towards prognostic tests aiming at the
prevention of such incidents. However, the discussion about
means to this end not only revealed many of the presently
evident gaps in the knowledge about the basic mechanisms of
trauma. In addition questions of practicability and validity of well established laboratory tests to the use in patients connected to artificial organs became evident. While
for obvious practical reasons simple tests were requested
by the surgeons and anaesthetists, the interpretability of
presently available routine-tests was seriously questioned
by the experts in the field of blood physiology and pathophysiology. The forum agreed that much more basic as well
as applied research in this field was necessary and that
concerted problem oriented research efforts are essential
in this field. The hope was dimmed that a simple transfer
of basic knowledge to practical application through tech-
nological development would soon solve the present problems.

It was therefore agreed that within the frame-work of the
concerted action the practical and theoretical problems of
heparin chemistry and pharmacology, heparin-dosage and
heparin neutralisation deserved utmost priority and should
be the subject of separate meetings in the near future. A
A close look into alternative methods of preventing coagulation (such as defibrinogenation and/or hemodilution)
was advocated, as well as the trial of more aggressive
pharmacological procedures aiming at interference with platelet activation (aggregation, adhesion and release). All
agreed that a meeting on these topics could be organized in
the near future.

During the discussion many tests were proposed and rejec-
ted, there was agreement that for most of them the verifi-
cation of their validity as prognostic tool remains to be
established. The proposed and undisputed tests and their
proponents are listed in table I, page    . It was attemp-

400

ted to differentiate between tests which should be persued with the aim of learning more about the unknown basic mechanism and those presently giving a reliable information in the operating and/or recovery room.

There is no disagreement to the proposal that at present already activated clotting times (kaoline activation), platelet counts, tests of platelet reactivity and tests for the so-called platelet factor III availability (liberated thromboplastic material coming from thrombocytes, damaged red cells, tissue and/or components of pumps and oxygenators) are of significant value to assess the overall function of the platelets. Likewise, fibrinogen contents, the concentration of free heparin, antithrombin III activity and the tests sensitive to the activation of factor VII can be taken as a measurement of the extent of activation of the coagulation cascade and the inhibitory activity of administered and/or natural antithrombotic antithrombin activity.

There was little disagreement that the hemolysis rate, hemolysis index correcting for perfused volume and time of extracorporeal circulation can be taken as a reliable index of red cell damage. Tests of red cell shape and red cell deformability were proposed to assess the so-called sub-hemolytic damage. There is no general agreement on future tests of granulocytes activity and of indices of the immediate state of the defense system. It was, however, not thought a problem of concern during the actual extracorporeal circulation but rather during the subsequent stages. The problems of protein denaturation by the artificial surface and/or the plasma protein interphase were not given high priority.

The meeting adjourned following multiple calls, first for better theoretical ellucidation of the underlying mechanisms that lead to activation and consumption of coagulation factors and secondly, for simple, reliable, automatized and rapid testing procedure immediately applicable near the patient by the physicians, surgeons, pump technicians and oxygenator technicians in the operating or recovery room.

| | PROPOSALS | PROPONENT |
|---|---|---|
| | **Coagulation system** | |
| ✡ | Activated coagulation Times | AGOSTONI |
| ✡ | Partial thromboplastin Time | WENZEL |
| | Fibrin-Polymerization-Time | '' |
| ✡ | a) Thrombin-Time | '' |
| ✡ | b) Reptilase-Time | '' |
| § | Platelet factor 4 | '' |
| § | Fibrinopeptide | HEMKER |
| § | Prothrombin breakdown products | '' |
| § | Activated Factor VII | '' , WENZEL |
| ✡ | Tests for Thromboplastic Material (Platelet factor 3) | HEMKER, SCHMID-SCHÖNBEIN |
| | **Platelets** | |
| ✡ | Platelet number | WILDEVUUR, DAWIDS, WENZEL |
| ✡ | Platelet volume | WENZEL |
| | Platelet function | |
| ✡ | a) spontaneous aggregability and shape change | SCHMID-SCHÖNBEIN |
| ✡ | b) ADP induced aggregation corrected for hemodilution | WILDEVUUR, BIRNBAUM, ENGELL |
| | **Red cells** | |
| ✡ | Corrected rate of hemolysis | MOTTAGHY |
| § | Red cell deformability | SCHMID-SCHÖNBEIN |
| § | Red cell shape and volume | BIRNBAUM |
| § | Adenosin Nucleotides in plasma | SCHMID-SCHÖNBEIN |
| | $\boxed{K^+}$ in plasma | '' |
| | **Plasma-Serum** | |
| § | Complement $C_5$ | AGOSTONI |
| ✡ | Haptoglobins | SCHMID-SCHÖNBEIN |
| ✡ | Immunoglobulins | HAKIM |
| ✡ | Fibrinogen-Concentration | WENZEL |
| § | Antithrombin III, | WENZEL, HEMKER |

Table I: List of proposed test parameters for blood trauma during
extracorporeal oxygenation

§ Primarily for Research
✡ Routine tests

AGOSTONI, A., University of Milan, Via Quadronno 11, 1 - Milano

ANGELKORT, B., Abteilung Innere Medizin II, Medizinische Fakultät der
  RWTH Aachen, Goethestr. 27/29, D - 5100 Aachen

BAURSCHMIDT, P., Zentralinstitut für Biomedizinische Technik der
  Friedrich-Alexander-Universität, Turnstr. 5 , D - 8520 Erlangen

BIRNBAUM, D.,Freie Universität Berlin, Universitätsklinikum
  Charlottenburg (FB 3), Spandauer Damm 130, D - 1000 Berlin 19

BLASBERG, P., Abteilung Physiologie, Medizinische Fakultät der RWTH
  Aachen, Melatenerstr. 211, D - 5100 Aachen

BORN, G.V.R., Department of Pharmacology, University of London
  King's College, Strand, GB - London WC2R 2LS

DAWIDS, S., Medical Department P. Rigshospitalet University Hospital,
  9 Blegdamsvej, DK - 2100 Copenhagen

DEGGELLER, K., Centraal Klinisch Chemisch Laboratorium, Academisch
  Ziekenhuis, Oostersingel 59, NL - Groningen

DRIESSEN, G., Abteilung Physiologie, Medizinische Fakultät der RWTH
  Aachen, Melatenerstr. 211, D - 5100 Aachen

ENGELL, H.C., Rigshospitalet,State University Hospital, 9 Blegdamsvej,
  DK - 2100 Copenhagen Ø

FEIJEN, J., Twente University of Technology, Department of Chemical
  Engineering, NL - Enschede

FISCHER, T.M., Abteilung Physiologie, Medizinische Fakultät der RWTH
  Aachen, Melatenerstr. 211, D - 5100 Aachen

FLEMING, J.S., Department of Surgery, University of London,
  Hammersmith Hospital, Ducane Road, GB London W12 OHS

FORST, R., Abteilung Physiologie, Medizinische Fakultät der RWTH Aachen,
  Melatenerstr. 211, D - 5100 Aachen

HAKIM, J., Laboratoire Central d'Immunologie et d'Hématologie,
  Hôpital Bichat, 170, Boulevard Ney, F - 75877 Paris Cédex 18

HÄUSSINGER, G., Helmholtz-Insitut für Biomedizinische Technik an der
  RWTH Aachen, Goethestr. 27/29, D - 5100 Aachen

HEMKER, H.C., Rijksuniversiteit Limburg, Faculty of Medicine,
  Beeldsnijdersdreef 101, NL 6200 MD Maastricht

JÜNGLING, E., Abteilung Physiologie, Medizinische Fakultät der RWTH
  Aachen, Melatenerstr. 211, D - 5100 Aachen

KRAUSE, E., Lehrstuhl für Strömungslehre und Aerodynamisches Institut
  der RWTH Aachen, Templergraben 55, D - 5100 Aachen

403

KRATZER, M., Institut für Biologie, Abteilung für Physiologie,
Gesellschaft für Strahlen- und Umweltforschung mbH,
Ingolstädter Landstr. 1, D - 8042 Neuherberg Post Oberschleißheim

LAURANT, D., Service de Physiologie et d'Explorations Fonctionnelles
Hôpital Henri Mondor, 51, Avenue du Marechal-de-Lattre-de-Tassigny
F - 94010 Créteil

MÜLLER-MOHNSSEN, H., Institut für Biologie, Abteilung für Physiologie
Gesellschaft für Strahlen- und Umweltforschung mbH,
Ingolstädter Landstr. 1, D - 8042 Neuherberg Post Oberschleißheim

MOTTAGHY, K., Abteilung Physiologie, Medizinische Fakultät der RWTH
Aachen, Melatenerstr. 211, D - 5100 Aachen

NAUMANN, A., Lehrstuhl für Strömungslehre und Aerodynamisches Institut
der RWTH Aachen, Templergraben 55, D - 5100 Aachen

OLIJSLAGER, J., Twente University of Technology, Department of Chemical
Engineering, NL - Enschede

ROHLING-WINKEL, I., Abteilung Physiologie, Medizinische Fakultät der
RWTH Aachen, Melatenerstr. 211, D - 5100 Aachen

SCHMID-SCHÖNBEIN, H., Abteilung Physiologie, Medizinische Fakultät
der RWTH Aachen, Melatenerstr. 211, D - 5100 Aachen

STÖHR-LIESEN, M., Abteilung Physiologie, Medizinische Fakultät der
RWTH Aachen, Melatenerstr. 211, D - 5100 Aachen

TEITEL, P., Abteilung Physiologie, Medizinische Fakultät der RWTH
Aachen, Melatenerstr. 211, D - 5100 Aachen

TILLMANN, W., Helmholtz-Institut für Biomedizinische Technik an der
RWTH Aachen, Goethestr. 27/29, D - 5100 Aachen

WEHNER, W., Battelle-Institut, D - 6000 Frankfurt a.M.

WENZEL, E., Abteilung für klinische Haemostaseologie und Transfusions-
medizin, Universität des Saarlandes, D - 6650 Homburg/Saar

WILLIAMS, A.R., University of Manchester, Department of Medical Biophysics, Stopford Building, Oxford Road, GB - M 139PT Manchester

WURZINGER, L.J., Abteilung Physiologie, Medizinische Fakultät der
RWTH Aachen, Melatenerstr. 211, D - 5100 Aachen